MURRAY'S BASIC MEDICAL MICROBIOLOGY

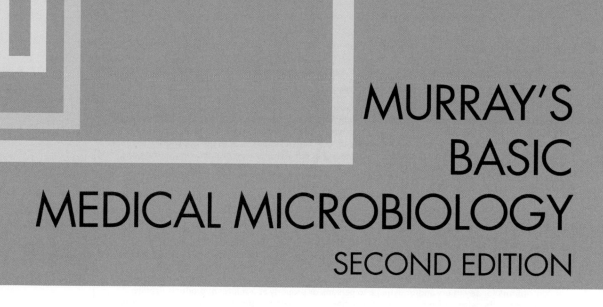

MURRAY'S BASIC MEDICAL MICROBIOLOGY

SECOND EDITION

PATRICK R. MURRAY, PhD

Emeritus Professor,
University of Maryland School of Medicine,
Baltimore, MD, United States

ELSEVIER

Elsevier
1600 John F. Kennedy Blvd.
Ste 1800
Philadelphia, PA 19103-2899

MURRAY'S BASIC MEDICAL MICROBIOLOGY, SECOND EDITION ISBN: 978-0-323-87810-4

Notice

Previous edition copyrighted 2018.

Publisher: Elyse O'Grady
Content Development Specialist: Shweta Pant
Content Development Manager: Somodatta Roy Choudhury
Publishing Services Manager: Shereen Jameel
Project Manager: Haritha Dharmarajan
Design Direction: Brian Salisbury

Printed in Canada

Last digit is the print number: 9 8 7 6 5 4 3 2 1

Working together to grow libraries in developing countries

www.elsevier.com • www.bookaid.org

By writing an introduction to the second edition of *Basic Medical Microbiology*, I have an opportunity to reflect on the important changes that have been made to the first edition for the benefit of the students who use this text as well as the materials that have been retained. In many ways, microbiology is an evolving science with newly discovered pathogens and diseases. This was dramatically illustrated by the global pandemic caused by SARS Coronavirus-2 and the subsequent variants. However, I think it is important to recognize that student learning also evolves. The challenges of remote learning during the COVID-19 pandemic brought this acutely into focus. The one thing that did not change when I prepared this edition of *Basic Medical Microbiology* was the underlying foundation for this textbook. So, I ask for forgiveness for retaining a portion of the original Preface; after this, I will explain the "why and how" of the changes in this second edition.

What is the bigger challenge for a student or the instructor in the understanding of what is important in medical microbiology? Many years ago, when I took my first graduate course in medical microbiology, I read thousands of pages of text, listened to 5 h of lectures a week, and performed lab exercises 6 h a week for 1 year. I was given a wonderful foundation in microbiology, but I frequently asked myself a question that was also voiced by other students: do I really need to know all this stuff? The answer to that question is certainly no, but the challenge is understanding what information is needed. Years later, when I set out to write my first textbook on microbiology, my goal was to give the students only what they need to know, described in a way that is informative, factual, and concise. I think I was successful in that effort, but I also realize that the discipline of microbiology continues to change as do approaches to presenting information to students. I am still firmly convinced that my efforts in my first textbook, *Medical Microbiology*, and subsequent editions are important, as they form the foundations of microbiology knowledge for a student. This cannot be replaced by a quick search of the internet or a published review because much of the subject matter presented in medical microbiology—epidemiology, virulence, clinical diseases, diagnostics,

and treatment—is a distillation of the review of numerous research articles and clinical and technical experience. Having stated that, students frequently turn to review books consisting of abbreviated summaries, illustrations (should I say cartoons), and various mnemonic aids for mastering this subject. As I have watched this evolution of learning microbiology, I am struck by the sacrifice that has been made. I believe microbiology is a beautiful subject, which balances health and disease defined by the biology of individual organisms and microbial communities. Without an understanding of biology, lists of facts are soon forgotten. But I am a realist and know the burden students face, mastering not only microbiology but also a number of other subjects. So the personal question I posed was—is there a better way to present to the student a summary of information that is easy to understand and remember? This book is my approach to answering this question. First, almost by definition, it is not comprehensive. Just as I have carefully selected organisms and diseases to present in this book, I have also intentionally not mentioned others—not because they are unimportant but because they are less common. I have also not presented a detailed discussion of microbial biology and virulence or the immune response of the patient to an infection, but simply presented the association between an organism and the disease it causes. Again, I felt those discussions should be reserved for *Medical Microbiology*. Finally, the organization of this book is focused on organisms—bacteria, viruses, fungi, and parasites—rather than diseases. This is because I think it is easier for a student to remember a limited number of diseases associated with an organism rather than a long list of organisms (or a significantly incomplete list) implicated in a specific disease such as pneumonia. Patients present with diseases, and the observer must develop a list of organisms that could be responsible; so to aid the student, I provide this differential diagnosis in the introductory chapter of each organism section. I also provide in these introductory chapters an overview of the classification of organisms (a structural framework to remember organisms) and a listing of antimicrobials that are used to treat infections. The individual chapters in Sections II–V are organized under a common theme: a brief discussion of the individual organisms, a summary of facts (properties, epidemiology, clinical disease, diagnosis, and treatment) provided in a concise table, and illustrations provided as a visual learning aid. The most significant change that was made in this second edition was the reorganization and expansion of the clinical cases in a series of eight clinical syndrome chapters in Section VI. My goal was to provide clinical situations that illustrate for the student how the foundational knowledge gained in the organism chapters can be used to make clinical diagnoses. Finally, examination questions are provided in Section VII to help students assess their ability to assimilate this material. Again, I will emphasize that this text should not be considered a comprehensive review of microbiology. On the other hand, I believe that if students master this material, they will have a firm foundation in the principles and applications of microbiology. I welcome comments on how successful my efforts are.

I would like to acknowledge the support and guidance from the Elsevier professionals who help bring this concept to reality, particularly Jim Merritt, Katie DeFrancesco, Elyse O'Grady, and Shweta Pant. I also want to thank the many students who have challenged me to think about the broad world of microbes and distil this into the essential microbiology material into a factual, coherent story for a novice in this field.

CONTENTS

SECTION I Introduction

1 Overview of Medical Microbiology, 1
Viruses, 2
Bacteria, 2
Fungi and Parasites, 3
Good Versus Bad Microbes, 3
Conclusion, 3

SECTION II Bacteria

2 Introduction to Bacteria, 5
A Word of Caution, 5
Overview, 5
Classification, 5
Role in Disease, 6
Antibacterial Agents, 8

3 Aerobic Gram-Positive Cocci, 12
Staphylococcus aureus, 15
ß-Hemolytic Streptococci, 17
Streptococcus pneumoniae, 20
Viridans Streptococci, 21
Enterococcus, 22
Supplemental Reading, 23

4 Aerobic Gram-Positive Rods, 24
Bacillus anthracis and *Bacillus cereus*, 25
Listeria monocytogenes, 27
Corynebacterium diphtheriae, 28
Supplemental Reading, 29

5 Acid-Fast Bacteria, 30
Acid-Fast Organisms, 30
Mycobacterium tuberculosis, 32
Mycobacterium leprae, 33
Mycobacterium avium Complex, 34
Nocardia Species, 34
Supplemental Reading, 36

6 Aerobic Gram-Negative Cocci and Coccobacilli, 37
Neisseria gonorrhoeae, 38
Neisseria meningitidis, 39
Eikenella corrodens, 40
Kingella kingae, 41
Moraxella catarrhalis, 41
Haemophilus influenzae, 42
Pasteurella multocida, 43
Acinetobacter baumannii, 44
Bordetella pertussis, 45
Francisella tularensis, 46
Brucella Species, 47
Supplemental Reading, 48

7 Aerobic Fermentative Gram-Negative Rods, 49
Escherichia coli, 51
Klebsiella pneumoniae, 52
Proteus mirabilis, 53
Salmonella species, 54
Shigella species, 55
Yersinia, 56
Vibrio cholerae, 57
Supplemental Reading, 58

8 Aerobic Nonfermentative Gram-Negative Rods, 59
Pseudomonas aeruginosa, 60
Burkholderia cepacia, 61
Stenotrophomonas maltophilia, 61
Supplemental Reading, 62

9 Anaerobic Bacteria, 63
Clostridium tetani, 64
Clostridium botulinum, 65
Clostridium perfringens, 66
Clostridioides difficile, 67
Bacteroides fragilis, 68
Supplemental Reading, 70

10 Spiral-Shaped Bacteria, 71
Campylobacter jejuni, 72
Helicobacter pylori, 73
Treponema pallidum, 74
Borrelia burgdorferi, 75
Leptospira species, 76
Supplemental Reading, 77

11 Intracellular Bacteria, 78
    Rickettsia rickettsii, 79
    Ehrlichia chaffeensis, 80
    Coxiella burnetii, 81
    Chlamydia trachomatis, 82
    Supplemental Reading, 83

SECTION III Viruses

12 Introduction to Viruses, 85
    Overview, 85
    Classification, 85
    Role in Disease, 87
    Antiviral Agents, 89

13 Human Immunodeficiency Viruses, 91
    Human Immunodeficiency Virus 1
        (HIV-1), 92
    Supplemental Reading, 93

14 Human Herpesviruses, 94
    Herpes Simplex Virus, Types 1 and 2, 95
    Varicella-Zoster Virus, 96
    Cytomegalovirus, 97
    Epstein-Barr Virus, 98
    Human Herpesviruses 6, 7, and 8, 99
    Supplemental Reading, 100

15 Respiratory Viruses, 101
    Rhinoviruses, 101
    Coronaviruses, 102
    Influenza Viruses, 103
    Paramyxoviridae, 104
    Parainfluenza Viruses (PIV), 104
    Respiratory Syncytial Virus (RSV), 105
    Human Metapneumovirus (HMV), 106
    Adenovirus, 107
    Supplemental Reading, 107

16 Hepatitis Viruses, 108
    Hepatitis A Virus, 109
    Hepatitis B and D Viruses, 109
    Hepatitis C Virus, 110
    Hepatitis E Virus, 111
    Supplemental Reading, 112

17 Gastrointestinal Viruses, 113
    Rotavirus, 113
    Norovirus and Sapovirus, 114
    Astrovirus, 115

    Adenovirus, 116
    Supplemental Reading, 116

18 Human Papillomavirus, 117
    Supplemental Reading, 118

SECTION IV Fungi

19 Introduction to Fungi, 119
    Overview, 119
    Classification, 119
    Role in Disease, 120
    Antifungal Agents, 121

20 Cutaneous and Subcutaneous
    Fungi, 123
    Dermatophytosis, 124
    Fungal Keratitis, 125
    Lymphocutaneous Sporotrichosis, 126
    Other Subcutaneous Infections, 127
    Supplemental Reading, 127

21 Systemic Dimorphic Fungi, 128
    Blastomyces dermatitidis, 129
    Coccidioides immitis and *Coccidioides
        posadasii*, 130
    Histoplasma capsulatum, 131
    Supplemental Reading, 133

22 Opportunistic Fungi, 134
    Candida albicans and Related Species, 134
    Cryptococcus neoformans, 136
    Miscellaneous Yeast-Like Fungi, 137
    Aspergillus fumigatus, 137
    Miscellaneous Opportunistic
    Molds, 138
    Supplemental Reading, 139

SECTION V Parasites

23 Introduction to Parasites, 141
    Overview, 141
    Classification, 141
    Role in Disease, 143
    Antiparasitic Agents, 144

24 Protozoa, 148
    Intestinal Amoeba, 148
    Coccidia, 149

Flagellates, 151
Free-Living Amoeba, 153
Blood Protozoa, 154
Tissue Protozoa, 156
Supplemental Reading, 159

25 Nematodes, 160
Intestinal Nematodes, 160
Blood Nematodes, 165
Tissue Nematodes, 167
Supplemental Reading, 167

26 Trematodes, 168
Intestinal Trematode, 169
Tissue Trematodes, 170
Blood Trematodes, 172
Supplemental Reading, 174

27 Cestodes, 175
Intestinal Cestodes, 176
Tissue Cestodes, 178
Supplemental Reading, 179

28 Arthropods, 180

SECTION VI Clinical Cases—Introduction
to Infectious Diseases

Section Overview, 181
References, 181

29 Upper Respiratory Tract Infections, 182

30 Lower Respiratory Tract Infections, 187

31 Gastrointestinal Tract Infections, 198

32 Genitourinary Tract Infections, 208

33 Central Nervous System Infections, 213

34 Skin and Soft Tissue Infections, 221

35 Sepsis and Cardiovascular Infections, 235

36 Miscellaneous Infections, 248

SECTION VII Review Questions

Questions, 255
Answers, 269
Index, 282

1

Overview of Medical Microbiology

Microbiology can certainly be overwhelming for the student confronted with the daunting task of learning about hundreds of medically important microbes. I remember well the first day of my introductory graduate course in medical microbiology; the course instructor handed each student a 1000-page syllabus consisting of lecture outlines, notes, and literature references. That became known not so lovingly as *the book of pain*. Not to be limited to lecture notes, we also had an assigned 2000-page textbook to guide our studies. In retrospect, much of the information in both the notes and the textbook was very interesting from a fundamental microbiology perspective but of very little relevance for a student studying medicine. However, I have always felt that the information that is important for a student to know can be presented in a clear, organized, logical way without unnecessary

digression into the minutia of this field. For example, microbiology is not so challenging if the subject matter—the microbes—is subdivided into groups and further subdivided into related units. Let me illustrate this in this introductory chapter.

Microbes are subdivided into one of the four groups:

- Viruses
- Bacteria
- Fungi
- Parasites

The structural complexity of these groups increases from viruses (the simplest structure) to parasites (the most complex). There is generally no confusion about which group a microbe should be placed in, although a few fungi were formerly classified as parasites. Each group of microbes is then further subdivided, generally based on a key feature of the group.

Microbial Classification		
Microbes	**Primary Classification**	**Secondary Classification**
Viruses	DNA virus	Single- versus double-stranded nucleic acid
	RNA virus	Outer envelope or no envelope
Bacteria	Gram-positive	Cocci versus rods
	Gram-negative	Aerobic versus anaerobic
		Spore-former versus no spores (only gram-positive bacteria)
	Acid-fast	Partial or complete acid-fast staining
	Miscellaneous	Spiral-shaped
		Obligate intracellular

Continued

Microbial Classification—cont'd		
Microbes	**Primary Classification**	**Secondary Classification**
Fungi	Yeast (single-celled)	
	Mold (multi-celled)	Pigment versus no pigment
		Nuclei separated by a wall (septum) or nonseptated
	Dimorphic (yeast and mold forms)	
Parasites	Protozoa (single-celled)	Amoeba
		Flagellates
		Sporozoa
	Worms (helminths)	Roundworms (nematodes)
		Flatworms (trematodes)
		Tapeworms (cestodes)
	Bugs (arthropods)	Mosquitos
		Ticks
		Fleas
		Lice
		Mites
		Flies

VIRUSES

Viruses are very simple microbes, consisting of nucleic acid, a few proteins, and (in some) a lipid envelope. These microbes are completely dependent on the cells they infect for their survival and replication. Medically important viruses are subdivided into 20 families defined by the structural properties of the members. The most important feature is the nucleic acid. Viruses contain either DNA or RNA but not both. The families of DNA viruses and RNA viruses are further subdivided into viruses with either single-stranded or double-stranded nucleic acids. Lastly, these viral families are further subdivided into viruses with an outer envelope and naked or nonenveloped viruses. Now the perceptive student would say that this gives us eight families of viruses and not 20. Well, the viruses are further subdivided by their shape (spherical or rodlike) and size (big or small ["pico"]). Thus, the key to understanding viruses is to place them into their respective families based on their structural features.

BACTERIA

Bacteria are a bit more complex, with both RNA and DNA, metabolic machinery for self-replication, and a complex cell wall structure. Bacteria are **prokaryotic** organisms, i.e., simple unicellular organisms with no nuclear membrane, mitochondria, Golgi bodies, or endoplasmic reticulum, and they reproduce by asexual division. The key feature that is used to classify most bacteria is their staining property, with the Gram stain and acid-fast stain being the most important. Most bacteria are either **gram-positive** (retain the blue dye) or **gram-negative** (lose the blue stain and stain with the red dye). These bacteria are then subdivided by their shape (either spherical [cocci] or rod-shaped), whether they grow aerobically or anaerobically (many bacteria grow in both atmospheres and are called **facultative anaerobes**), and whether they form resilient **spores** or not (only gram-positive rods are spore-formers). The other important bacterial stain is the **acid-fast** stain that is retained only by a few bacteria that have a characteristic lipid-rich cell wall. This group is further subdivided by how difficult it is to remove the acid-fast stain (the stain is named because an acid solution removes the stain from most other bacteria). Finally, there are groups of organisms that do not stain with these procedures so they are separated by other features, such as shape (spiral-shaped bacteria) or their need to grow inside a host cell (e.g., leukocyte) or cell cultures in the laboratory.

FUNGI AND PARASITES

Fungi and parasites are more complex **eukaryotic** organisms that contain a well-defined nucleus, mitochondria, Golgi bodies, and endoplasmic reticulum. Single-celled and multi-celled organisms are members of both groups. As can be seen, the line separating these two groups is not as well defined as that separating these organisms from bacteria or viruses, but the classification is still well-recognized.

Fungi

Fungi are subdivided into single-celled organisms (**yeasts**) or multi-celled organisms (**molds**), with a few medically important members existing in both forms (**dimorphic fungi**). Molds are complex organisms with cells organized into threadlike tubular structures (**hyphae**) and specialized asexual reproductive forms (**conidia**). The molds are then further subdivided by the structure of the hyphae (pigmented or nonpigmented, separated into individual cells [septated molds] or not) and the arrangement of the conidia.

Parasites

Parasites are also subdivided into single-celled organisms (**protozoa**) or multi-celled organisms (**worms** and **bugs**). Members of the family Protozoa are then further divided into amebae, flagellates (think of them as hairy protozoa), and coccidia (some are shaped like cocci but many are not). The worms (technically called **helminths**) are nicely classified by their shape: roundworms, flatworms, and tapeworms—pretty simple, although many have very complex lifecycles that unfortunately are important for understanding how the parasites infect humans and cause disease. The **bugs** are simply "bugs." These include mosquitos, ticks, fleas, lice, mites, and flies. They are important because they are vectors of a number of viruses and bacteria (but not fungi) that are responsible for diseases. Other bugs obviously exist (such as spiders), but these generally are not vectors for other pathogenic microbes.

GOOD VERSUS BAD MICROBES

Microbes, particularly the bacteria, have unjustly earned a bad reputation. Most have historically been viewed as bad and recognized only for their ability to cause diseases. We have coined the derogatory term *germs*, and great efforts are made to eliminate our exposure to these organisms. The reality is most microbes are not only good but critical for our health. The surfaces of the skin, nose, mouth, gut, and genitourinary tract are covered with bacteria, as well as some fungi and parasites. These organisms are critical for the maturation of our immune system, important metabolic functions such as the digestion of food products, and protection from infection with unwanted pathogens. These organisms are referred to as our **normal flora** or **microbiome**. If these organisms are maintained in their proper balance, then health can be maintained. If they are disrupted either naturally or through man-made interventions (e.g., antibiotics, skin peels, enemas), then we risk disease. Infectious diseases are also initiated when the members of the microbiome are introduced into normally sterile sites (e.g., abdominal cavity, tissues, lungs, urinary tract) through trauma or disease. This is referred to as an **endogenous** infection or an infection caused by the normal microbial population. Finally, infections can be caused by **exogenous** organisms; that is, those introduced from outside. Only a few of the microbes that we encounter in our environment are pathogens, but some of the most serious infections are caused by these exogenous pathogens. So the important lesson is that most microbes are good and not associated with disease. A subset of our endogenous organisms can cause disease when introduced into normally sterile areas, but most endogenous organisms do not have the virulent properties to cause disease. Likewise, most of the exogenous organisms we are exposed to cause no problems at all, but some can cause quite significant disease. It is important to understand which organisms have the necessary properties (**virulence**) to cause disease and under what circumstances this will occur. It is also important to understand which organisms are not associated with disease.

CONCLUSION

The perceived complexity of microbiology is simplified if we understand the relationships between the members of each of the four groups of microbes. This is further simplified if we separate pathogens from nonpathogens and then understand the conditions under which pathogens produce disease. The following chapters are designed to develop these themes for the individual groups of organisms.

2

Introduction to Bacteria

A WORD OF CAUTION

Alright, there is way too much information in the next few pages. I certainly do not expect the student to master these details before he or she moves on to the rest of the bacteriology chapters. Rather, a quick scan of the information should be done first. Then, as each subsequent chapter is digested, this chapter can provide a framework for linking each of the bacteriology chapters.

OVERVIEW

Bacteria are prokaryotic (*pro*, before; *karyon*, kernel) organisms that are relatively simple in structure. They are unicellular and have no nuclear membrane, mitochondria, Golgi bodies, or endoplasmic reticulum, and they reproduce by asexual division. The bacterial cell wall is complex, consisting of one of two basic forms defined by their staining ability with the **Gram stain**: a gram-positive cell wall with a thick peptidoglycan layer and a gram-negative cell wall with a thin peptidoglycan layer and an overlying **outer membrane**. Some bacteria lack this cell wall structure and compensate by surviving only inside host cells in a hypertonic environment. The human body is inhabited by thousands of different bacterial species (called the "**microbiome**"), some living transiently and others in a permanent synergistic relationship. Likewise, the environment that surrounds us, including the air we breathe, the water we drink, and the food we eat, is populated with bacteria, many of which are relatively harmless and some of which are capable of causing life-threatening disease. Disease can result from the toxic effects of bacte-

rial products (e.g., toxins) or when bacteria invade normally sterile body tissues and fluids.

CLASSIFICATION

The size (1–20μm or larger), shape (spheres [cocci], rods [bacilli], or spirals), and spatial arrangement (single cells, pairs, chains, or clusters) of the cells, as well as specific growth properties (e.g., **aerobic** [require oxygen], **anaerobic** [cannot grow in the presence of oxygen], or **facultative anaerobes** [grow in the presence or absence of oxygen]), are used for the preliminary classification of bacteria. This is a useful exercise that can provide some order to an otherwise confusing list of organisms. The following tables are not comprehensive; rather, these are a listing of the most commonly isolated or clinically important bacteria.

Gram-Positive Bacteria		
Aerobic Gram-Positive Cocci: • *Staphylococcus* • *Streptococcus* • *Enterococcus*	**Anaerobic Gram-Positive Cocci:** • Many genera	**Aerobic Acid-Fast Rods:** • *Mycobacterium* • *Nocardia* • *Rhodococcus*
Aerobic Gram-Positive Rods: • *Bacillus* • *Listeria* • *Corynebacterium*	**Anaerobic Gram-Positive Rods:** • *Clostridium* • *Actinomyces* • *Lactobacillus* • *Cutibacterium*	

Gram-Negative Bacteria

Aerobic Gram-Negative Cocci and Coccobacilli:	Aerobic Gram-Negative Rods:	Anaerobic Gram-Negative Cocci:
• *Neisseria*	• Enterobacteriales (many genera)	• *Veillonella*
• *Moraxella*	• *Vibrio*	**Anaerobic Gram-Negative Rods:**
• *Eikenella*	• *Pseudomonas*	
• *Kingella*	• *Burkholderia*	
• *Haemophilus*	• *Stenotro-phomonas*	• *Bacteroides*
• *Acinetobacter*		• *Fusobac-terium*
• *Bordetella*		
• *Brucella*		
• *Francisella*		

Other Bacteria

Spiral-Shaped Bacteria:	Obligate Intracellular Organisms:
• *Campylobacter*	• *Rickettsia*
• *Helicobacter*	• *Orientia*
• *Treponema*	• *Ehrlichia*
• *Borrelia*	• *Anaplasma*
• *Leptospira*	• *Coxiella*
	• *Chlamydia*

ROLE IN DISEASE

Occasionally, some diseases have a characteristic presentation and are associated with a single organism. Unfortunately, multiple organisms can produce a similar clinical picture (e.g., sepsis, pneumonia, gastroenteritis, meningitis, urinary tract infection, genital infection). The clinical management of infections is predicted by the ability to develop an accurate differential diagnosis defined by the most common organisms associated with the clinical picture, selection of the appropriate diagnostic tests, and initiation of effective empirical therapy. Once the diagnosis is confirmed, empirical therapy can be modified to provide narrow-spectrum, directed therapy. The following is a list of the most common organisms associated with specific clinical syndromes.

Common Organisms and Their Associated Clinical Syndromes

Disease	Most Common Pathogens
Sepsis	
General sepsis	*Staphylococcus aureus*, coagulase-negative *Staphylococcus*, *Escherichia coli*, *Klebsiella pneumoniae*, *Pseudomonas aeruginosa*
Catheter-related sepsis	Coagulase-negative *Staphylococcus*
Septic thrombophlebitis	*S. aureus*, *P. aeruginosa*
Cardiovascular Infections	
Endocarditis	Viridans *Streptococcus*, *S. aureus*, coagulase-negative *Staphylococcus*, HACEK organisms (*Haemophilus*, *Aggregatibacterium*, *Cardiobacterium*, *Eikenella*, *Kingella*), *Coxiella*
Myocarditis	*S. aureus*, *Borrelia burgdorferi*
Pericarditis	*S. aureus*, *Streptococcus pneumoniae*
Upper Respiratory Infections	
Pharyngitis	*Streptococcus pyogenes* (group A)
Sinusitis	*S. pneumoniae*, *Haemophilus influenzae*, *Moraxella catarrhalis*, mixed aerobic and anaerobic
Ear Infections	
Otitis externa	*Pseudomonas aeruginosa*, *S. aureus*
Otitis media	*S. pneumoniae*, *H. influenzae*, *M. catarrhalis*

Common Organisms and Their Associated Clinical Syndromes—cont'd

Disease	Most Common Pathogens
Eye Infections	
Conjunctivitis	*S. aureus, S. pneumoniae, Haemophilus aegyptius*
Keratitis	*S. aureus, S. pneumoniae, P. aeruginosa*
Endophthalmitis	*Bacillus cereus, S. aureus, P. aeruginosa*
Pleuropulmonary and Bronchial Infections	
Bronchitis	*M. catarrhalis, Mycoplasma pneumoniae*
Empyema	*S. aureus, S. pneumoniae, S. pyogenes* (group A)
Pneumonia	*S. pneumoniae, S. aureus, K. pneumoniae,* other Enterobacteriales, *P. aeruginosa, Legionella pneumophila*
Central Nervous System Infections	
Meningitis	*Streptococcus agalactiae* (group B), *E. coli, H. influenzae, S. pneumoniae, Neisseria meningitidis, Listeria monocytogenes*
Encephalitis	Rarely bacterial
Brain abscess	*S. aureus, Fusobacterium* species, anaerobic species
Subdural empyema	*S. aureus, S. pneumoniae*
Intra-abdominal Infections	
Peritonitis	*E. coli, B. fragilis, Enterococcus* species
Dialysis-associated peritonitis	Coagulase-negative *Staphylococcus*
Gastrointestinal Infections	
Gastritis	*Helicobacter pylori*
Gastroenteritis	*Salmonella* species, *Shigella* species, *Campylobacter jejuni, Campylobacter coli, E. coli, Vibrio cholera, Vibrio parahaemolyticus, B. cereus, P. aeruginosa*
Antibiotic-associated diarrhea	*Clostridioides difficile*
Food intoxication	*S. aureus, B. cereus*
Proctitis	*Neisseria gonorrhoeae, Chlamydia trachomatis*
Genital Infections	
Genital ulcers	*Treponema pallidum, Haemophilus ducreyi*
Urethritis	*N. gonorrhoeae, C. trachomatis, Mycoplasma genitalium*
Vaginitis	*Mycoplasma hominis, Mobiluncus* species, other anaerobic species
Cervicitis	*N. gonorrhoeae, C. trachomatis, M. genitalium*
Urinary Tract Infections	
Cystitis and pyelonephritis	*E. coli, Proteus mirabilis,* other Enterobacteriales, *Staphylococcus saprophyticus*
Renal calculi	*P. mirabilis, S. saprophyticus*
Renal abscess	*S. aureus*
Prostatitis	*E. coli, P. aeruginosa, Enterococcus* species
Skin and Soft-Tissue Infections	
Impetigo	*S. pyogenes* (group A), *S. aureus*
Folliculitis	*S. aureus, P. aeruginosa*
Furuncles and carbuncles	*S. aureus*
Paronychia	*S. aureus, S. pyogenes* (group A), *P. aeruginosa*
Erysipelas	*S. pyogenes* (group A)
Cellulitis	*S. pyogenes* (group A), *S. aureus*

Continued

Common Organisms and Their Associated Clinical Syndromes—cont'd

Disease	Most Common Pathogens
Necrotizing cellulitis and fasciitis	*S. pyogenes* (group A), *Clostridium perfringens*, *B. fragilis*
Bacillary angiomatosis	*Bartonella henselae, Bartonella quintana*
Infections of burns	*S. aureus, P. aeruginosa, Enterococcus* species, Enterobacteriales
Surgical wounds	*S. aureus*, coagulase-negative *Staphylococcus*
Bite wounds	*Eikenella corrodens, Pasteurella multocida*, mixed aerobes and anaerobes
Traumatic wounds	*Bacillus* species, *S. aureus*
Bone and Joint Infections	
Osteomyelitis	*S. aureus*, coagulase-negative *Staphylococcus, P. aeruginosa*, Enterobacteriales
Arthritis	*S. aureus, N. gonorrhoeae*
Prosthetic-associated infection	*S. aureus*, coagulase-negative *Staphylococcus*
Granulomatous Infections	
General	*Mycoplasma tuberculosis, Nocardia* species, *T. pallidum*

ANTIBACTERIAL AGENTS

This section presents an overview of the most commonly used antibacterial agents, their mode of action, and spectrum of activity. By its nature, this is not a comprehensive summary of antibacterial therapy. Additionally, in the following chapters, the recommended therapies for individual organisms are listed.

Commonly Used Antibacterial Agents, Their Mode of Action, and Spectrum of Activity

Mode of Action	Antibiotic	Spectrum of Activity
DISRUPTION OF CELL WALL		
Binds proteins (Penicillin-binding proteins) and enzymes responsible for peptidoglycan synthesis	Natural penicillins (penicillin G)	Active against all β-hemolytic streptococci and most other streptococci; very limited activity against staphylococci; active against meningococci and most gram-positive anaerobes; poor activity against gram-negative rods
	Penicillinase-resistant penicillins (methicillin, nafcillin, oxacillin, cloxacillin, dicloxacillin)	Similar to the natural penicillins except for enhanced activity against staphylococci
	Extended-spectrum penicillins (ampicillin, amoxicillin, piperacillin)	Active against gram-positive cocci equivalent to the natural penicillins; active against some gram-negative rods
	Narrow-spectrum cephalosporins and cephamycins (cephalexin, cephalothin, cefazolin, cefadroxil)	Activity equivalent to oxacillin against gram-positive bacteria; some gram-negative activity (e.g., *E. coli, Klebsiella, P. mirabilis*)
	Expanded-spectrum cephalosporins and cephamycins (cefuroxime, cefotetan, cefoxitin, cefprozil)	Activity equivalent to oxacillin against gram-positive bacteria; improved gram-negative activity to include *Enterobacter, Citrobacter*, and additional *Proteus* species

Commonly Used Antibacterial Agents, Their Mode of Action, and Spectrum of Activity—cont'd

Mode of Action	Antibiotic	Spectrum of Activity
	DISRUPTION OF CELL WALL—cont'd	
	Broad-spectrum cephalosporins (cefixime, cefotaxime, ceftriaxone, ceftazidime, cefpodoxime, cefepime, cefpirome)	Activity equivalent to oxacillin against gram-positive bacteria; improved gram-negative activity to include *Pseudomonas*
	Carbapenems (imipenem, meropenem, ertapenem, doripenem)	Broad-spectrum antibiotics active against most aerobic and anaerobic gram-positive and gram-negative bacteria except for oxacillin-resistant staphylococci, most *Enterococcus faecium*, and selected gram-negative rods (*Pseudomonas, Stenotrophomonas, Burkholderia*)
	Narrow-spectrum monobactam (aztreonam)	Active against selected aerobic gram-negative rods but inactive against anaerobes and gram-positive cocci
Binds β-lactamases and prevents enzymatic inactivation of β-lactam	β-Lactams with β-lactamase inhibitor (ampicillin-sulbactam, amoxicillin-clavulanate, piperacillin-tazobactam, ceftazidime-avibactam, ceftolozane-tazobactam, meropenem-vaborbactam)	Activity similar to natural penicillins plus improved activity against β-lactamase-producing staphylococci and selected gram-negative rods including some carbapenem-resistant gram-negative rods (the last three listed represent the newest class of antibiotics)
Inhibits cross-linkage of peptidoglycan layers	Glycopeptides (vancomycin)	Active against all staphylococci and streptococci; inactive against many enterococci, gram-positive rods, and all gram-negative bacteria
Inhibits bacterial cytoplasmic membrane formation and movement of peptidoglycan precursors	Polypeptide (bacitracin)	Topical agent active against staphylococci and streptococci; inactive against gram-negative bacteria
Disrupts bacterial outer membrane permeability	Polypeptide (colistin, polymyxin B)	Active against most gram-negative bacteria but not gram-positive bacteria (no outer membrane)
Blocks N-acetylmuramic acid synthesis and early cell wall synthesis	Fosfomycin	Broad spectrum of activity for treatment of urinary tract infections caused by gram-positive and gram-negative bacteria
Inhibits mycolic acid synthesis	Isoniazid, ethionamide	Active against mycobacteria
Inhibits synthesis of arabinogalactan	Ethambutol	
Inhibits cross-linkage of peptidoglycan precursors	Cycloserine	

Continued

Commonly Used Antibacterial Agents, Their Mode of Action, and Spectrum of Activity—cont'd

Mode of Action	Antibiotic	Spectrum of Activity
INHIBITION OF PROTEIN SYNTHESIS		
Produces premature release of peptide chains from 30S ribosome	Aminoglycosides (neomycin, streptomycin, kanamycin, gentamicin, tobramycin, amikacin)	Primarily used to treat infections with gram-negative rods; neomycin used topically; kanamycin with limited activity; tobramycin slightly more active than gentamicin vs *Pseudomonas*; amikacin most active
Prevents polypeptide elongation at 30S ribosome	Tetracyclines (tetracycline, doxycycline, minocycline)	Broad-spectrum antibiotics active against gram-positive and some gram-negative bacteria (*Neisseria*, some Enterobacteriales), mycoplasmas, chlamydiae, and rickettsiae
Binds to 30S ribosome and prevents initiation of protein synthesis	Glycylcyclines (tigecycline)	Spectrum similar to tetracyclines but more active against gram-negative bacteria and rapidly growing mycobacteria
Prevents initiation of protein synthesis at 50S ribosome	Oxazolidinone (linezolid)	Active against *Staphylococcus*, *Enterococcus*, *Streptococcus*, gram-positive rods, *Clostridium*, and anaerobic cocci; not active against gram-negative bacteria
Prevents polypeptide elongation at 50S ribosome	Macrolides (erythromycin, azithromycin, clarithromycin)	Broad-spectrum antibiotics active against gram-positive and some gram-negative bacteria, *Neisseria*, *Legionella*, *Mycoplasma*, *Chlamydia*, *Treponema*, and *Rickettsia*; clarithromycin and azithromycin active against some mycobacteria
	Lincosamide (clindamycin)	Broad spectrum of activity against aerobic gram-positive cocci and anaerobes
	Streptogramins (quinupristin-dalfopristin)	Primarily active against gram-positive bacteria; good activity against methicillin-susceptible and methicillin-resistant staphylococci, streptococci, *E. faecium* (no activity against *Enterococcus faecalis*), *Haemophilus*, *Moraxella*, and anaerobes; not active against Enterobacteriales or other gram-negative rods
Inhibition of RNA polymerase by binding to DNA-RNA polymerase complex	Fidaxomicin	Bactericidal macrolide used for the treatment of *Clostridioides difficile* infections
INHIBITION OF NUCLEIC ACID SYNTHESIS		
Binds α-subunit of DNA gyrase	Narrow-spectrum quinolone (nalidixic acid)	Active against selected gram-negative rods; no useful gram-positive activity
	Broad-spectrum quinolone (ciprofloxacin, levofloxacin)	Broad-spectrum antibiotics with activity against gram-positive and gram-negative bacteria
	Extended-spectrum quinolones (moxifloxacin, gatifloxacin, delafloxacin, gemifloxacin)	Broad-spectrum antibiotic with enhanced activity against gram-positive bacteria; activity against gram-negative rods similar to that of ciprofloxacin

Commonly Used Antibacterial Agents, Their Mode of Action, and Spectrum of Activity—cont'd

Mode of Action	Antibiotic	Spectrum of Activity
INHIBITION OF NUCLEIC ACID SYNTHESIS—cont'd		
Prevents transcription by binding DNA-dependent RNA polymerase	Rifampin, rifabutin	Active against aerobic gram-positive bacteria including mycobacteria; no gram-negative activity
Disrupts bacteria DNA	Metronidazole	Active against anaerobic bacteria but not against aerobic or facultative anaerobes
ANTIMETABOLITE		
Inhibits dihydropteroate synthase and disrupts folic acid synthesis	Sulfonamides	Effective against a broad range of gram-positive and gram-negative organisms and a drug of choice for Urinary tract infections
Inhibits dihydropteroate reductase and disrupts folic acid synthesis	Trimethoprim	
Inhibits dihydropteroate synthase	Dapsone	Active against mycobacteria

Aerobic Gram-Positive Cocci

The aerobic gram-positive cocci are a heterogeneous collection of spherical bacteria that are commonly present in the mouth, gastrointestinal tract and genitourinary tract, and on the skin surface. The most important genera are *Staphylococcus*, *Streptococcus*, and *Enterococcus*.

The staphylococci, streptococci, and enterococci are gram-positive cocci, typically arranged in clusters (*Staphylococcus*), chains (*Streptococcus*), or pairs (*S. pneumoniae, Enterococcus*), and generally grow well aerobically and anaerobically. The thick cell wall allows these bacteria to survive for a prolonged period of time on dry surfaces, such as hospital linens, tables, and door knobs, and these can serve as a source of infection to those who touch the surfaces. Virulence of the bacteria is determined by their ability to evade the host immune system, adhere to host cells, and produce toxins and/or hydrolytic enzymes responsible for tissue destruction. The species with the greatest potential for disease are *Staphylococcus aureus*, *Streptococcus pyogenes*, *Streptococcus agalactiae*, and *Streptococcus pneumoniae*, illustrated by the wide variety of virulence factors expressed by each. Particularly noteworthy are a group of toxins: staphylococcal enterotoxins, exfoliative toxins, and toxic shock syndrome toxins, as well as *S. pyogenes* pyrogenic exotoxins. These toxins are termed **"superantigens"** because they stimulate a massive release of cytokines by the patient with resulting pathology.

Staphylococcus, Streptococcus, and Enterococcus

Genus	Historical Derivation of the Name
Staphylococcus	*Staphyle*, bunch of grapes; *coccus*, grain or berry; round, berrylike bacterial cells arranged in grapelike clusters
Streptococcus	*Streptus*, pliant; *coccus*, grain or berry; refers to the appearance of long, flexible chains of cocci
Enterococcus	*Enteron*, intestine; *coccus*, berry; intestinal cocci

Although staphylococci, streptococci, and enterococci are among the most common bacteria implicated in disease, it is important to remember that these are also common residents in the human body. Simply recovering these bacteria in a clinical specimen does not define disease. Disease is found in specific populations of patients and under well-defined clinical conditions, so it is important to understand this epidemiology.

Diagnosis of *S. aureus* infections is generally not difficult because the organism grows readily in culture, and nucleic acid amplification tests are widely used for the rapid detection of both methicillin-susceptible (MSSA) and methicillin-resistant (MRSA) *S. aureus* in clinical specimens. Likewise, diagnosis of infections caused by streptococci and enterococci is not difficult; however, because many of these bacteria are part of the normal microbial population in the body, care must be taken to collect uncontaminated specimens.

Treatment of staphylococcal infections is difficult because the majority are MRSA strains. MRSA strains are resistant not only to methicillin but also to all β-lactam antibiotics (including penicillins, cephalosporins, and carbapenems). Most streptococcal infections can be treated with penicillins, cephalosporins, or macrolides, although resistance is observed with *S. pneumoniae* and some other species of streptococci. Serious enterococcal infections are difficult to manage because resistance to most antibiotics is common.

Prevention of infections with all these bacteria is also difficult because most infections originate from the patient's own microbial population or through routine daily interactions such as touching a contaminated surface.

One exception to this is the neonatal disease caused by *S. agalactiae* because the infant acquires the infection from the mother. Pregnant women are screened for vaginal carriage with this organism shortly before delivery, and colonized women are treated with antibiotic prophylaxis. Polyvalent vaccines are currently only available for *S. pneumoniae* infections.

The most common species of *Staphylococcus* associated with disease is *S. aureus*, which will be the primary focus in the discussion of this genus. Other species, commonly referred to as **coagulase-negative staphylococci**, are primarily opportunistic pathogens, but three species are noteworthy: *Staphylococcus epidermidis*, *Staphylococcus saprophyticus*, and *Staphylococcus lugdunensis*.

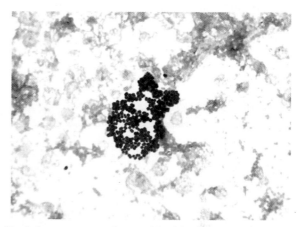

Staphylococcus aureus in a positive blood culture. Note the arrangement of gram-positive cocci in grapelike clusters.

Important Staphylococci

Species	Historical Derivation of the Name	Diseases
S. aureus	*Aureus*, golden or yellow; *S. aureus* colonies can turn yellow with age	Pyogenic infections; toxin-mediated infections
S. epidermidis	*Epidermidis*, epidermidis (outer skin)	Opportunistic infections (e.g., catheter-associated infections, surgical site infections where a foreign body is present such as an artificial heart valve [subacute endocarditis])
S. saprophyticus	*Saprophyticus: sapros*, putrid; *phyton*, plant (saprophytic or growing on dead tissue)	Urinary tract infections, particularly in sexually active young women
S. lugdunensis	*Lugdunensis: Lugdunun*, Latin name for Lyon where the organism was first isolated	Acute endocarditis in patients with native heart valves

The classification of the streptococci is confusing because three different schemes have been used: hemolytic patterns on blood agar, serologic properties, and biochemical properties. The following is an oversimplification but may help sort through the confusion. The streptococci can be divided into two groups: (1) β-**hemolytic** (complete hemolysis on blood agar) species that are subclassified by serologic properties (grouped from A to W) and (2) the **viridans streptococci** group that consists of α-hemolytic (partial hemolysis of blood) and γ-hemolytic (no hemolysis) species. Some species of viridans streptococci such as members of the *Streptococcus anginosus* group (with three species) are classified in both the β-hemolytic group and the viridans group because they are biochemically the same but have different hemolytic patterns. Disease caused by the *S. anginosus* group is the same regardless of their hemolytic properties. The following are the most important representatives of the β-hemolytic and viridans group streptococci.

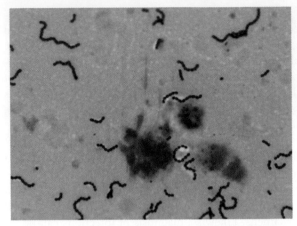

Streptococcus mitis (viridans group) in positive blood culture. Note the long chain of gram-positive cocci.

Important β-Hemolytic Streptococci

Group	Representative Species	Historical Derivation	Diseases
A	S. pyogenes	*Pyus*, pus; *gennaio*, producing (producing pus)	Pharyngitis, skin and soft-tissue infections, rheumatic fever, acute glomerulonephritis
	S. anginosus group	*Anginosus*, pertaining to angina	Abscesses
B	S. agalactiae	*Agalactia*, want of milk (original isolate associated with bovine mastitis)	Neonatal disease, endometritis, wound infections, urinary tract infections, pneumonia, skin and soft-tissue infections
C	S. dysgalactiae	*Dys*, ill; *galactia*, pertaining to milk (associated with bovine mastitis and loss of milk)	Pharyngitis, acute glomerulonephritis

Important Viridans Streptococci

Group	Representative Species	Historical Derivation	Diseases
Anginosus	S. anginosus group	*Anginosus*, pertaining to angina	Abscesses
Mitis	Streptococcus mitis	*Mitis*, mild (incorrectly thought to cause mild disease)	Subacute endocarditis, sepsis in neutropenic patients
	S. pneumoniae	*Pneumon*, the lungs (causes pneumonia)	Pneumonia, meningitis, sinusitis, otitis media, fulminant septicemia
Mutans	S. mutans	*Mutans*, changing (cocci that may appear rodlike)	Dental caries, subacute endocarditis

Important Viridans Streptococci—cont'd

Group	Representative Species	Historical Derivation	Diseases
Salivarius	*Streptococcus salivarius*	*Salivarius*, salivary (found in the mouth in saliva)	Subacute endocarditis
Bovis	*Streptococcus gallolyticus*	*Gallatum*, gallate; *lyticus*, to loosen (able to digest or hydrolyze methyl gallate)	Bacteremia associated with gastrointestinal cancer, meningitis

Members of the genus *Enterococcus* were classified originally as *Streptococcus* but were reclassified in 1984. Two species of enterococci are particularly important because they cause similar diseases and are frequently resistant to most antibiotics.

Important Enterococci

Representative Species	Historical Derivation	Diseases
E. faecalis	*Faecalis*, relating to feces	Urinary tract infections, peritonitis, wound infections, endocarditis
E. faecium	*Faecium*, of feces	

The following are summaries of the major groups of gram-positive cocci.

STAPHYLOCOCCUS AUREUS

Diseases caused by *S. aureus* are divided into two groups: (1) localized pyogenic or "pus-producing" diseases that are characterized by tissue destruction mediated by hydrolytic enzymes and cytotoxins and (2) diseases mediated by toxins that function as superantigens producing systemic diseases.

STAPHYLOCOCCUS AUREUS

Properties	• Ability to grow aerobically and anaerobically, over a wide range of temperatures, and in the presence of a high concentration of salt; the latter is important because these bacteria are a common cause of food poisoning
	• Polysaccharide capsule that protects the bacteria from phagocytosis
	• Cell surface proteins (**protein A**, clumping factor proteins) that mediate adherence of the bacteria to host tissues
	• **Catalase** that protects staphylococci from peroxides produced by neutrophils and macrophages
	• **Coagulase** converts fibrinogen to insoluble fibrin that forms clots and can protect S. aureus from phagocytosis
	• **Hydrolytic enzymes and cytotoxins**:
	• Lipases, nucleases, and hyaluronidase that cause tissue destruction
	• Cytotoxins (alpha, beta, delta, gamma, leukocidin) that lyse erythrocytes, neutrophils, macrophages, and other host cells
	• Toxins:
	• **Enterotoxins** (many antigenically distinct) are relatively resistant to cooking temperatures and resistant to gastric acids; toxins responsible for food poisoning
	• **Exfoliative toxins** A and B cause the superficial layers of skin to peel off (scalded skin syndrome)
	• **Toxic shock syndrome toxin** is a heat- and protease-resistant toxin that mediates multiorgan pathology
Epidemiology	• Common cause of infections both in the community and in the hospital because the bacteria are easily spread person to person and through direct contact or exposure to contaminated bed linens, clothing, and other surfaces
	• Antibiotic-resistant strains (e.g., MRSA) are widely distributed in both the hospital and the community

Continued

STAPHYLOCOCCUS AUREUS—cont'd

Clinical Disease	**S. aureus Pyogenic Diseases** • **Impetigo**: localized skin infection characterized by pus-filled vesicles on a reddened or erythematous base; seen mostly in children on their face and limbs • **Folliculitis**: impetigo involving hair follicles, such as the beard area • **Furuncles (boils) and carbuncles**: large, pus-filled skin nodules; can progress to deeper layers of the skin and spread into the blood and other areas of the body • **Wound infections**: characterized by erythema and pus at the site of trauma or surgery; more difficult to treat if a foreign body is present (e.g., splinter, surgical suture); majority of infections both in the community and the hospital are caused by MRSA; recurrent bouts of infections are common • **Pneumonia**: abscess formation in the lungs; observed primarily in the very young and old and frequently following viral infections of the respiratory tract (e.g., influenza) • **Endocarditis**: infection of the endothelial lining of the heart; disease can progress rapidly and is associated with a high mortality rate • **Osteomyelitis**: destruction of bones, particularly the highly vascularized areas of long bones in children • **Septic arthritis**: infection of joint spaces characterized by a swollen, reddened joint with accumulation of pus; the most common cause of septic arthritis in children **S. aureus-Toxin-Mediated Diseases** • **Food poisoning**: after consumption of food contaminated with the **heat-stable enterotoxin**, there is a rapid (2–4 h) onset of severe vomiting, diarrhea, and stomach cramps that typically resolve within 24 h. This is because the intoxication is caused by the preformed toxin present in the food rather than an infection where the bacteria would have to grow and produce toxin in the intestine, and the toxin is rapidly flushed from the intestines with vomiting and diarrhea • **Scalded skin syndrome**: bacteria in a localized infection (e.g., newborn umbilicus) produce the toxin that spreads through the blood and causes the outermost layer of the skin to blister and peel off; almost exclusively seen in very young children • **Toxic shock syndrome**: bacteria in a localized infection (e.g., vagina, wound) produce the toxin that affects multiple organs; characterized initially by fever, hypotension, and a diffuse, macular, erythematous rash. There is a very high mortality rate associated with this disease unless antibiotics are promptly administered and the local infection is managed

Diagnosis	• **Microscopy**: useful for pyogenic infections but not for bacteremia (too few organisms present), food poisoning (intoxication), or scalded skin syndrome and toxic shock syndrome (toxin production at the localized site of infection and the bacteria are typically not in affected organ tissues)
	• **Culture**: organisms are recovered on most laboratory media
	• **Nucleic acid amplification tests**: sensitive method for rapid detection of MSSA and MRSA in clinical specimens
	• **Identification tests**:
	  • **Catalase**: separates *Staphylococcus* (+) from *Streptococcus* and *Enterococcus* (−)
	  • **Coagulase**: separates *S. aureus* (+) from other species of *Staphylococcus* (−)
	  • **Protein A**: separates *S. aureus* (+) from other species of *Staphylococcus* (−)

Treatment, Control, and Prevention	• Localized infections managed by incision and drainage
	• Antibiotic therapy indicated for systemic infections; empiric therapy should include antibiotics active against MRSA
	  • Oral therapy can include trimethoprim-sulfamethoxazole, clindamycin, or doxycycline
	  • Vancomycin is the drug of choice for intravenous therapy
	• Treatment is symptomatic for patients with food poisoning although the source of infection should be identified so other individuals will not be exposed
	• Proper cleansing of wounds and use of disinfectants help prevent infections
	• Thorough hand washing and covering the exposed skin help medical personnel prevent infection or spread to other patients
	• No vaccine is currently available

β-HEMOLYTIC STREPTOCOCCI

Two species of β-hemolytic streptococci will be discussed here: *S. pyogenes* and *S. agalactiae*, but other important species will be mentioned briefly. *S. anginosus* and related bacteria are classified with both the β-hemolytic streptococci and the viridans streptococci and are discussed below; however, it should be recognized that these are important causes of deep tissue abscesses. *Streptococcus dysgalactiae* is an uncommon cause of pharyngitis. This is mentioned because the disease resembles pharyngitis caused by *S. pyogenes* and can be complicated with acute glomerulonephritis but not rheumatic fever (both complications are seen with some *S. pyogenes* isolates).

Diseases caused by *S. pyogenes* are subdivided into suppurative (characterized by the formation of pus) and nonsuppurative. **Suppurative diseases** range from pharyngitis to localized skin and soft-tissue infections to necrotizing fasciitis ("flesh eating" bacterial infection) and streptococcal toxic shock syndrome. **Nonsuppurative diseases** are an autoimmune complication following streptococcal pharyngitis (rheumatic fever, acute glomerulonephritis) and pyodermal infections (only acute glomerulonephritis). Antibodies directed against specific *S. pyogenes* proteins (M proteins) cross-react with host tissues in nonsuppurative diseases.

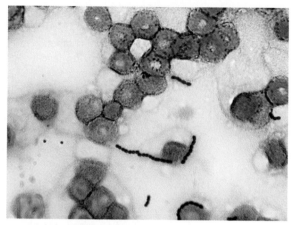

Streptococcus pyogenes in positive blood culture.

STREPTOCOCCUS PYOGENES

Properties	• Outer hyaluronic acid **capsule** (single serotype) protects *S. pyogenes* from phagocytic clearance (nonimmunogenic because bacterial and host hyaluronic acid are identical)
	• Cell wall proteins (**M proteins, M-like proteins,** and **C5a peptidase**) block complement-mediated phagocytosis
	• M proteins and F proteins facilitate adherence and invasion into epithelial cells
	• Hydrolytic enzymes:
	  • **Streptolysin S** and **streptolysin O** lyse erythrocytes, leukocytes, platelets, and cultured cells
	  • **Streptokinase** lyse blood clots and fibrin deposits, facilitating rapid spread
	  • **DNases** lyse free DNA in abscesses, facilitating rapid spread
	• Toxins:
	  • Four distinct heat-labile **streptococcal pyrogenic exotoxins** enhance the release of proinflammatory cytokines responsible for the clinical manifestations of severe streptococcal diseases

Epidemiology	• Person-to-person spread by respiratory droplets (pharyngitis) or through breaks in the skin after direct contact with the infected person, fomite, or arthropod vector • Pharyngitis and soft-tissue infections typically caused by strains with different M proteins • **Most common cause of bacterial pharyngitis** • Individuals at a higher risk of disease include children aged 5–15 years (pharyngitis); children aged 2–5 years with poor personal hygiene (pyoderma); patients with soft-tissue infection (streptococcal toxic shock syndrome); patients with prior streptococcal pharyngitis (rheumatic fever, glomerulonephritis) or soft-tissue infection (glomerulonephritis) • Pharyngitis is most common in the cold months; no seasonal incidence for soft-tissue infections

Continued

STREPTOCOCCUS PYOGENES—cont'd

Clinical Disease	• **Pharyngitis**: reddened pharynx with exudates generally present; cervical lymphadenopathy can be prominent • **Scarlet fever**: complication of streptococcal pharyngitis; diffuse erythematous rash beginning on the chest and spreading to the extremities • **Pyoderma**: localized skin infection with vesicles progressing to pustules; no evidence of systemic disease • **Erysipelas**: localized skin infection with pain, inflammation, lymph node enlargement, and systemic symptoms • **Cellulitis**: infection of the skin that involves subcutaneous tissues • **Necrotizing fasciitis**: deep infection of the skin that involves destruction of muscle and fat layers • **Streptococcal toxic shock syndrome**: multiorgan systemic infection resembling staphylococcal toxic shock syndrome; however, most patients are bacteremic (not seen with staphylococcal disease) and with evidence of fasciitis • **Rheumatic fever**: nonsuppurative complication of streptococcal pharyngitis characterized by inflammatory changes of the heart (pancarditis), joints (arthralgias to arthritis), blood vessels, and subcutaneous tissues • **Acute glomerulonephritis**: nonsuppurative complication of streptococcal pharyngitis or soft-tissue infections characterized by acute inflammation of the renal glomeruli with edema, hypertension, hematuria, and proteinuria
Diagnosis	• Microscopy is useful in soft-tissue infections but not in pharyngitis or nonsuppurative complications • Direct tests for the group A antigen are useful for the diagnosis of streptococcal pharyngitis • Isolates identified by catalase (negative), positive l-pyrrolidonyl arylamidase reaction, susceptibility to bacitracin, and presence of group-specific antigen (group A antigen) • Antistreptolysin O (ASO) test is useful for confirming rheumatic fever or glomerulonephritis associated with streptococcal pharyngitis; anti-DNase B test (not antistreptolysin O) should be performed for glomerulonephritis associated with pharyngitis or soft-tissue infections
Treatment, Control, and Prevention	• Penicillin V or amoxicillin used to treat pharyngitis; oral cephalosporin or macrolides for penicillin-allergic patients; intravenous penicillin plus clindamycin used for systemic infections • Oropharyngeal carriage occurring after treatment can be retreated; treatment is not indicated for prolonged asymptomatic carriage because antibiotics disrupt normal protective flora • Starting antibiotic therapy within 10 days in patients with pharyngitis prevents rheumatic fever • In patients with a history of valvular heart disease caused by rheumatic fever, antibiotic prophylaxis is required before procedures (e.g., dental) that can induce bacteremias leading to endocarditis • For glomerulonephritis, no specific antibiotic treatment or prophylaxis is indicated

S. agalactiae infections are most common in newborns, acquired either *in utero* or during the first week of life, and are associated with high mortality or significant neurologic sequelae.

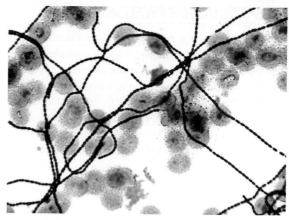

Streptococcus agalactiae in positive blood culture.

STREPTOCOCCUS AGALACTIAE	
Properties	• Outer polysaccharide **capsule** (multiple serotypes) protects from phagocytic clearance • **Sialic acid** blocks complement-mediated phagocytosis
Epidemiology	• Asymptomatic colonization of the upper respiratory tract and genitourinary tract • Early-onset disease acquired by neonates from the mother during pregnancy or at the time of birth • Women with genital colonization are at risk of postpartum disease • Neonates are at a higher risk of infection if: (1) there is premature rupture of membranes, prolonged labor, preterm birth, or disseminated maternal group B streptococcal disease; and (2) the mother is without type-specific antibodies and has low complement levels • Men and nonpregnant women with diabetes mellitus, cancer, or alcoholism are at an increased risk of disease • No seasonal incidence
Clinical Disease	• **Early-onset neonatal disease**: within 7 days of birth, infected newborns develop signs and symptoms of pneumonia, meningitis, and sepsis • **Late-onset neonatal disease**: more than 1 week after birth, neonates develop signs and symptoms of meningitis with bacteremia • **Infections in pregnant women**: most often present as postpartum endometritis, wound infections, and urinary tract infections; disseminated complications may occur • **Infections in other adult patients**: most common diseases include pneumonia, bone and joint infections, and skin and soft-tissue infections
Diagnosis	• Microscopy useful for meningitis (cerebrospinal fluid), pneumonia (lower respiratory secretions), and wound infections (exudates) • Antigen tests are less sensitive than microscopy and should not be used • Culture is a sensitive test for detection of vaginal carriage in pregnant women if a selective broth (i.e., LIM) is used • Nucleic acid amplification tests are commercially available and are rapid and more sensitive than culture • Isolates are identified by demonstration of group-specific cell wall carbohydrate or positive nucleic acid amplification test
Treatment, Control, and Prevention	• Penicillin G is the drug of choice; combination of penicillin and aminoglycoside is used in patients with serious infections; a cephalosporin or vancomycin is used for patients allergic to penicillin • For high-risk babies, penicillin is given at least 4h before delivery • No vaccine is currently available

STREPTOCOCCUS PNEUMONIAE

S. pneumoniae is the most important member of the viridans streptococci and is typically considered separately because it is one of the most common causes of a spectrum of diseases: pneumonia, meningitis, otitis, and sinusitis. Recurrent infections with this bacterium are common because immunity to infection is mediated by the presence of antibodies to the polysaccharide capsule, and nearly 100 unique serotypes have been described.

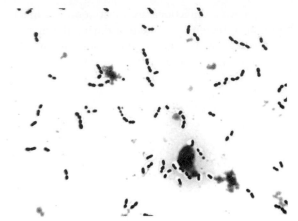

Streptococcus pneumoniae in positive blood culture. Note the arrangement of cocci in pairs and short chains.

STREPTOCOCCUS PNEUMONIAE	
Properties	• Outer **polysaccharide capsule** (multiple serotypes) protects from phagocytic clearance • Surface protein adhesins bind bacteria to epithelial cells • Phosphorylcholine binds to receptors on the surface of endothelial cells, leukocytes, and platelets; upon entering the cells, the bacteria are protected from opsonization and phagocytosis • Immunoglobulin (Ig) A protease prevents inactivation of bacteria trapped in mucus by secretory IgA • Pneumolysis is a cytotoxin similar to streptolysin O; binds to cholesterol in host cell wall and creates pores, destroying epithelial and phagocytic cells
Epidemiology	• The most virulent member of the viridans streptococci • Most infections are caused by endogenous spread from the colonized nasopharynx or oropharynx to the distal site (e.g., lungs, sinuses, ears, meninges) • Person-to-person spread through infectious droplets is rare • Colonization is highest in young children and their contacts • Individuals with antecedent viral respiratory tract disease or other conditions that interfere with bacterial clearance from the respiratory tract are at an increased risk of pneumonia, otitis media (young children), and sinusitis (all ages) • Children and the elderly are at the greatest risk of meningitis • People with hematologic disorder (e.g., malignancy, sickle cell disease) or functional asplenia are at risk of fulminant sepsis • Although the organism is ubiquitous, disease is more common in cool months
Clinical Disease	• **Pneumonia**: acute onset of chills and sustained fever; productive cough with blood-tinged sputum; lobar consolidation • **Meningitis**: severe infection involving the meninges, with headache, fever, and sepsis; high mortality and severe neurologic deficits in survivors • **Sinusitis and otitis media**: common cause of acute infections of the paranasal sinuses and ear; typically preceded by a viral infection of the upper respiratory tract with leukocyte infiltration and obstruction of the sinuses and ear canal • **Fulminant sepsis**: bacteremia is more common in patients with pneumonia and meningitis than with sinusitis or otitis media; fulminant sepsis in asplenic patients

STREPTOCOCCUS PNEUMONIAE—cont'd	
Diagnosis	• Microscopy is highly sensitive, as is culture, unless the patient has been treated with antibiotics • Specific antigen tests for pneumococcal C polysaccharide are sensitive with cerebrospinal fluid for the diagnosis of meningitis but should not be used with other specimen types or infections • Nucleic acid amplification tests are not commonly used for diagnosis except for meningitis • Culture requires the use of enriched-nutrient media (e.g., sheep blood agar); organism is susceptible to many antibiotics, so culture can be negative in partially treated patients • Isolates identified by catalase (negative), susceptibility to optochin (common disk test performed for identification), and solubility in bile (rapid test where colonies dissolve in a drop of bile within a few minutes)
Treatment, Control, and Prevention	• Penicillin is the drug of choice for susceptible strains, although resistance is increasingly common • Vancomycin combined with ceftriaxone is used for empiric therapy; monotherapy with a cephalosporin, fluoroquinolone, or vancomycin can be used in patients with susceptible isolates • Immunization with 13-valent **conjugated vaccine** is recommended for all children younger than 2 years of age; a 23-valent **polysaccharide vaccine** is recommended for adults at risk of the disease

VIRIDANS STREPTOCOCCI

The viridans streptococci are commonly thought of as a homogeneous collection of streptococci, but in truth, the individual species of bacteria are associated with distinct infections (e.g., abscess formation, dental caries, subacute endocarditis, septicemia, and meningitis), so it is important to know the specific disease associations.

VIRIDANS STREPTOCOCCI	
Properties	• Although relatively avirulent, individual species have a predilection of producing disease in specific anatomic sites (abscess formation, endocarditis, meningitis)
Epidemiology	• Ubiquitous colonizers of mucosal surfaces (mouth, gastrointestinal tract, genitourinary tract); not commonly found on the skin surface • Most are opportunistic pathogens • No seasonal incidence of disease
Clinical Disease	• Abscess formation in deep tissues: associated with the *S. anginosus* group • Septicemia in neutropenic patients: associated with *S. mitis* • Subacute endocarditis: associated with *S. mitis*, *S. mutans*, and *S. salivarius* • Dental caries: associated with *S. mutans* • Malignancies of gastrointestinal tract: associated with *S. gallolyticus* subsp. *gallolyticus* • Meningitis: associated with *S. gallolyticus* subsp. *pasteurianus* and *S. mitis*
Diagnosis	• Diagnosis of most viridans group infections is based on clinical presentation and isolation of the organism in blood or surgically collected specimens • Biochemical identification of most species is not accurate, so either sequencing or mass spectroscopy must be done
Treatment, Control, and Prevention	• With the exception of the *S. mitis* group, most viridans streptococci are highly susceptible to penicillins and cephalosporins • Vancomycin should be used for resistant bacteria or in penicillin-allergic patients

ENTEROCOCCUS

Enterococci are one of the most common causes of nosocomial (hospital-acquired) infections, particularly in patients treated with broad-spectrum cephalosporins (antibiotics that are inherently inactive against enterococci).

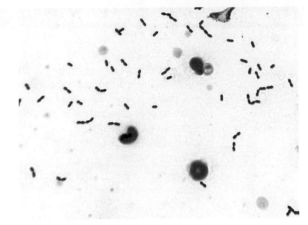

Enterococcus faecium in positive blood culture. Note the arrangement of pairs of cocci resemble *Streptococcus pneumoniae*.

ENTEROCOCCUS FAECALIS AND ENTEROCOCCUS FAECIUM

Properties	• **Antibiotic resistance** limits effective antibiotic therapy
Epidemiology	• Colonizes the gastrointestinal tracts of humans and animals; spreads to other mucosal surfaces if broad-spectrum antibiotics eliminate the normal bacterial population • Cell wall structure typical of gram-positive bacteria, which allows survival on environmental surfaces for prolonged periods • Most infections are endogenous (from the patient's bacterial flora); some are caused by patient-to-patient spread • Patients at increased risk include those hospitalized for prolonged periods and treated with broad-spectrum antibiotics (particularly cephalosporins, to which enterococci are naturally resistant)
Clinical Disease	• **Urinary tract infection**: dysuria and pyuria, most common in hospitalized patients with an indwelling urinary catheter and receiving broad-spectrum cephalosporin antibiotics • **Peritonitis**: abdominal swelling and tenderness after abdominal trauma or surgery; patients are typically acutely ill and febrile; most infections are polymicrobial • **Bacteremia and endocarditis**: bacteremia associated with localized infection or endocarditis; endocarditis can be acute or chronic, involving the heart endothelium or valves
Diagnosis	• Grows readily on common, nonselective media • Differentiated from related organisms by simple tests (catalase negative, l-pyrrolidonyl arylamidase-positive, resistant to bile and optochin)
Treatment, Control, and Prevention	• Therapy for serious infections requires a combination of an aminoglycoside with a cell-wall-active antibiotic (penicillin, ampicillin, or vancomycin); newer agents used for antibiotic-resistant strains include linezolid, daptomycin, tigecycline, and quinupristin/dalfopristin • Antibiotic resistance to each of these drugs is becoming increasingly common, and infections with many isolates (particularly *E. faecium*) are not treatable with any antibiotics • Prevention and control of infections require careful restriction of antibiotic use and implementation of appropriate infection-control practices

CLINICAL CASES (REFER TO SECTION VI)

Upper Respiratory Tract Infections
- *Streptococcal pyogenes* pharyngitis with scarlet fever

Lower Respiratory Tract Infections
- *Staphylococcus aureus* pneumonia
- *Streptococcus pneumoniae* pneumonia

Gastrointestinal Tract Infections
- Staphylococcal food poisoning

Genitourinary Tract Infections
- *Staphylococcus saprophyticus* urinary tract infection

Central Nervous System Infections
- *Streptococcus pneumoniae* meningitis
- *Streptococcus agalactiae* disease in a neonate

Skin and Soft-Tissue Infections
- *Staphylococcus aureus* furuncle and septic shock
- *Staphylococcus aureus* scalded skin syndrome
- *Streptococcus pyogenes* necrotizing fasciitis and septic shock
- *Streptococcal anginosus* abscess
- *Enterococcus faecalis* intraabdominal infection

Sepsis and Cardiovascular Infections
- *Staphylococcus aureus* endocarditis
- Staphylococcal toxic shock syndrome
- *Staphylococcus epidermidis* endocarditis
- *Staphylococcus lugdunensis* endocarditis
- *Streptococcus pyogenes* acute rheumatic fever
- *Streptococcus pneumoniae* fulminant septicemia
- *Streptococcus mutans* endocarditis
- *Enterococcus faecalis* subacute endocarditis

SUPPLEMENTAL READING

1. Lowy FD. *Staphylococcus aureus* infections. *N Engl J Med.* 1998;339:520–532.
2. Becker K, HeilmannC PG. Coagulase-negative staphylococci. *Clin Microbiol Rev.* 2014;276.
3. Dietrich ML, Steele RW. Group A *Streptococcus. Pediatr Rev.* 2018;39(8):379–391.
4. Raabe VN, Shane AL. Group B *Streptococcus (Streptococcus agalactiae). Microbiol Spectr.* 2019;7(2). https://doi.org/10.1128/microbiolspec.GPP3-0007-2018.
5. Ortqvist A, Hedlund J, Kalin M. *Streptococcus pneumoniae* epidemiology, risk factors, and clinical features. *Semin Respir Crit Care Med.* 2005;26(6):563–574.
6. Miller WR, Murray BE, Rice LB, Arias CA. Vancomycin-resistant enterococci: therapeutic challenges in the 21st century. *Infect Dis Clin North Am.* 2016;30(2):415–439.

4

Aerobic Gram-Positive Rods

INTERESTING FACTS

- Anthrax is primarily a disease of herbivores (e.g., cattle, sheep) acquired by ingestion or inhalation of the spores of *Bacillus anthracis*. Humans are accidental victims, with infections most commonly acquired by contact with contaminated animal products.
- It is estimated that *Bacillus cereus* is responsible for almost 65,000 episodes of acute food poisoning every year in the USA, characterized by nausea and vomiting and indistinguishable from *Staphylococcus aureus* food poisoning.

- The most common food products associated with *Listeria monocytogenes* infections are processed meats, including hot dogs and turkey franks, soft cheeses, unpasteurized milk, and uncooked vegetables. The bacteria tolerate salt and grow in refrigerator temperatures down to freezing.
- Before vaccination, between 100,000 and 200,000 people in the USA were infected with *Corynebacterium diphtheriae*; however, only two cases have been reported since 2002.

The aerobic gram-positive rods can be subdivided into spore-forming rods (*Bacillus* is the most common) and non-spore-forming rods (*Listeria* and *Corynebacterium* are the most common). In this chapter, I will focus on four clinically important species, recognizing that there are many other species that may be isolated in clinical specimens.

Clinically Important Species

Species	Derivation	Diseases
B. anthracis	*Bacillum*, a small rod; *anthrax*, charcoal (refers to the black, necrotic wound associated with cutaneous anthrax)	Anthrax (cutaneous, gastrointestinal, inhalation)
B. cereus	*Cereus*, waxen (refers to a typical dull surface of colonies)	Gastroenteritis; ocular infections; anthrax-like pulmonary disease
L. monocytogenes	*Listeria*, named after the English surgeon, Lord Joseph Lister; *monocytum*, monocyte; *gennaio*, produce (stimulates monocyte production in rabbits although not seen in human infections)	Neonatal disease with abscesses, granulomas, and meningitis; influenza-like illness in healthy adults; primary septicemia and meningitis in pregnant women and immunocompromised adults
C. diphtheriae	*Coryne*, a club (club-shaped rods); *diphthera*, leather or skin (reference to the leathery membrane that forms over the pharynx)	Diphtheria (respiratory, cutaneous)

BACILLUS ANTHRACIS AND BACILLUS CEREUS

Because *Bacillus* produces endospores (heat-resistant, dormant bacterial forms), they can survive for years in harsh environments. Many species of *Bacillus* have been discovered, but two are clinically important for very different reasons: *B. anthracis* causes the disease anthrax, and *B. cereus* is an opportunistic pathogen. For *B. anthracis* to cause disease, it must carry genes for capsule production and three individual proteins (protective antigen, edema factor, and lethal factor) that combine to form two toxins (edema toxin and lethal toxin). *B. cereus* carries genes for heat-stable and heat-labile enterotoxins, which are responsible for gastrointestinal infections, as well as cytotoxic enzymes that cause tissue destruction in opportunistic infections.

Anthrax is primarily an animal (zoonotic) disease, and humans are accidental victims. Animal herds in industrial countries are vaccinated for anthrax, so this is primarily a disease of resource-limited countries. However, it was also recognized that this is an ideal biological weapon because the spores are extremely stable and can be used to expose a large population to infectious aerosols. In contrast with *B. anthracis*, *B. cereus* is ubiquitous in the environment, so food poisoning with this organism is common. For this reason, it is important to recognize the symptoms of disease and the public health implications of improperly prepared and stored foods.

Diagnosis of *B. anthracis* and *B. cereus* infections is challenging due to different reasons. *B. anthracis* is rarely seen, so it may not be initially suspected and the microbiologist would generally have little or no experience identifying this organism. Obviously, this would change if there was a recognized bioterrorism outbreak. In contrast, *B. cereus* is commonly isolated in the laboratory and is easy to identify; however, because most isolates are clinically insignificant contaminants, the importance of the organism may not be initially recognized.

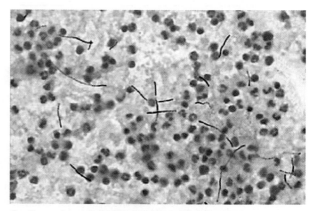

Bacillus anthracis in the blood of a patient with inhalation anthrax.

BACILLUS ANTHRACIS	
Properties	• **Polypeptide capsule** consisting of poly-D-glutamic acid; inhibits phagocytosis • **Edema toxin** (protective antigen + edema factor) with adenylate cyclase activity that is responsible for fluid accumulation • **Lethal toxin** (protective antigen + lethal factor) stimulates macrophages to release TNF-α, IL-1β, and other proinflammatory cytokines
Epidemiology	• *B. anthracis* primarily infects herbivores, with humans as accidental hosts • Rarely isolated in industrial countries but is prevalent in impoverished areas where vaccination of animals is not practiced • The greatest danger of anthrax in industrial countries is the use of *B. anthracis* as an agent of bioterrorism
Clinical Disease	• **Cutaneous anthrax** (most common natural exposure in humans): painless papule progresses to ulceration with surrounding vesicles and then to eschar formation; painful lymphadenopathy, edema, and systemic signs may develop • **Gastrointestinal anthrax** (most common in herbivores): ulcers form at the site of invasion (e.g., mouth, esophagus, intestine) leading to regional lymphadenopathy, edema, and sepsis • **Inhalation anthrax (bioterrorism)**: initial nonspecific signs followed by the rapid onset of sepsis with fever, edema, and lymphadenopathy (mediastinal lymph nodes); meningeal symptoms in half of the patients, and most patients will die unless treatment is initiated immediately

Continued

BACILLUS ANTHRACIS—cont'd

Diagnosis	• Microscopy of wound specimens and blood typically positive; grows readily in culture • Preliminary identification is based on microscopic (gram-positive, nonmotile rods) and colonial (non-hemolytic, adherent colonies) morphology; confirmed by demonstrating capsule and either a positive direct fluorescent antibody test for the specific cell wall polysaccharide or positive nucleic acid amplification test for the toxin genes
Treatment, Control, and Prevention	• Inhalation or gastrointestinal anthrax should be treated with ciprofloxacin or doxycycline, combined with one or two additional antibiotics (e.g., rifampin, vancomycin, penicillin, imipenem, clindamycin, clarithromycin) • Naturally acquired cutaneous anthrax can be treated with amoxicillin • Vaccination of animal herds and people in endemic areas can control disease, but spores are difficult to eliminate from contaminated soils • Vaccination of animal herds and at-risk humans is effective, although the development of a less toxic vaccine is desired

BACILLUS CEREUS

Properties	• **Heat-stable enterotoxin** produces emetic form of disease (vomiting) and **heat-labile enterotoxin** produces diarrheal form of disease • **Cereolysin** and **phospholipase C** with hemolysin and lecithinase activity, respectively; responsible for pathology associated with eye infections and tissue destruction
Epidemiology	• Ubiquitous in soils throughout the world • Infection is associated with consumption of food contaminated with the bacterium (e.g., rice [most common source], pasta, meat, vegetables, sauces); penetrating injuries (e.g., to the eye); individuals receiving potentially nonsterile injections
Clinical Disease	• **Gastroenteritis**: emetic form characterized by a rapid onset (a few hours) of vomiting and abdominal pain and a short duration (generally <24 h); diarrheal form characterized by a longer onset (8–12 h) and duration (1–2 days) of diarrhea and abdominal cramps • **Traumatic eye infection**: rapid, progressive destruction of the eye after traumatic introduction of the bacteria into the eye • **Opportunistic infections**: sepsis associated with contaminated intravenous catheter • **Anthrax-like pulmonary disease**: severe pulmonary disease in immunocompetent patients infected with strains that have acquired genes for capsule formation and edema and lethal toxins (rare but important for biosafety concerns)
Diagnosis	• Diagnosis of enteric infections most commonly based on clinical and epidemiological history; organism can be isolated in the implicated food • Isolation of the organism in nonfecal specimens (e.g., eye, wound)
Treatment, Control, and Prevention	• Gastrointestinal infections are treated symptomatically • Ocular infectious or other invasive diseases require removal of foreign bodies and aggressive treatment with vancomycin, clindamycin, ciprofloxacin, or gentamicin • Gastrointestinal disease is prevented by proper preparation of food (e.g., foods should be consumed immediately after preparation or refrigerated)

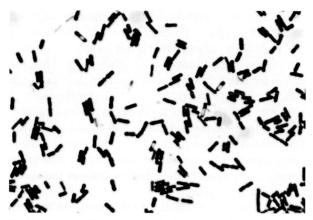

Bacillus cereus. The spores typically do not take up the Gram stain and appear as clear areas in the rods.

LISTERIA MONOCYTOGENES

L. monocytogenes is a short gram-positive rod that grows aerobically and anaerobically over a broad temperature range (including refrigerator temperatures), in high salt concentrations, and when exposed to gastric pH, digestive enzymes, and bile salts. Human exposure is primarily through ingestion of contaminated food products. *Listeria* is a facultative intracellular pathogen, so it must penetrate cells, survive intracellular killing, replicate, and migrate from cell to cell while avoiding the host's immune response.

Listeria is of public health concern because many infections are in fact outbreaks, involving many individuals over a potentially wide geographic distribution (e.g., multistate outbreaks involving improperly prepared commercial food products).

Diagnosis of *Listeria* is challenging because the bacteria are slow-growing organisms that may initially resemble either streptococci or nonpathogenic *Corynebacterium* species on Gram staining. These other organisms are commonly isolated and considered part of the normal bacterial population on the skin; therefore, the significance of this isolate may also not be recognized.

LISTERIA MONOCYTOGENES	
Properties	• Bacterial **surface proteins** (internalins A, B) interact with host surface receptor • **Hemolysins** (listeriolysin O, two phospholipase C enzymes) allow intracellular survival and growth of bacteria
Epidemiology	• Isolated in soil, water, and vegetation and from a variety of animals, including humans (transient gastrointestinal carriage) • Disease associated with consumption of contaminated food products (e.g., milk and soft cheese, processed meats such as turkey franks, raw vegetables [especially cabbage]) or transplacental spread from mother to neonate; sporadic cases and epidemics occur throughout the year • Neonates, the elderly, pregnant women, and patients with defects in cellular immunity are at increased risk of disease
Clinical Disease	• **Early-onset neonatal disease**—acquired transplacentally *in utero* and is characterized by disseminated abscesses and granulomas in multiple organs • **Late-onset neonatal disease**—acquired at or shortly after birth and presents as meningitis or meningoencephalitis with septicemia • Disease in pregnant women or adults with cell-mediated immune defects—can present as primary febrile bacteremia or as disseminated disease with hypotension and meningitis • Disease in healthy adults—typically an influenza-like illness with or without gastroenteritis
Diagnosis	• Microscopy is insensitive; culture may require incubation for 2 to 3 days or enrichment at 4°C (refrigerate specimen so *Listeria* grows slowly while other insignificant organisms die) • Characteristic properties include motility at room temperature, weak β-hemolysis, and growth at 4°C and in high salt concentrations
Treatment, Control, and Prevention	• The treatment of choice for severe disease is penicillin or ampicillin, alone or in combination with gentamicin • People at high risk should avoid eating raw or partially cooked foods of animal origin, soft cheese, and unwashed raw vegetables

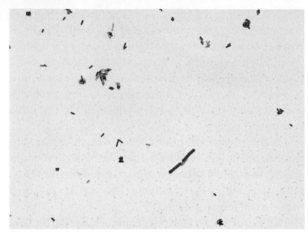

Listeria monocytogenes. Note the gram-positive rods are very small compared with the much larger pair of gram-negative rods.

CORYNEBACTERIUM DIPHTHERIAE

There are many corynebacteria species on the human skin and mucosal membranes, most of which only cause opportunistic infections (e.g., catheter-related bacteremia) or are recovered as contaminants of blood collected for culture. The exception is *C. diphtheriae*, a strictly human pathogen that is not commonly isolated but causes a significant disease, **diphtheria**. This disease is mediated by diphtheria toxin, an **A–B exotoxin** that is introduced into strains of *C. diphtheriae* by a lysogenic bacteriophage, β-phage (so not all strains of *C. diphtheriae* have the toxin). A–B toxins consist of: (1) a catalytic region (active toxin molecule) on the A subunit and (2) a receptor-binding region (binds to the target) and a translocation region (moves the active toxin into the cell) on the B subunit. A–B toxins are observed in other bacteria, but this is one of the first described.

Diphtheria has fortunately been eliminated in most industrial countries through vaccination, but it is still an important disease in resource-limited countries where vaccination is not widespread. Diagnosis of these infections is also a challenge. *C. diphtheriae* is a well-known pathogen, but many other species of corynebacteria colonize the mouth, so the pathogen may not be initially recognized unless infection was suspected.

CORYNEBACTERIUM DIPHTHERIAE	
Properties	• **Diphtheria exotoxin** is an A-B toxin that inhibits protein synthesis by inactivating protein chain elongation factor-2
Epidemiology	• Worldwide distribution maintained in asymptomatic carriers and infected patients • Humans are the only known reservoir, with carriage in the oropharynx or on the skin • Spread person to person by exposure to respiratory droplets or skin contact • Disease observed in unvaccinated or partially immune children or adults traveling to countries with endemic disease • Diphtheria is very uncommon in the USA and other countries with active vaccination programs
Clinical Disease	• **Respiratory diphtheria**: sudden onset with exudative pharyngitis, sore throat, low-grade fever, and malaise; a thick pseudomembrane develops over the pharynx; in critically ill patients, cardiac and neurologic complications are most significant • **Cutaneous diphtheria**: a papule can develop on the skin, which progresses to a nonhealing ulcer; systemic signs can develop
Diagnosis	• Microscopy is nonspecific • Culture should be performed on nonselective (blood agar) and selective media developed for recovery of *C. diphtheriae* • Definitive identification is by biochemical tests or species-specific gene sequencing • Demonstration of exotoxin is performed by Elek test or nucleic acid amplification test for the encoding gene
Treatment, Control, and Prevention	• Infections are treated with a combination of: (1) diphtheria antitoxin to neutralize exotoxin; (2) penicillin or erythromycin to eliminate *C. diphtheriae* and terminate toxin production; and (3) immunization of convalescing patients with diphtheria toxoid to stimulate protective antibodies • Diphtheria vaccine and booster shots should be administered to susceptible population

CLINICAL CASES (REFER TO SECTION VI)

Upper Respiratory Tract Infections
- Respiratory diphtheria
- Fatal *Corynebacterium diphtheriae* infection

Gastrointestinal Tract Infections
- *Bacillus cereus* food poisoning
- *Listeria monocytogenes* gastroenteritis and bacteremia

Central Nervous System Infections
- *Listeria monocytogenes* meningitis in immunocompromised people

Sepsis and Cardiovascular Infections
- Inhalation anthrax
- *Bacillus anthracis* disease with sepsis

Miscellaneous Infections
- *Bacillus cereus* traumatic endophthalmitis

SUPPLEMENTAL READING

1. Pilo P, Frey J. Pathogenicity, population genetics and dissemination of *Bacillus anthracis*. *Infect Genet Evol* 2018;64:115–125.
2. Tuipulotu DE, Mathur A, Ngo C, Man SM. *Bacillus cereus*: epidemiology, virulence factors, and host–pathogen interactions. *Trends Microbiol* 2021;29(5):458–471.
3. Lecuit M. *Listeria monocytogenes*, a model in infection biology. *Cell Microbiol* 2020;22(4), e13186.
4. Sharma NC, Efstratiou A, Mokrousov I, et al. Diphtheria. *Nat Rev Dis Primers* 2019;5(1):81. https://doi.org/10.1038/s41572-019-0131-y.
5. Bernard K. The genus *Corynebacterium* and other medically relevant coryneform-like bacteria. *J Clin Microbiol* 2012;50(10):3152–3158.

5

Acid-Fast Bacteria

The bacteria discussed in this chapter are nonmotile, non-spore-forming, aerobic gram-positive rods that stain "**acid-fast**." This means these bacteria are resistant to decolorization with acid solutions due to the presence of medium to long chains of **mycolic acids** in their cell wall. This staining property is important because only five genera of acid-fast bacteria are medically important: *Mycobacterium*, *Nocardia*, *Rhodococcus*, *Gordonia*, and *Tsukamurella*. Mycobacteria and *Nocardia* will be the focus of this chapter. *Rhodococcus* is a pathogen of immunocompromised patients, primarily causing invasive pulmonary disease, and *Gordonia* and *Tsukamurella* are uncommon opportunistic pathogens, responsible for pulmonary infections in immunocompromised patients and intravenous catheter infections. The latter three genera will not be discussed further.

All acid-fast organisms are relatively slow growing, requiring incubation for 3–7 days (*Nocardia* and some mycobacterial species), to as long as 4 weeks or more (*Mycobacterium* species such as *Mycobacterium tuberculosis*). *Mycobacterium leprae*, the etiologic agent of leprosy, has not been grown in culture. Acid-fast organisms are resistant to many disinfectants, survive in relatively harsh environmental conditions, and are resistant to many antibiotics that are used to treat other bacterial infections. Although more than 350 species of acid-fast bacteria have been described, only a few will be discussed in this chapter. A few species of mycobacteria are closely related to *M. avium* and produce similar human diseases, so they will be referred to as the *M. avium* complex. Likewise, I am not distinguishing between the many species of *Nocardia*.

ACID-FAST ORGANISMS

Some "rapid-growing" mycobacteria (e.g., *Mycobacterium fortuitum*, *Mycobacterium chelonae*, *Mycobacterium abscessus*, and *Mycobacterium mucogenicum*) are common opportunistic pathogens, and some "slow-growing" mycobacteria (e.g., *Mycobacterium kansasii* and *Mycobacterium marinum*) are also relatively common pathogens. I will not discuss these pathogens in this chapter but will present clinical cases in Section VI to illustrate diseases caused by these mycobacteria.

It is difficult to list virulence properties for acid-fast bacteria, because much of the pathology results from the infected host's response to the organism. *M. tuberculosis* is an intracellular pathogen that is able to establish a lifelong infection. Maintenance of persistent infections, without progression to disease, involves a delicate host-parasite relationship: balance between the growth of the bacteria and the immunologic control by the host. When the host regulation is disrupted, progressive mycobacterial growth occurs and subsequently disease develops. At the time of exposure, *M. tuberculosis* enters the respiratory airways and penetrates the alveoli, where the bacteria are phagocytized by alveolar macrophages. The bacteria prevent fusion of the phagosome with lysosomes and evade macrophage killing. However, in response to infection with *M. tuberculosis*, macrophages secrete cytokines that in turn recruit T cells and natural killer cells into the area of the infected macrophages, activate the macrophages, and stimulate intracellular killing. The subsequent mass of necrotic cells (termed **granuloma**) will contain the infection, but also permits some surviving bacteria. These are the bacteria that will subsequently cause disease when the immune process is disrupted.

The ability of *M. leprae* to produce disease is also a manifestation of the slow growth properties of the organism and the host immunologic response. This organism is acquired through the inhalation of infectious aerosols or skin contact with respiratory secretions or wound exudates. The bacteria replicate very slowly, and disease may take years before it is clinically apparent. Two forms of disease develop in direct response to the host immune response: (1) **tuberculoid leprosy**, where

there is a strong cellular immune reaction with the induction of cytokine production that mediates macrophage activation, phagocytosis, and bacillary clearance; and (2) **lepromatous leprosy**, where a strong antibody response is observed, but the cellular response is defective. Mycobacterial diseases are primarily controlled by cellular immunity; as a result, the lepromatous form is characterized by the presence of abundant acid-fast bacteria and extensive tissue destruction, the most commonly described form of leprosy.

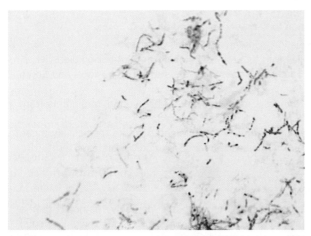

Acid-fast stain of *Mycobacterium tuberculosis* in sputum specimen. Note the "beaded" appearance of the individual rods.

Acid-Fast Organisms Discussed in This Chapter

Species	Derivation	Diseases
M. tuber-culosis	*Myces*, a fungus; *bakterion*, a small rod (fungus-like rod); *tuberculum*, a small swelling or tubercle (characterized by tubercles in lungs of infected patients)	Tuberculosis (pulmonary, disseminated)
M. leprae	*Lepra*, of leprosy	Leprosy, also called **Hansen's disease** (tuberculoid, lepromatous)
M. avium complex	*Avis*, of birds (original isolate from birds with tuberculosis-like illness)	Pulmonary disease in immunocompetent patients; cervical adenitis in children; disseminated disease in immunocompromised patients
Nocardia species	*Nocard*, named after the French veterinarian Edmond Nocard	Pulmonary disease; primary or secondary cutaneous infections; meningitis; brain abscesses

M. avium is an intracellular pathogen that produces either a slowly progressive disease in patients with compromised pulmonary function or a rapidly progressive, disseminated disease in patients with severe depression of cellular immunity.

Nocardia, like its mycobacterial relatives, is an intracellular pathogen that effectively produces disease by avoiding the host immune response.

Mycobacterial and nocardial infections are **exogenous**—caused by organisms that are not normally part of the normal human microbial population. *M. tuberculosis* and *M. leprae* are transmitted from person to person, while all other members of these genera are acquired directly from the environment. Isolation of acid-fast bacteria in a clinical specimen is always noteworthy, but the significance of an isolate, with the exception of *M. tuberculosis* and *M. leprae*, must be proven; i.e., the isolate could represent transient colonization with an environmental contaminant.

Diseases with these pathogens are well characterized, so demonstration of the significance of an isolate should not be difficult. The possible exception to this would be with *M. avium*. It may be necessary to isolate the organism from multiple sputum specimens in elderly patients with chronic pulmonary disease.

Diagnosis of these infections is by a combination of microscopy (observation of acid-fast bacteria in clinical specimens), culture, and molecular tests such as nucleic acid amplification tests. Detection of cellular immune response to infection (most commonly by reactivity in a specific skin test) is useful for *M. tuberculosis* and the tuberculoid form of *M. leprae* disease, but this does not distinguish between active disease and past exposure.

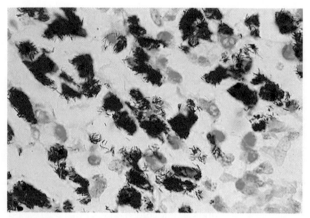

Mycobacterium avium complex in tissue from an AIDS patient. The abundant Bacilli in the tissue of immunocompromised patients are typical.

MYCOBACTERIUM TUBERCULOSIS

MYCOBACTERIUM TUBERCULOSIS	
Properties	• Acid-fast rods frequently observed in clumps • Growth in culture is slow, typically incubation for 2–6 weeks is required
Epidemiology	• Worldwide; one-fourth of the world's population is infected with this organism • In 2019, an estimated 10 million people fell ill with tuberculosis globally and 1.4 million died • Disease is most common in China, India, Eastern Europe, Pakistan, sub-Saharan Africa, and South Africa • Fewer than 9,000 new cases in the USA annually; most infections observed in immigrants from countries with endemic disease • Populations at the greatest risk of disease are immunocompromised patients (particularly those with HIV infection), drug or alcohol abusers, homeless persons, and individuals exposed to diseased patients • Humans are the only natural reservoir • Person-to-person spread by infectious aerosols
Clinical Disease	• **Pulmonary tuberculosis**: infections in immunocompetent patients primarily restricted to the lungs; typically present with nonspecific symptoms (malaise, weight loss, cough, night sweats) with sputum production (bloody and purulent with cavitary disease) • **Extrapulmonary tuberculosis**: disseminated disease following hematogenous spread; kidneys, bones, spleen, and meninges most common foci of the disseminated disease

MYCOBACTERIUM TUBERCULOSIS—cont'd

Diagnosis	• **Tuberculin skin test** and **interferon-γ release assay (IGRA)** are sensitive markers for exposure to the organism • Microscopy and culture are sensitive and specific • Direct detection of *M. tuberculosis* in clinical specimens commonly performed by nucleic acid amplification tests • Identification of clinical isolates most commonly made using species-specific molecular probes
Treatment, Control, and Prevention	• Treatment regimens are rapidly evolving, so refer to regional guidance • Currently, drug-susceptible infections are treated with four drugs (isoniazid, rifampicin, ethambutol, and pyrazinamide) for 6 months • Treatment for multidrug-resistant infections is guided by in vitro susceptibility results; prolonged treatment is required to prevent the development of drug-resistant strains • Prophylaxis for exposure to tuberculosis can include a weekly dose of rifapentine and isoniazid for 3 months • Immunoprophylaxis with **Bacille Calmette-Guérin (BCG)** vaccination is used in countries with endemic disease, but its effectiveness is limited • Control of disease is through active surveillance, prophylactic and therapeutic intervention, and careful case monitoring

MYCOBACTERIUM LEPRAE

MYCOBACTERIUM LEPRAE

Properties	• Acid-fast rods
Epidemiology	• 200,000 new cases were reported in 2019, with most cases in India, Brazil, and Indonesia • 100–200 new cases reported annually in the USA • Lepromatous form of the disease, but not the tuberculoid form, is highly infectious • Person-to-person spread by direct contact or inhalation of infectious aerosols
Clinical Disease	• **Tuberculoid leprosy**: skin lesions characterized by scant erythematous or hypopigmented plaques with flat centers and raised, demarcated borders; peripheral nerve damage with complete sensory loss; visible enlargement of nerves • **Lepromatous leprosy**: skin lesions with many erythematous macules, papules, or nodules; extensive tissue destruction (e.g., nasal cartilage, bones, ears); diffuse nerve involvement with patchy sensory loss; lack of nerve enlargement
Diagnosis	• Microscopy is sensitive for the lepromatous form but not for the tuberculoid form • *M. leprae* does **not grow in culture** • Suspected tuberculoid leprosy infections confirmed with **skin test**; poorly reactive in lepromatous leprosy
Treatment, Control, and Prevention	• Tuberculoid form is treated with rifampicin, dapsone, and clofazimine for 6 months; treatment of the lepromatous form is extended to a minimum of 12 months • Disease is controlled through the prompt recognition and treatment of infected people

MYCOBACTERIUM AVIUM COMPLEX

MYCOBACTERIUM AVIUM COMPLEX	
Properties	• Small acid-fast rods
Epidemiology	• Worldwide distribution, but disease is recognized most commonly in countries where tuberculosis is less prevalent • Acquired primarily through ingestion of contaminated water or food; inhalation of infectious aerosols is believed to play a minor role in transmission • Patients at the greatest risk of disease are those who are immunocompromised (particularly patients with AIDS) or those with long-standing pulmonary disease
Clinical Disease	• **Pulmonary disease** in immunocompetent patients: slowly progressive chronic pulmonary disease that resembles tuberculosis or may present as chronic bronchiectasis • **Cervical adenitis** in children: development of a solitary enlarged lymph node • **Disseminated disease** in immunocompromised patients: overwhelming disseminated infection in AIDS patients with CD4 T lymphocytes < 10 cells/mm^3
Diagnosis	• Microscopy and culture are sensitive and specific • Identification of clinical isolates most commonly made using species-specific molecular probes
Treatment, Control, and Prevention	• Infections treated for a prolonged period with clarithromycin or azithromycin, combined with ethambutol and rifabutin • Prophylaxis in AIDS patients who have a low CD4 cell count consists of clarithromycin, azithromycin, or rifabutin, and such treatment has greatly reduced the incidence of disease

NOCARDIA SPECIES

NOCARDIA SPECIES	
Properties	• **Partially acid-fast** bacteria typically arranged in long branching filaments
Epidemiology	• Worldwide distribution in soil rich in organic matter • Exogenous infections acquired by inhalation (pulmonary) or traumatic introduction (cutaneous) • Opportunistic pathogen causing disease most commonly in immunocompromised patients with T-cell deficiencies (transplant recipients, patients with malignancies, HIV patients, patients receiving corticosteroids) or in healthy individuals with traumatic infections
Clinical Disease	• **Bronchopulmonary disease**: indolent pulmonary disease with necrosis and abscess formation; dissemination most common to the central nervous system or skin • **Mycetoma**: chronic progressive, destructive disease, generally of the extremities, characterized by suppurative granulomas, progressive fibrosis and necrosis, and sinus tract formation • **Lymphocutaneous disease**: primary infection or secondary spread to the cutaneous site characterized by chronic granuloma formation and erythematous subcutaneous nodules, with eventual ulcer formation • **Cellulitis and subcutaneous abscesses**: granulomatous ulcer formation with surrounding erythema, but minimal or no involvement of the draining lymph nodes • **Brain abscess**: chronic infection with fever, headache, and focal deficits related to the location of the slowly developing abscesses

NOCARDIA SPECIES—cont'd

Diagnosis	• Microscopy is sensitive and relatively specific when branching, partially acid-fast organisms are seen • Culture is slow, requiring incubation for up to 1 week; selective media (e.g., buffered charcoal yeast extract agar) may be required for isolating *Nocardia* in mixed cultures • Identification at the genus level can be made by microscopic and macroscopic appearances (branching, weakly acid-fast rods, forming colonies with fuzzy aerial hyphae) • Identification at the species level requires genomic analysis for most isolates; the species cannot be reliably identified by biochemical tests
Treatment, Control, and Prevention	• Infections are treated with antibiotics and proper wound care • Trimethoprim-sulfamethoxazole used as initial empiric therapy for cutaneous infections in immunocompetent patients; therapy for severe infections and cutaneous infections in immunocompromised patients should include trimethoprim-sulfamethoxazole plus amikacin for pulmonary or cutaneous infections and trimethoprim-sulfamethoxazole plus imipenem or a cephalosporin for central nervous system infections; prolonged treatment (up to 12 months) is recommended • Exposure cannot be avoided because nocardiae are ubiquitous

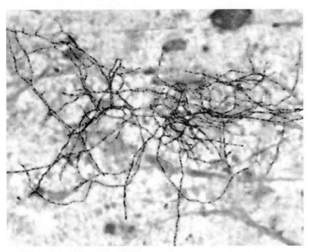

Gram stain of *Nocardia* in expectorated sputum. The long delicate filaments and irregular staining are characteristic of *Nocardia*.

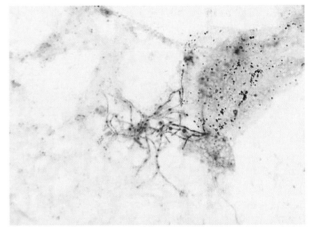

Acid-fast stain of *Nocardia* in expectorated sputum. Note the branching filaments that partially retain the acid-fast stain.

CLINICAL CASES (REFER TO SECTION VI)

Lower Respiratory Tract Infections
• Drug-resistant *Mycobacterium tuberculosis*
• *Mycobacterium avium* infection in an AIDS patient
• *Rhodococcus equi* pulmonary infection in an immunocompromised patient

Central Nervous System Infections
• Disseminated nocardiosis

Skin and Soft-Tissue Infections
• *Mycobacterium leprae* infection

Sepsis and Cardiovascular Infections
• Mycobacterial infections associated with nail salons
• *Mycobacterium* catheter-associated bacteremia
• *Tsukamurella* bacteremia

SUPPLEMENTAL READING

1. Lin W, Kruse R, Yang K, Musher D. Diagnosis and management of pulmonary infection due to *Rhodococcus equi*. *Clin Microbiol Infect*. 2019;25(3):310–315.

2. Suzuki J, Sasahara T, Toshima M, Morisawa Y. Peripherally inserted central catheter-related bloodstream infection due to *Tsukamurella pulmonis*: a case report and literature review. *BMC Infect Dis*. 2017;17:677–680.

3. Banuls A, Sanou A, Anh N, Godreuil S. *Mycobacterium tuberculosis*: ecology and evolution of a human bacterium. *J Med Microbiol*. 2015;64:1261–1269.

4. Britton WJ, Lockwood DN. Leprosy. *Lancet*. 2004;363: 1209–1219.

5. To K, Cao R, Yegiazaryan A, et al. General overview of nontuberculous mycobacteria opportunistic pathogens: *Mycobacterium avium* and *Mycobacterium abscessus*. *J Clin Med*. 2020;9(8):2541. https://doi.org/10.3390/jcm9082541.

6. Wilson J. Nocardiosis: updates and clinical overview. *Mayo Clin Proc*. 2012;87(4):403–407.

6

Aerobic Gram-Negative Cocci and Coccobacilli

INTERESTING FACTS

- Gonorrhea is the second most commonly reported notifiable disease in the USA (chlamydia being the most common), with more than 600,000 reported in the USA in 2019, an increase of almost 100% over the past 10 years.
- In contrast with viral meningitis, bacterial meningitis caused by *Neisseria meningitidis* and *Haemophilus influenzae* is contagious, so person-to-person spread with the development of meningitis can occur.
- Although pediatric disease with *Haemophilus influenzae* has been virtually eliminated with the HIB vaccine, this is a significant pathogen in countries where vaccination is not widely used.
- *Acinetobacter baumannii* was largely ignored until multidrug-resistant strains were observed in military hospitals during the Iraq and Afghanistan conflicts. Now these bacteria are widely disseminated worldwide, and treatment is increasingly challenging.
- Although the highest incidence of pertussis and complications is in children < 1 year of age, disease in older children and adults is frequently not appreciated, and these patients serve as an unrecognized reservoir for *Bordetella pertussis*.

The focus of this chapter is on a broad collection of bacteria that are gram-negative cocci or coccobacilli (short rods). The one true gram-negative cocci in this collection are the *Neisseria*. There are many species of *Neisseria*, but the two most important are *Neisseria gonorrhoeae* and *Neisseria meningitidis*. Two genera, *Eikenella* and *Kingella*, are members of the same family of bacteria as *Neisseria*, with a single important species in each genus, *Eikenella corrodens* and *Kingella kingae*. Both bacteria are normal residents of the human mouth, as are two other genera, *Moraxella* and *Haemophilus*. I will discuss *Moraxella catarrhalis* and *H. influenzae* as representatives of their genera. I should point out that *M. catarrhalis* was formerly classified as *Neisseria*, because both organisms are typically arranged in pairs (diplococci) with the adjacent sides flattened together (resembling coffee beans). Five additional genera are considered in this chapter. Members of the genus *Pasteurella* are commonly found in the mouths of dogs and cats and are associated with bite wounds. The genus *Acinetobacter* contains many species, but *A. baumannii* is the most important, because many strains that cause opportunistic infections in hospitalized patients are multidrug resistant and virtually untreatable. *Bordetella*, *Francisella*, and *Brucella* all cause specific diseases (pertussis, tularemia, and brucellosis, respectively) that are of significant public health interest. Each of these bacteria and their diseases are distinct; therefore, each will be considered individually.

Aerobic Gram-Negative Cocci and Coccobacilli

Bacteria	Historical Derivation
Neisseria gonorrhoeae	Named after the German physician Albert Neisser, who originally described the organism responsible for gonorrhea; *gone*, seed; *rhoia*, a flow (a flow of seeds in reference to the purulent exudate produced in the disease gonorrhea)
Neisseria meningitidis	*Meningis*, the covering of the brain; *itis*, inflammation (inflammation of the meninges as in meningitis)
Eikenella corrodens	Named after M. Eiken who first described the organism and observed the ability of the organism to pit or "corrode" agar

Aerobic Gram-Negative Cocci and Coccobacilli—cont'd

Bacteria	Historical Derivation
Kingella kingae	Named after Elizabeth King who described the organism
Moraxella catarrhalis	Named after Morax who first described the organism; catarrhus, catarrh (refers to inflammation of respiratory membranes)
Haemophilus influenzae	Haemo, blood; hilos, lover (blood lover, requires blood for growth in culture); originally thought to cause influenza
Pasteurella multocida	Named after Louis Pasteur; multus, many; cidus, to kill; pathogenic for many species of animals
Acinetobacter baumannii	Akinetos, unable to move; bactrum, rod (nonmotile rods); baumannii, named after the microbiologist Baumann
Bordetella pertussis	Named after Bordet who first isolated the organism; per, severe; tussis, cough (a severe cough)
Francisella tularensis	Named after Francis who first described the disease; tularensis, pertaining to Tulare County, California, where the disease was first described
Brucella melitensis	Named after Bruce who first recognized the organism as a cause of "undulant fever"

NEISSERIA GONORRHOEAE

Despite the fact *N. gonorrhoeae* survives poorly when exposed to cold temperatures and requires humidity and carbon dioxide when grown in laboratory cultures, it has managed to become the second most common cause of sexually transmitted bacterial diseases worldwide. In fact, it is interesting that the three most common bacteria responsible for sexually transmitted diseases—*N. gonorrhoeae*, *Treponema pallidum* (syphilis), and *Chlamydia trachomatis*—all survive poorly outside their human hosts. Maybe this illustrates how important close physical contact is for the maintenance of these diseases.

Neisseria gonorrhoeae in urethral exudate. Note the gram-negative cocci are arranged in pairs with flattened sides (gram-negative diplococci).

NEISSERIA GONORRHOEAE

Properties	• Pilin protein mediates initial attachment to nonciliated epithelial cells in the vagina, fallopian tube, and buccal cavity; interferes with neutrophil killing • Porin proteins promote intracellular survival by preventing phagolysosome fusion and subsequent bacterial death in neutrophils • Opacity proteins mediate firm attachment to host cells • Transferrin, lactoferrin, and other hemoglobin-binding proteins mediate acquisition of iron for bacterial metabolism and growth • Cell wall lipooligosaccharide (LOS) has endotoxin activity • β-lactamase mediates resistance to penicillin

NEISSERIA GONORRHOEAE—cont'd

Epidemiology	• Humans are the only natural hosts • Carriage can be asymptomatic, particularly in women, facilitating transmission • Transmission is primarily by sexual contact • The most common cause of septic arthritis in sexually active adults • More than 615,000 cases reported in the USA in 2019 (true incidence of disease believed to be at least twice that); estimated 100 million new cases worldwide annually • Incidence of disease is highest in people aged 15–24 years, males, blacks, residents of the southeastern USA, and people who have multiple sexual encounters • Higher risk of disseminated disease in patients with deficiencies in late components of the complement
Clinical Disease	• **Gonorrhea**: characterized by purulent discharge from an involved site (e.g., urethra, cervix, epididymis, prostate, rectum) after a 2- to 5-day incubation period • **Disseminated infections**: spread of infection from the genitourinary tract through the blood to skin or joints; characterized by pustular rash with erythematous base and suppurative arthritis in involved joints • **Ophthalmia neonatorum**: purulent ocular infection acquired by neonate at birth
Diagnosis	• Gram stain of urethral specimens (presence of gram-negative diplococci) is accurate only for symptomatic males • Gram stain of synovial fluid is diagnostic for septic arthritis • Culture of genital specimens is sensitive and specific but has been replaced with nucleic acid amplification tests (NAATs) in most laboratories • Culture is the test of choice for all other specimens
Treatment, Control, and Prevention	• Ceftriaxone with azithromycin is currently the treatment of choice, although high-level resistance to cephalosporins, as well as to penicillins and fluoroquinolones, has been observed • For neonates, prophylaxis with 1% silver nitrate; ophthalmia neonatorum is treated with ceftriaxone • Prevention consists of patient education, use of condoms or spermicides with nonoxynol-9 (only partially effective), and aggressive follow-up of sexual partners of infected patients • Effective vaccines are not available

NEISSERIA MENINGITIDIS

Rarely does a bacterial pathogen strike as much fear in a community as *N. meningitidis*, for it can produce meningitis and overwhelming sepsis in healthy children and adults and rapidly spreads to the contacts of the initial victims.

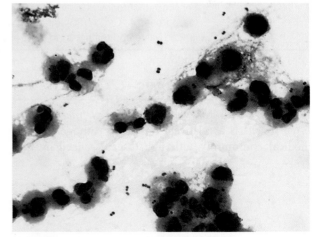

Neisseria meningitidis in cerebrospinal fluid of a child with meningitis. Note the morphology is identical to *Neisseria gonorrhoeae*.

NEISSERIA MENINGITIDIS

Properties	• Pilin protein mediates initial attachment to host cells; interferes with neutrophil killing • Polysaccharide capsule protects bacteria from antibody-mediated phagocytosis; a number of immunologic distinct serogroups have been described • Cell wall LOS has endotoxin activity
Epidemiology	• Humans are the only natural hosts • Person-to-person spread occurs via aerosolization of respiratory tract secretions • The highest incidence of disease is in children younger than 5 years (particularly infants <6 months of age), young adults in college or military settings, institutionalized people, and patients with late complement deficiencies • Endemic and epidemic disease is most commonly caused by serogroups A, B, C, W135, and Y (meningitis by serogroups A, B, C; pneumonia by serogroups W135 and Y); serogroup A and W135 infections are most common in resource-limited countries, while serogroup B infections are most common in industrial countries • Disease occurs worldwide, most commonly in the dry, cold months of the year
Clinical Disease	• **Meningitis**: purulent inflammation of meninges associated with headache, meningeal signs, and fever; high mortality rate unless promptly treated with effective antibiotics • **Meningococcemia**: disseminated infection characterized by thrombosis of small blood vessels and multiorgan involvement; small, petechial skin lesions coalesce into larger hemorrhagic lesions • **Pneumonia**: milder form of meningococcal disease characterized by bronchopneumonia in patients with underlying pulmonary disease
Diagnosis	• Gram stain of CSF (gram-negative diplococci) is sensitive and specific but is of limited value for blood specimens (too few organisms are generally present, except in overwhelming sepsis) • Culture is definitive, but the organism is fastidious and dies rapidly when exposed to cold or dry conditions • Tests to detect meningococcal antigens in CSF are insensitive and nonspecific • NAATs are available in multiplex assays for the diagnosis of meningitis
Treatment, Control, and Prevention	• Empiric treatment of patients with suspected meningitis or bacteremia should be initiated with ceftriaxone, cefotaxime, meropenem, or (for patients with severe allergies to ß-lactams) moxifloxacin • Chemoprophylaxis for contact with persons with the disease is with rifampin, ciprofloxacin, or ceftriaxone • Breast-feeding infants have passive immunity (first 6 months) • For immunoprophylaxis, vaccination is an adjunct to chemoprophylaxis; tetravalent vaccines (serogroups A, C, Y, W135) are now widely used; however, vaccines for serogroup B have proved of limited value and restricted to control of outbreaks

EIKENELLA CORRODENS

In contrast with *N. gonorrhoeae* and *N. meningitidis*, *E. corrodens* is a relatively unknown pathogen to the medical community, although disease caused by this organism, particularly bite-related infections, is well-documented. Basic knowledge of this organism is important, because antibiotic treatment of these infections is different from traditional gram-negative infections.

EIKENELLA CORRODENS	
Properties	• Opportunistic pathogen
Epidemiology	• Normal resident of the human mouth
Clinical Disease	• **Human bite wound** or fist fight injury • **Subacute endocarditis** in patients with preexisting heart disease • **Opportunistic infections** (pneumonia, lung or brain abscesses, sinusitis) in immunocompromised patients or patients with trauma of the oral cavity
Diagnosis	• Slow-growing facultative anaerobe that requires 2 or more days of incubation • Preliminary identification of the cultured organism is possible based on the Gram stain morphology and whether the colonies pit the agar ("corrodes" agar; about half the isolates will do this) and produce a bleach-like odor (very common) • Definitive identification by biochemical tests or mass spectroscopy
Treatment, Control, and Prevention	• Monomicrobic infections treated with ampicillin; polymicrobic infections with amoxicillin-clavulanate; endocarditis treated with ceftriaxone

KINGELLA KINGAE

This organism also remains in the shadows, unknown to many medical practitioners. This fact is emphasized because the organism most commonly produces disease with a nonspecific but insidious presentation and is frequently difficult to recover in culture unless extended incubation is used.

KINGELLA KINGAE	
Properties	• Opportunistic pathogen
Epidemiology	• Normal resident of the human mouth, particularly in children
Clinical Disease	• **Septic arthritis** in children • **Subacute endocarditis** in patients with preexisting heart disease
Diagnosis	• Slow-growing facultative anaerobe that requires 3 or more days of incubation • Definitive identification by biochemical tests or mass spectroscopy
Treatment, Control, and Prevention	• Susceptible to ß-lactams, macrolides, tetracycline, fluoroquinolones

MORAXELLA CATARRHALIS

For many years, *M. catarrhalis* was considered a relatively insignificant member of the genus *Neisseria*. This changed when it was realized that the only thing the two genera had in common was their gram-negative diplococci morphology. Additionally, you only have to look at a Gram stain of sputum collected from a patient with *M. catarrhalis* pneumonia to recognize the presence of abundant organisms, surrounded by equally numerous inflammatory cells. Any organism capable of triggering such a vigorous immune response has to be significant.

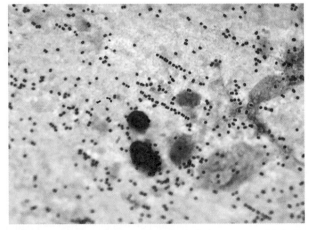

Typical appearance of *Moraxella catarrhalis* in sputum with large numbers of gram-negative diplococci and host inflammatory cells. *M. catarrhalis* resembles and is frequently mistaken for *Neisseria*.

MORAXELLA CATARRHALIS

Properties	• Opportunistic pathogen
Epidemiology	• Normal resident of the human mouth
Clinical Disease	• **Bronchitis or bronchopneumonia** in patients with chronic pulmonary disease • **Sinusitis** and **otitis** in previously healthy individuals
Diagnosis	• Gram stain (gram-negative diplococci) is suggestive of *Moraxella* but cannot be differentiated from *Neisseria* • Strict aerobic growth in 1–2 days on most nonselective laboratory media • Identification by biochemical tests or mass spectroscopy
Treatment, Control, and Prevention	• Most isolates product β-lactamase and are resistant to all penicillins • Susceptible to most other antibiotics including cephalosporins, erythromycin, tetracyclines, trimethoprim-sulfamethoxazole

HAEMOPHILUS INFLUENZAE

H. influenzae is a bacterium almost relegated to historical value. I say "almost" because despite the fact that the disease has been virtually eliminated in vaccinated populations of children, vaccination has not been universally adopted globally. This remains the challenge—and promise—for the future. A few other species of *Haemophilus* should be mentioned here:

- *Haemophilus aegyptius,* an important cause of acute purulent **conjunctivitis** ("pinkeye"); associated with epidemics during the warm months of the year
- *Haemophilus ducreyi*, the etiologic agent of the sexually transmitted disease soft chancre, or **chancroid**; characterized by a tender papule with an erythematous base that progresses to painful ulceration with associated lymphadenopathy
- Other species of Haemophilus are opportunistic pathogens primarily responsible for **sinusitis, otitis, or bronchitis**

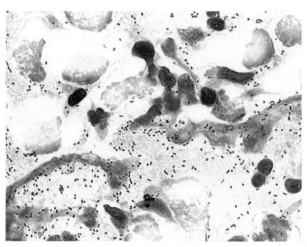

Haemophilus influenzae in sputum. Bacteria typically appear as very small coccobacilli, arranged as single cells or occasionally in pairs.

HAEMOPHILUS INFLUENZAE

Properties	• *H. influenzae* subdivided serologically based on capsular antigens (types a to f); **serotype b** is clinically the most virulent • The major virulence factor in ***H. influenzae* type b (HIB)** is the antiphagocytic **polysaccharide capsule**, which contains ribose, ribitol, and phosphate; commonly referred to as polyribitol phosphate or PRP; antigen is used in vaccines • Antibodies developed against PRP are protective • Bacterial cell wall lipopolysaccharide lipid A induces meningeal inflammation
Epidemiology	• *Haemophilus* species are normal residents of the human mouth although *H. influenzae* type b is relatively uncommon • Disease caused by *H. influenzae* type b is primarily a pediatric problem (<5 years of age) although vaccination has eliminated this pathogen in many populations • Patients at the greatest risk of the disease are those with inadequate levels of protective antibodies, those with depleted complement, and those who have undergone splenectomy

HAEMOPHILUS INFLUENZAE—cont'd

Clinical Disease	• **Meningitis**: the most common cause of pediatric meningitis in unvaccinated populations; starts with mild upper respiratory symptoms and then progresses to meningeal signs • **Epiglottitis**: cellulitis and swelling of the supraglottic tissues; represents a life-threatening emergency in young children with naturally narrow airways • **Cellulitis**: development of reddish-blue patches on the cheeks or periorbital areas; accompanied by fever • **Arthritis**: prior to vaccination, this was the most common cause of arthritis in children younger than 2 years of age
Diagnosis	• Gram stain and culture of CSF or synovial fluid is diagnostic • Blood cultures typically positive for most *Haemophilus* diseases • Immunoassays for PRP antigen are sensitive with CSF or urine specimens (antigen concentrated in urine), but rarely used today following the introduction of the vaccine in the community
Treatment, Control, and Prevention	• Broad-spectrum cephalosporins are used for initial empiric therapy; use of alternative antibiotics should be guided by in vitro susceptibility tests • Primary approach to prevent *H. influenzae* type b disease is through immunization with a **conjugated PRP vaccine** (combined with protein to stimulate an immune response in very young children); vaccine administered before 6 months of age, followed by booster vaccination between age 12 and 15 months; vaccine only effective against type b strains of *H. influenzae*

PASTEURELLA MULTOCIDA

Pasteurella are gram-negative coccobacilli that are commonly found in the mouth of healthy animals. *Pasteurella multocida* is the most common human pathogen, often associated with animal bites, scratches, and other close contacts such as sharing food. Infections caused by cat bites are particularly problematic because the organisms can be introduced deep into the tissue where superficial cleaning and antibacterial ointment can be ineffective.

PASTEURELLA MULTOCIDA

Properties	• Opportunistic pathogen
Epidemiology	• Normal resident in animal mouths (e.g., dogs, cats)
Clinical Disease	• Localized cellulitis and lymphadenitis after an animal bite or scratch • Exacerbation of chronic respiratory disease in patients with underlying pulmonary dysfunction • Systemic infection in immunocompromised patients, particularly those with underlying hepatic disease
Diagnosis	• Grows well on blood agar and chocolate agar but not MacConkey agar or other media selective for gram-negative rods • Characteristic large buttery colonies with musty odor after overnight incubation • Identification by biochemical tests or mass spectroscopy
Treatment, Control, and Prevention	• Monomicrobic infections can be treated with penicillin and expanded spectrum cephalosporins, macrolides, tetracyclines, or fluoroquinolones are acceptable alternatives • Resistant to oxacillin and first-generation cephalosporins • Good wound care important because some animal bites (i.e., cat bites) may be deep

ACINETOBACTER BAUMANNII

For many years, *A. baumannii* and other species of *Acinetobacter* occupied the relatively common niche of opportunistic pathogens that infrequently caused significant disease. This has changed in recent years, because these bacteria, particularly *A. baumannii*, added one additional property to their assets: resistance to virtually all antimicrobials. This ability has not only made treatment a challenge, it has also handicapped the control of the spread of these bacteria in hospitals. This became most evident during the military conflicts in Iraq and Afghanistan. Injured soldiers developed wound infections, pneumonia, and overwhelming sepsis in the military hospitals where infection control practices were inadequate, and then they became reservoirs for infections when they were transferred back to their home countries. The organisms now persist in many hospitals worldwide and certainly will remain a challenge for many years to come.

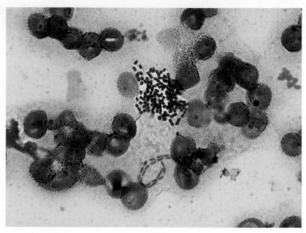

Acinetobacter baumannii in a positive blood culture with *Pseudomonas aeruginosa*. This gram-negative coccobacillus resembles fat gram-positive cocci, arranged as single cells or in pairs. In contrast, *P. aeruginosa* are gram-negative rods arranged in a chain.

ACINETOBACTER BAUMANNII	
Properties	• Opportunistic pathogen • Many strains are **multidrug resistant**
Epidemiology	• *Acinetobacter* species are ubiquitous saprophytes present in the environment inside and outside the hospital; able to survive both on moist surfaces such as mechanical ventilation equipment and on dry surfaces such as the human skin • Although other *Acinetobacter* species can colonize the human mouth, *A. baumannii* is not considered a normal resident, so isolation in clinical specimens is typically considered significant • Patients at risk of infection include those receiving broad-spectrum antibiotics, recovering from surgery, on respiratory ventilation, or exposed to patients with *Acinetobacter* infections
Clinical Disease	• **Opportunistic pathogen** causing infections in the respiratory tract, urinary tract, wounds, and sepsis
Diagnosis	• Gram stain morphology is characteristic—large, plump coccobacilli that may appear gram-positive and typically in pairs (larger and more round than *Streptococcus* pneumoniae or *Enterococcus* so this should not cause confusion)
	• Growth on nonselective media is typically seen after 1 day of incubation • Identification of *A. baumannii* can be made using biochemical tests, but these are generally unreliable for other *Acinetobacter* species; gene sequencing is used for identification of these organisms
Treatment, Control, and Prevention	• Treatment must be guided by in vitro susceptibility tests because multidrug resistance is common • Colistin may be the only active antibiotic and can be used with combination therapy (e.g., ampicillin-sulbactam) • Proper infection control practices are required to prevent the spread of this organism in critically ill hospitalized patients, particularly for wound care and use of mechanical respiratory devices

BORDETELLA PERTUSSIS

One should question why we are seeing a resurgence of infections with an organism whose biology, epidemiology, and pathogenesis are so well known and where vaccines to control the disease are readily available. The reality is we know much about this organism because it is such an important pathogen. The use of effective, nontoxic vaccines has only recently replaced older vaccines, and disease in adult patients persists because the initial vaccines did not provide lasting immunity. Elimination of pertussis will only be achieved by an aggressive vaccine program and vigilance in monitoring for subclinical disease. Until this is accomplished, understanding the importance of this organism will remain paramount.

BORDETELLA PERTUSSIS	
Properties	• **Filamentous hemagglutinin** and **pertactin** bind to the membranes of ciliated cells in the trachea; these proteins are highly immunogenic and are used in the current vaccines • **Pertussis toxin** binds to ciliated epithelial cells of the oropharynx as well as to the surface of phagocytic cells • **Pertussis toxin** (A–B toxin) inactivates G1α, a protein that controls adenylate cyclase activity, resulting in increased levels of cyclic adenosine monophosphate (AMP) with a subsequent increase in respiratory secretions and mucus production; also inhibits phagocytic killing and monocyte migration • **Adenylate cyclase/hemolysin toxin** increases cyclic AMP levels; also inhibits phagocytic killing and monocyte migration • **Tracheal cytotoxin** kills ciliated respiratory cells and stimulates the release of interleukin-1 resulting in febrile response
Epidemiology	• Strict human pathogen • Worldwide distribution • Unvaccinated individuals are at the greatest risk of disease • Disease was traditionally restricted primarily to children younger than 1 year; however, disease is now commonly observed in older children and adults, most likely due to waning immunity • Disease spreads person to person by infectious aerosols
Clinical Disease	• **Pertussis**: develops after a 7- to 10-day incubation period; characterized in children by: (1) **catarrhal** stage (resembles a common cold); progressing to the (2) **paroxysmal** stage (repetitive coughs followed by inspiratory whoops); and then the (3) **convalescence** stage (diminishing paroxysms and secondary complications) • Paroxysmal stage may be less prominent in older children and adults because their airways may not be obstructed as in infants
Diagnosis	• Microscopy is insensitive and nonspecific • Culture on selective media is specific but insensitive and generally not widely available • NAATs are the most sensitive and specific tests and have generally replaced microscopy and culture • Serology can be used as a confirmatory test but is not widely used
Treatment, Control, and Prevention	• Treatment with a macrolide (i.e., azithromycin, clarithromycin) is effective • Macrolides are used for prophylaxis • Vaccines containing inactivated pertussin toxin, filamentous hemagglutinin, and pertactin are highly effective • Pediatric vaccine is administered in five doses (ages 2, 4, 6, 15–18 months, and 4–6 years); adult vaccine is administered at ages 11–12 years and 19–65 years

FRANCISELLA TULARENSIS

F. tularensis has reached the "lofty" status of **Select Agent**, an organism of potential bioterrorism. The importance of this organism and the high degree of infectivity were not wasted on me as a young microbiologist when I started my career in St. Louis and recovered this organism in culture every summer (it is well established in the area's rabbit population). My staff quickly realized how dangerous this organism was and exercised extreme caution when the almost submicroscopic gram-negative coccobacilli were observed in a positive blood culture. The ease with which this can be transmitted to a technologist in the laboratory is similar to the ease of transmission from infected animal tissues or a tick bite.

FRANCISELLA TULARENSIS	
Properties	• Polysaccharide capsule protects bacteria for antibody-mediated phagocytosis • Intracellular pathogen resistant to killing in serum and by phagocytes
Epidemiology	• Humans are accidental hosts • Wild mammals, domestic animals, and blood-sucking arthropods are reservoirs; **rabbits**, cats, **hard ticks**, and biting flies are most commonly associated with human disease • Worldwide distribution, with disease in the USA most common in Oklahoma, Missouri, and Arkansas • Infectious dose is small (as few as 10–50 bacteria) when exposure is by arthropod, through skin penetration, or by inhalation; larger numbers of organisms must be ingested for disease by this route • Ticks must feed for a prolonged time before transmission of the bacteria in their feces
Clinical Disease	• **Ulceroglandular tularemia**: characterized by the development of a painful papule that is initially observed at the site of inoculation and then progresses to ulceration with localized lymphadenopathy • **Oculoglandular tularemia**: after inoculation into the eye (e.g., rubbing the eye with a contaminated finger), infection is characterized by the development of conjunctivitis with regional lymphadenopathy • **Pneumonic tularemia**: pneumonitis with signs of sepsis develops rapidly after exposure to contaminated aerosols; high mortality unless disease is promptly diagnosed and treated
Diagnosis	• Microscopy is insensitive because the organism is very small (this morphology is similar to *Brucella* and is quite characteristic for both organisms) • Growth of the organism must be on cysteine-supplemented media (e.g., chocolate agar, buffered charcoal yeast extract agar), and prolonged incubation (3 or more days) is required; culture is insensitive unless the organism is suspected and culture plates incubated longer than what is typical
	• *Francisella* is highly contagious, so care must be taken if the organism is isolated in culture • Serology can be used to confirm the diagnosis, but antibodies persist for years and cross-react with *Brucella* infections
Treatment, Control, and Prevention	• Gentamicin is the antibiotic of choice; fluoroquinolones and doxycycline have good activity; penicillins and some cephalosporins are ineffective • Disease prevented by avoiding the reservoirs and vectors of infections • Prompt removal of infected ticks is usually effective • Live attenuated vaccine is available but rarely used for preventing human disease

BRUCELLA SPECIES

Much like *Francisella*, *Brucella* species are extremely small gram-negative coccobacilli that are now classified as **Select Agents**. The most common species responsible for human disease is *Brucella melitensis*, an organism that unfortunately finds its way into the USA primarily via unpasteurized dairy products from Mexico. This is the species that is also responsible for the most acute, severe systemic disease and associated complications.

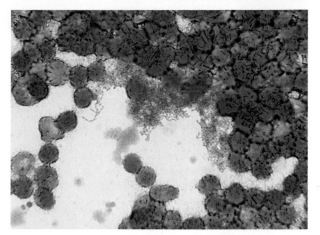

Brucella melitensis in a positive blood culture. The bacteria are extremely small, poorly staining coccobacilli, arranged in clumps around the much larger erythrocytes. Individual cells of the bacteria would be very difficult to detect due to their size and staining properties. *Francisella* has a very similar morphology.

BRUCELLA SPECIES	
Properties	• Intracellular pathogen of the reticuloendothelial system and is able to resist being killed in serum and by phagocytes
Epidemiology	• Animal reservoirs: goats and sheep (*B. melitensis*); cattle and American bison (*Brucella abortus*); swine, reindeer, and caribou (*Brucella suis*); and dogs, foxes, and coyotes (*Brucella canis*) • Humans are accidental hosts that can develop disease from any of the *Brucella* species • Infects animal tissues rich in erythritol (e.g., breast, uterus, placenta, epididymis), with the shedding of organisms in high numbers in milk, urine, and birth products • Worldwide distribution; vaccination of herds has controlled disease in the USA • Most disease in the USA is reported in California and Texas, and in travelers from Mexico • Individuals at the greatest risk of disease are people who consume unpasteurized dairy products such as milk and cheeses, people in direct contact with infected animals, and laboratory workers
Clinical Disease	• **Brucellosis**: initially presents with nonspecific symptoms of malaise, chills, sweats, fatigue, myalgias, weight loss, arthralgias, and fever; typically progresses to systemic symptoms and involvement of the gastrointestinal tract, bones or joints, respiratory tract, or other organs • Fever can be intermittent (termed "**undulant fever**")
Diagnosis	• Microscopy is insensitive because the organism is very small, although characteristic when observed • Culture (blood, bone marrow, infected tissue) is sensitive if prolonged incubation is used (3 days to 2 weeks) • Serology can be used to confirm the clinical diagnosis, but high titers can persist for months to years, and cross-reactivity is observed with other infections
Treatment, Control, and Prevention	• Recommended treatment is with doxycycline combined with gentamicin or streptomycin • Human disease is controlled by eradication of the disease in the animal reservoir through vaccination, and serologic monitoring of the animals for evidence of disease; pasteurization of dairy products; and use of proper safety practices in clinical laboratories working with this organism

CLINICAL CASES (REFER TO SECTION VI)

Upper Respiratory Tract Infections
- *Haemophilus influenzae* epiglottitis
- *Bordetella pertussis* respiratory outbreak in health care workers
- *Bordetella pertussis* whooping cough in children

Lower Respiratory Tract Infections
- *Neisseria meningitidis* pneumonia
- *Moraxella catarrhalis* bronchopneumonia
- *Haemophilus influenzae* pneumonia
- *Acinetobacter baumannii* pneumonia
- *Francisella tularensis* pneumonia

Genitourinary Tract Infections
- *Neisseria gonorrhoeae* urethritis

Central Nervous System Infections
- *Haemophilus influenzae* meningitis

Skin and Soft-Tissue Infections
- *Eikenella corrodens* bite wound infection
- *Pasteurella multocida* necrotizing fasciitis
- Cat-associated *Francisella tularensis* ulceroglandular tularemia
- *Francisella tularensis* ulceroglandular tularemia

Sepsis and Cardiovascular Infections
- *Neisseria meningitidis* sepsis
- *Kingella kingae* endocarditis
- *Brucella melitensis* sepsis

Miscellaneous Infections
- *Neisseria gonorrhoeae* arthritis
- *Neisseria gonorrhoeae* arthritis

SUPPLEMENTAL READING

1. Unemo M, Seifert H, Hook E, et al. Gonorrhoea. *Nat Rev Dis Primers.* 2019;21(5):79. https://doi.org/10.1038/s41572-019-0128-6.
2. Hollingshead S, Tang C. An overview of *Neisseria meningitidis. Methods Mol Biol.* 2019;1969:1–16.
3. Sharara S, Tayyar R, Kanafani Z, Kanj S. HACEK endocarditis: a review. *Exp Rev Anti Infect Ther.* 2016;14(6):539–545.
4. Karalus R, Campagnari A. *Moraxella cararrhalis*: a review of an important human mucosal pathogen. *Microbes Infect.* 2000;2(5):547–559.
5. Jordens J, Slack M. *Haemophilus influenzae*: then and now. *Eur J Clin Microbiol Infect Dis.* 1995;14(11):935–948.
6. Wilkie I, Harper M, Boyce J, Adler B. *Pasteurella multocida*: diseases and pathogenesis. *Curr Top Microbiol Immunol.* 2012;361L1-22.
7. Autunes L, Visca P, Towner K. *Acinetobacter baumannii*: evolution of a global pathogen. *Pathog Dis.* 2014;71(3):292–301.
8. Nieves D, Heininger U. *Bordetella pertussis. Microbiol Spectr.* 2016;4:3. https://doi.org/10.1128/microbiolspec.El10-0008-2015.
9. Ellis J, Oyston P, Green M, Titball R. Tularemia. *Clin Microbiol Rev.* 2002;15(4):631–646.
10. Franco M, Mulder M, Gilman R, Smits H. Human brucellosis. *Lancet Infect Dis.* 2007;7(12):775–786.

Aerobic Fermentative Gram-Negative Rods

In the first edition of this book, I discussed two large and important families of bacteria in this chapter: **Enterobacteriaceae** and **Vibrionaceae**. Unfortunately, the family of Enterobacteriaceae was subsequently subdivided into seven families and placed in the Order Enterobacteriales. Although these classification changes are appropriate from a taxonomic perspective, I recognize this only causes confusion for the student. So, in this chapter, instead of referring to the seven individual families, I will simply refer to them as the Enterobacteriales.

First and foremost, it is important to understand that these gram-negative bacteria are among the most common human pathogens, responsible for diseases well documented in history, including cholera, plague, and typhoid fever, as well as common diseases such as pneumonia, gastroenteritis, and urinary tract infections. It is not practical to discuss individual members of these families without first understanding the common properties found in all family members that contribute to their virulence, epidemiology, and diseases they produce.

The Enterobacteriales are the largest, most heterogeneous collection of medically important gram-negative rods. The bacteria are **ubiquitous**, found worldwide in soil, water, and vegetation, and are part of the normal intestinal flora of most animals, including humans. All members can grow rapidly, aerobically and anaerobically, on a variety of nonselective (e.g., blood agar) and selective (e.g., MacConkey agar) media. The Enterobacteriales have simple nutritional requirements; they ferment glucose and are oxidase negative. The absence of cytochrome oxidase activity is an important characteristic because it can be measured rapidly with a simple test and is used to distinguish these bacteria from many other fermentative (e.g., *Vibrio*) and nonfermentative (e.g., *Pseudomonas*) gram-negative rods. The appearance of the bacteria on culture media has been used to differentiate common members. For example,

fermentation of lactose (detected by color changes in lactose-containing media such as the commonly used MacConkey agar) has been used to differentiate some enteric pathogens that do not ferment lactose (e.g., *Salmonella*, *Shigella*; colorless colonies on MacConkey agar) from lactose-fermenting species (e.g., *Escherichia*, *Klebsiella*; pink-purple colonies on MacConkey agar). **Resistance to bile salts** in some selective media has also been used to separate enteric pathogens (e.g., *Shigella*, *Salmonella*) from commensal organisms that are inhibited by bile salts. In this example, using culture media that assess lactose fermentation and resistance to bile salts is a rapid screening test for enteric pathogens that would be otherwise difficult to detect in diarrheal stool specimens where many different organisms may be present. Some Enterobacteriales, such as *Klebsiella*, are also characteristically mucoid (wet, heaped, viscous colonies with prominent **capsules**), whereas a loose-fitting, diffusible slime layer surrounds other species.

The heat-stable **lipopolysaccharide (LPS)** is a major cell wall antigen and consists of three components: the outermost somatic **O polysaccharide,** a core polysaccharide common to all Enterobacteriales (**enterobacterial common antigen**), and **lipid A**. The lipid A component of LPS is responsible for endotoxin activity, and many of the systemic manifestations of gram-negative bacterial infections are initiated by endotoxin—activation of complement, release of cytokines, leukocytosis, thrombocytopenia, disseminated intravascular coagulation, fever, decreased peripheral circulation, shock, and death.

The epidemiologic (serologic) classification of the Enterobacteriales is based on three major groups of antigens: **somatic O polysaccharides, K antigens** in the capsule (type-specific polysaccharides), and **H proteins** in the bacterial flagella. Detection of these various antigens has important clinical significance beyond epidemiologic investigations, as some pathogenic species of bacteria are associated with specific O and H serotypes (e.g., *E. coli* O157:H7 is associated with hemorrhagic colitis).

The family Vibrionaceae is large, consisting of more than 100 species, with *V. cholerae* being the most important. All of the species can grow on a variety of simple media but require salt for growth (halophilic or "salt loving"). These species can also tolerate a wide range of temperatures and pH but are susceptible to gastric acid. For this reason, exposure to a large inoculum is required for disease. As with the Enterobacteriales, the cell wall of Vibrionaceae contains LPS consisting of the outer O polysaccharide, core polysaccharide, and inner lipid A components. The O polysaccharide is used to subdivide *Vibrio* species into serogroups. There are more than 200 serogroups of *V. cholerae*, with *V. cholerae* O1 being the most important. This is the serogroup responsible for worldwide pandemics of cholera.

Although the discussion of *Vibrio* species in this chapter focuses on *V. cholerae*, two other species deserve mention: *Vibrio parahaemolyticus* and *Vibrio vulnificus*. Following ingestion of contaminated seafood, *V. parahaemolyticus* can cause **diarrheal disease**, ranging from self-limited, watery diarrhea to a mild form of cholera. The illness lasts 3 days or more but results in an uneventful recovery. In contrast, *V. vulnificus* is a particularly virulent species, with the most common presentation being **primary septicemia** after consumption of contaminated raw oysters or a rapidly **progressive wound infection** after exposure to contaminated seawater. Mortality can be 50% in septic patients and 20%–30% in patients with wound infections. Immunocompromised patients are at particular risk, as well as those with preexisting hepatic disease, hematopoietic disease, or chronic renal failure.

Enterobacteriales and Vibrionaceae	
Bacteria	**Historical Derivation**
Order Enterobacteriales	
Escherichia coli	*Escherichia*, named after the discoverer Theodor Escherich; *coli*, of the colon
Klebsiella pneumoniae	*Klebsiella*, named after the German microbiologist Edwin Klebs; *pneumoniae*, inflammation of the lungs
Proteus mirabilis	*Proteus*, a god able to change himself into different shapes; *mirabilis*, surprising (refers to pleomorphic colony forms)
Salmonella typhi	*Salmonella*, named after Daniel Salmon, chairman of the department where the discoverer, Theobald Smith, worked; *typhi*, of typhoid (referring to the disease typhoid fever)
Shigella dysenteriae	*Shigella*, named after the discoverer Kiyoshi Shiga; *dysenteriae*, dysentery

Enterobacteriales and Vibrionaceae—cont'd	
Bacteria	**Historical Derivation**
Yersinia pestis	*Yersinia*, named after Yersin who identified the first isolate; *pestis*, plague
Family Vibrionaceae	
Vibrio cholerae	*Vibrio*, move rapidly or vibrate (rapid movement caused by the polar flagella); *cholerae*, cholera or an intestinal disease

Discussion of the Enterobacteriales and Vibrionaceae cannot be comprehensive due to a large number of species responsible for disease; however, I believe the species I have selected are representative of these families.

ESCHERICHIA COLI

E. coli is the most common and important member of the Enterobacteriales. This organism is associated with a variety of diseases, including gastroenteritis and extraintestinal infections such as cystitis and pyelonephritis, intraabdominal infection, meningitis, and sepsis. A multitude of strains are capable of causing disease. For example, specific strains are responsible for urinary tract infections, others for meningitis, and gastroenteritis is caused by five different groups of *E. coli*: enterotoxigenic *E. coli* (ETEC), enteropathogenic *E. coli* (EPEC), enteroaggregative *E. coli* (EAEC), enteroinvasive *E. coli* (EIEC), and Shiga toxin-producing *E. coli* (STEC). Some serotypes are associated with greater virulence, such as *E. coli* O157, which is the most common cause of hemorrhagic colitis and hemolytic uremic syndrome. Finally, *E. coli* is the most common gram-negative bacteria responsible for bacteremia.

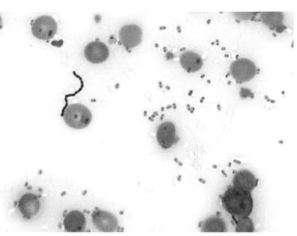

Escherichia coli and *Streptococcus* spp. in a positive blood culture. All members of the Enterobacteriaceae have bipolar staining; that is, the ends of the rods stain more intensely than the center of the cell, giving the initial appearance of diplococci.

ESCHERICHIA COLI

Properties	• Enterotoxigenic *E. coli* (ETEC) attach to the small intestine by colonization factor antigens and produce heat-labile and heat-stable toxins • Enteropathogenic *E. coli* (EPEC) attach to the small intestine by adhesins (bundle-forming pili, intimin) and disrupt the surface • Enteroaggregative *E. coli* (EAEC) attach to the small intestine by aggregative adherence fimbriae (AAF) and also disrupt the surface • Enteroinvasive *E. coli* (EIEC) invade and destroy the colonic epithelium • Shiga Toxin-Producing *E. coli* (STEC) initially attach to intestines by bundle-forming pili and intimin and then produce Shiga toxins Stx1 and Stx2 that damage the colonic epithelium • Uropathogenic *E. coli* strains bind to cells of the urinary bladder and upper urinary tract by adhesins (P pili, AAF, others). Hemolysin HlyA is produced that lyses the cells, leading to cytokine release, stimulation of the inflammatory response, and subsequent tissue damage • Majority of strains that cause neonatal meningitis possess the K1 capsular antigen
Epidemiology	• Most common aerobic gram-negative rods in the gastrointestinal tract • Urinary tract infections, intraabdominal infections, and sepsis are primarily endogenous (the patient's microbial flora); strains causing gastroenteritis are generally acquired exogenously • Meningitis primarily restricted to neonates • Intraabdominal infections related to spillage of intestinal bacteria into the abdomen during trauma or surgery; infections typically polymicrobial

Continued

ESCHERICHIA COLI—cont'd	

Clinical Disease	• **Gastroenteritis**: caused by a variety of strains with specific virulence factors; clinical illness reflection of the site of infection and pathology
	  • Infections of the small intestine (ETEC, EPEC, EAEC): characterized by watery diarrhea, vomiting, and low-grade fever
	  • Infections of the large intestine (STEC, EIEC): characterized by bloody diarrhea (hemorrhagic colitis) and abdominal cramps
	• **Hemolytic uremic syndrome**: a complication of STEC and EIEC infections
	• **Urinary tract infections**: may be restricted to inflammation of the bladder or may involve the upper tract, primarily the kidneys, with associated flank pain and fever
	• Polymicrobial **intraabdominal infection**: characterized by abscess formation (caused by associated bacteria) and septicemia
	• **Meningitis**: in neonates cannot be differentiated from other causes of meningitis (e.g., group B *Streptococcus*)

Diagnosis	• Gram stains of all Enterobacteriales stain most intensely at the ends with the center being pale (characteristic "bipolar" appearance) • Organisms grow rapidly on most culture media • Enteric pathogens, with the exception of STEC, are detected primarily by commercial nucleic acid amplification tests (NAATs) • STEC-producing strains detected by culture on selective media, immunoassays for detection of the toxins, or NAATs for toxin-specific genes
Treatment, Control, and Prevention	• Enteric pathogens are treated symptomatically unless disseminated disease (bacteremia) occurs • Antibiotic therapy is guided by *in vitro* susceptibility tests because of increased resistance to penicillins, cephalosporins, and carbapenems, mediated by extended-spectrum β-lactamases and carbapenemases • Appropriate infection control practices are used to reduce the risk of nosocomial infections (e.g., restricting the use of antibiotics, avoiding unnecessary use of urinary tract catheters) • Maintenance of high hygienic standards to reduce the risk of exposure to gastroenteritis strains, particularly for travelers to less developed regions • Proper cooking of beef products such as hamburgers to reduce the risk of STEC infections

KLEBSIELLA PNEUMONIAE

The most important member of the genus *Klebsiella* is *K. pneumoniae*, a prominent cause of **pneumonia**. Members of the genus are covered with a prominent mucoid capsule, which makes recognition of the bacteria by Gram stain (large rods surrounded by a large capsule) and culture relatively easy. The bacteria in this genus cause both community- and hospital-acquired pneumonia, with the destruction of the alveolar spaces, formation of cavities, and production of blood-tinged sputum prominent. The treatment of disease caused by this organism has also become a challenge, because many strains are resistant to all β-lactam antibiotics through the production of carbapenemases. The term "KPC" or *K. pneumoniae*-producing carbapenemases has unfortunately become an all-too-familiar part of our conversation today.

Klebsiella pneumoniae are large rods frequently surrounded by a prominent capsule. Note in this slide that many of the rods are surrounded by a clear area (particularly noticeable in the pair of rods in the center of the image). The clear area is the capsule that excludes the stain.

KLEBSIELLA PNEUMONIAE

Properties	• Prominent mucoid polysaccharide capsule • Production of carbapenemases and other β-lactamases
Epidemiology	• Widely distributed in nature and low-level colonization of healthy individuals • Disease primarily in patients with depressed pulmonary function or control of respiratory secretions (e.g., alcoholics, moribund hospitalized patients)
Clinical Disease	• **Pneumonia**: prominently involving one or more lobes ("lobar pneumonia") with cavity formation and production of bloody sputum
Diagnosis	• Gram stain of sputum with characteristic bacteria associated with a vigorous cellular immune response • Relatively easy to grow in culture
Treatment, Control, and Prevention	• Treatment must be guided by *in vitro* susceptibility tests because multidrug-resistant strains are common, particularly in hospital settings • Appropriate infection control practices are used to reduce the risk of nosocomial infections, including screening asymptomatic patients for carriage of resistant strains and limited use of antibiotics

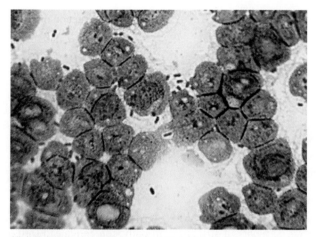

Klebsiella pneumoniae in a positive blood culture. Note the clear area around the gram-negative rods. This is due to the thick mucoid bacterial capsule that stains poorly.

PROTEUS MIRABILIS

The most commonly isolated member of the genus *Proteus* is *P. mirabilis*, which is an important cause of **urinary tract infections** in previously healthy adults. *P. mirabilis* produces large quantities of urease, an enzyme that splits urea into carbon dioxide and ammonia. This process raises the urine pH, precipitating magnesium and calcium in the form of struvite and apatite crystals, respectively, and results in the formation of renal stones. Other bacteria that infect the urinary tract and produce urease can produce the same effect (e.g., *Staphylococcus saprophyticus*).

PROTEUS MIRABILIS

Properties	• Urease production
Epidemiology	• Present in the gastrointestinal tract and can migrate to the urinary tract to produce disease • Patients with a history of infections with this organism are at increased risk of reinfections
Clinical Disease	• **Urinary tract infections** including cystitis (bladder) and pylenephritis (kidney) with stone formation
Diagnosis	• Grows readily in culture and has characteristic swarming motility on the surface of the agar plates (colony will rapidly spread and cover the entire plate surface with a thin sheet of bacteria) • Definitive identification by biochemical tests or mass spectroscopy
Treatment, Control, and Prevention	• Generally susceptible to ampicillin and cephalosporins; resistant to tetracycline • Restricted use of urinary tract catheters will reduce the risk of hospital-acquired infections

SALMONELLA SPECIES

More than 2500 serotypes of *Salmonella* are described and frequently listed as individual species, with the most common being *Salmonella typhi*, *Salmonella enteritidis*, *Salmonella choleraesuis*, and *Salmonella typhimurium*. In reality, most of these serotypes are members of a single species, *Salmonella enterica*. I don't believe the student is particularly interested in these taxonomic debates, but there is some confusion in the literature that should be recognized. To simplify this presentation, I will focus on the most important member of this genus, *S. typhi*, and provide a general commentary on the other species.

Salmonella species can colonize all animals, particularly poultry. Many species are restricted to their primary host, while some can crossover and cause disease in humans. *S. typhi* and closely related serotypes are unique because they are strictly human pathogens, producing severe acute disease initially presenting as bacteremia and then progressing to gastroenteritis. These bacteria are also capable of survival in the gallbladder, establishing chronic carriage and a source of new infections for contacts.

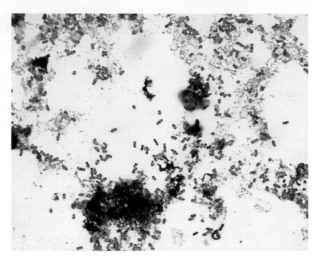

Salmonella typhi in a positive blood culture. Note the prominent bipolar staining.

SALMONELLA SPECIES	
Properties	• Virulence of *S. typhi* is regulated by genes on two large pathogenicity islands that facilitate the attachment, intracellular engulfment, and replication of bacteria in intestinal cells and macrophages • Bacteria are transported from the intestines to liver, spleen, and bone marrow by macrophages
Epidemiology	• In contrast with most *Salmonella* species that are acquired by eating contaminated food products (e.g., poultry, eggs, dairy products), *S. typhi* is a **strict human pathogen** and is acquired by person-to-person contact or ingestion of food or water contaminated by infected individuals • 400 to 500 *S. typhi* infections occur annually in the USA, most of which are acquired during foreign travel; more than 27 million cases worldwide with an estimated 200,000 deaths annually • Infectious dose is low facilitating person-to-person spread • Asymptomatic long-term colonization occurs commonly
Clinical Disease	• **Enteric fever**: 10 to 14 days after ingestion of *S. typhi*, patients experience gradually increasing fever with nonspecific complaints of headache, myalgias, fever, and anorexia; symptoms persist for 1 week or more followed by gastrointestinal symptoms • **Asymptomatic colonization**: chronic low-grade infection with *S. typhi*, localized to the gallbladder
Diagnosis	• *S. typhi* present in the **blood** during the first phase of illness and then recovered in **stool specimens** after infection is localized in the gallbladder • Culture is frequently negative because the bacteremic phase is transient and low numbers of organisms present in the stool specimen may be difficult to detect • Although serologic tests have been used historically to document present or past infections, these tests are considered insensitive and nonspecific

SALMONELLA SPECIES—cont'd

Treatment, Control, and Prevention	• Infections with *S. typhi* or disseminated infections with other organisms should be treated with an effective antibiotic (selected by *in vitro* susceptibility tests); fluoroquinolones (e.g., ciprofloxacin), chloramphenicol, trimethoprim-sulfamethoxazole, or a broad-spectrum cephalosporin may be used, but regional antibiotic resistance is common due to unrestricted use of antibiotics in some communities • Carriers of *S. typhi* should be identified and treated • Vaccination against *S. typhi* can reduce the risk of disease for travelers to endemic areas

SHIGELLA SPECIES

Species in the genus *Shigella* are actually biochemical variants (biogroups) of *E. coli*; however, they remain in a separate genus for historical reasons. It is probably easiest to think of *Shigella* species as variants of Enteroinvasive *E. coli* (EIEC) and STEC. Four species of *Shigella* are recognized, with *Shigella sonnei* responsible for the vast majority of infections in the USA and *Shigella flexneri* predominating in developing countries. Although *Shigella dysenteriae* infections are less common, primarily observed in West Africa and Central America, this is the most virulent species of *Shigella* and is associated with mortality rates of 5%–15%. The fourth species, *Shigella boydii*, is infrequently isolated.

SHIGELLA SPECIES

Properties	• Attach, invade, and replicate in cells lining the colon • Replicate in the cytoplasm of phagocytic cells and move cell to cell without extracellular exposure, thus protected from immune-mediated clearance • Induce programed cell death of macrophages, resulting in the release of interleukin-1β with resulting stimulation of localized inflammatory response and subsequent damage to lining of the colon • A-B exotoxin (**Shiga toxin** similar to STEC toxin) produced by *S. dysenteriae* disrupts protein synthesis and produces endothelial damage • Shiga toxin can also mediate damage to the glomerular endothelial cells, resulting in renal failure: **hemolytic uremic syndrome**
Epidemiology	• Estimated 500,000 cases of *Shigella* infections occur annually in the USA; 90 million cases worldwide (one of the most common causes of bacterial gastroenteritis) • **Humans are the only reservoir** for these bacteria • Disease spreads person to person by the fecal-oral route • Primarily a pediatric disease with young children in day-care centers, nurseries, and custodial institutions at the highest risk of disease; also at risk are siblings and parents of these children; communities with poor hygienic standards; and male homosexuals • Relatively few organisms can produce disease (highly infectious) • Disease occurs worldwide with no seasonal incidence (consistent with person-to-person spread involving a low inoculum)
Clinical Disease	• **Shigellosis** presents initially as watery diarrhea progressing within 1 to 2 days to abdominal cramps and tenesmus (cramping rectal pain) with or without bloody stools • **Bacterial dysentery** is a severe form of the disease, caused by *S. dysenteriae* • **Asymptomatic carriage** develops in a small number of patients (reservoir for future infections)

Continued

SHIGELLA SPECIES—cont'd

Diagnosis	• Microscopy is not useful because *Shigella* cannot be differentiated from *E. coli* and other gram-negative rods present in stool specimens from healthy individuals • Culture using selective media designed for the recovery of *Shigella* is useful, but care is needed in handling positive cultures because this organism is highly infectious (laboratory-acquired infections are not uncommon) • Multiplex NAATs (simultaneously testing for multiple enteric pathogens) are common and in many laboratories have replaced culture
Treatment, Control, and Prevention	• Antibiotic therapy shortens the course of symptomatic disease, fecal shedding, and infectivity for contacts • Treatment should be guided by *in vitro* susceptibility tests • Empirical therapy can be initiated with a fluoroquinolone or trimethoprim-sulfamethoxazole • Appropriate infection control measures should be instituted to prevent spread of the organism, including hand washing and proper disposal of soiled linens

YERSINIA

The best-known human pathogens in this genus are *Y. pestis* and *Y. enterocolitica*. *Y. pestis* causes the highly fatal systemic disease known historically as **plague** and will be the focus of this section. *Y. enterocolitica* is responsible for **gastroenteritis** in cold weather climates in Northern Europe and North America, as well as two additional diseases: (1) chronic inflammation of the terminal ileum with enlargement of the mesenteric lymph nodes resulting in "**pseudoappendicitis**" (primarily a disease in children) and (2) **blood transfusion-related bacteremia**. *Y. enterocolitica* can grow at 4°C, so this organism can multiply to high concentrations in refrigerated blood products.

YERSINIA PESTIS

Properties	• *Y. pestis* is covered with a protein capsule that interferes with phagocytosis • Produces a protease that degrades: (1) complement component C3b preventing opsonization; (2) complement C5a preventing phagocytic migration; and (3) fibrin clots permitting spread of the bacteria • Induces macrophage killing and suppression of cytokine production, resulting in diminished inflammatory response to infection • *Y. pestis* is resistant to serum killing enabling high-grade bacteremia
Epidemiology	• Plague was one of the most devastating diseases in history, with major epidemics recorded in the Old Testament, worldwide from 540 AD to mid-700 AD, in Europe in the 1320s (30%–40% of the population died), and beginning in China in the 1860s; epidemics and sporadic cases continue to occur • *Y. pestis* is a zoonotic infection with humans being the accidental host • Two epidemiologic forms of disease: (1) **urban plague** with rats as reservoir; (2) **sylvatic plague** with squirrels, rabbits, and domestic animals as reservoirs • Disease is spread by bites from the flea vector (spread within the reservoir host population or from host to humans), direct contact with infected tissues, or person to person by inhalation of infectious aerosols from a patient with pulmonary disease (patients with pulmonary disease are highly infectious) • Fewer than 10 cases are reported annually in the USA with disease primarily being sylvatic plague

YERSINIA PESTIS—cont'd	
Clinical Disease	• Two clinical manifestations: bubonic plague and pneumonic plague • **Bubonic plague**: characterized by incubation period of less than 1 week, followed by development of high fever and painful swelling or **bubo** of regional lymph nodes (groin or axilla) with bacteremia; high mortality rate unless promptly treated • **Pneumonic plague**: characterized by development of fever and pulmonary symptoms within 1 to 2 days after inhalation of bacteria; high mortality rate
Diagnosis	• Microscopy of bubo or pulmonary secretions suggestive if disease is clinically suspected but not specific (resembles other Enterobacteriales) • Organisms grow on most culture media but may require 2 days of incubation • Identification by biochemical testing or mass spectroscopy
Treatment, Control, and Prevention	• *Y. pestis* infections are treated with streptomycin; tetracyclines, chloramphenicol, or trimethoprim-sulfamethoxazole can be administered as alternative therapy • Enteric infections with other *Yersinia* species are usually self-limited; if antibiotic therapy is indicated, most organisms are susceptible to broad-spectrum cephalosporins, aminoglycosides, chloramphenicol, tetracyclines, and trimethoprim-sulfamethoxazole • Plague is controlled by reduction in the rodent population • Vaccine is no longer available in the USA

VIBRIO CHOLERAE

Much like *Y. pestis*, *V. cholerae* is responsible for one of the most feared diseases in history—**cholera**. We are currently in the midst of the seventh pandemic (worldwide epidemic) of cholera since 1817, with disease reported in most coastal countries with poor hygiene. *V. cholerae* is present in most oceans and seas, so most exposures result in no disease or self-limited diarrhea. Significant disease occurs only following ingestion of a large number of organisms, so control of epidemics is simple in principle but difficult to realize.

VIBRIO CHOLERAE	
Properties	• Cholera toxin is an A-B toxin that binds to receptors on intestinal epithelial cells, which results in hypersecretion of electrolytes and water • Toxin-coregulated pilus serves as the receptor site for the bacteriophage that transfers the two toxin genes into the bacteria; also mediates bacterial adherence to intestinal mucosal cells • Accessory cholera enterotoxin increases intestinal fluid secretion • Zonula occludens toxin increases intestinal permeability
Epidemiology	• Seven major pandemics of cholera have occurred since 1817, including the current pandemic that began in Asia and has spread worldwide • **Serotype 01** is responsible for major pandemics, with significant mortality in countries with substandard hygiene • Organisms are found in marine environments worldwide; associated with shellfish • Bacterial levels increase in warm months, so infections are seasonal • Infections most commonly acquired by consumption of contaminated water or shellfish • Person-to-person spread is rare because the infectious dose is high

Continued

***VIBRIO CHOLERAE*—cont'd**	
Clinical Disease	• **Cholera**: begins with an abrupt onset of watery diarrhea and vomiting and can progress rapidly to severe dehydration, metabolic acidosis and hypokalemia, and hypovolemic shock • **Gastroenteritis**: milder forms of diarrheal disease can occur in toxin-negative strains of *V. cholerae* O1 and in non-O1 serotypes
Diagnosis	• Microscopic examination of stool can be useful in acute infections, but rapidly become negative as the disease progresses because organisms are "flushed" out of the intestines with the profuse watery diarrhea • Immunoassays for cholera toxin or O1 antigen are useful although the analytic performance can be quite variable • Culture should be performed early in the course of disease with fresh stool specimens; delays in processing the specimen may result in a shift to acidic pH, which will result in loss of viable bacteria • Multiplex NAATs (simultaneously testing for multiple enteric pathogens) are becoming common and have replaced culture in many laboratories where resources are available
Treatment, Control, and Prevention	• Fluid and electrolyte replacement are crucial • Antibiotics (e.g., azithromycin) reduce the bacterial burden and exotoxin production, but play a secondary role in patient management • Improved community hygiene is critical for control of disease • Oral, inactivated cholera vaccines provide limited protection

CLINICAL CASES (REFER TO SECTION VI)

Lower Respiratory Tract Infections
• *Klebsiella pneumoniae* pneumonia

Gastrointestinal Tract Infections
• Shiga toxin *Escherichia coli* (STEC) outbreak
• Enterotoxigenic *Escherichia coli* (ETEC) gastroenteritis
• Enterohemorrhagic *Escherichia coli* hemolytic uremic syndrome
• *Salmonella* gastroenteritis
• *Shigella* infections in day-care centers
• *Shigella* gastroenteritis in gay males
• *Vibrio cholerae* gastroenteritis
• *Vibrio parahaemolyticus* gastroenteritis

Genitourinary Tract Infections
• *Escherichia coli* urinary tract infection
• *Proteus mirabilis* urinary tract infection

Central Nervous System Infections
• *Escherichia coli* meningitis in neonates

Sepsis and Cardiovascular Infections
• *Escherichia coli* bacteremia
• *Salmonella typhi* infection
• *Yersinia pestis* sepsis
• *Vibrio vulnificus* sepsis

SUPPLEMENTAL READING

1. Kaper J, Nataro J, Mobley H. Pathogenic *Escherichia coli*. *Nat Rev Microbiol*. 2004;2(2):123–140.
2. Paczosa M, Mecsas J. *Klebsiella pneumoniae*: going on the offense with a strong defense. *Microbiol Mol Biol Rev*. 2016;80(3):629–661.
3. Armbruster C, Mobley H, Pearson M. Pathogenesis of *Proteus mirabilis* infection. *EcoSal Plus*. 2018;8(1). https://doi.org/10.1128//ecosalplus.ESP-0009-2017.
4. Knodler L, Elfenbein J. *Salmonella enterica*. *Trends Microbiol*. 2019;27(11):964–965.
5. Wain J, Hendriksen R, Mikoleit M, et al. Typhoid fever. *Lancet*. 2015;385(9973):1136–1145.
6. Kotloff K, Riddle M, Platts-Mills J, et al. Shigellosis. *Lancet*. 2018;391(10122):801–812.
7. Yang R. Plague: recognition, treatment, and prevention. *J Clin Microbiol*. 2018;56(1). e01519-17.
8. Baker-Austin C, Oliver J, Alam M, et al. *Vibrio* spp infections. *Nat Rev Dis Primers*. 2018;4(1):8. https://doi.org/10.1038/s41572-018-0005-8.

Aerobic Nonfermentative Gram-Negative Rods

The nonfermentative gram-negative rods discussed in this chapter are opportunistic pathogens of plants, animals, and humans. It should be recognized there are many species of bacteria in this group that are opportunistic pathogens, but I am going to focus only on the three most common genera and their most important species. The organisms I will discuss were originally classified in the genus *Pseudomonas*, based on their inability to ferment carbohydrates and their morphologic appearance—small rods typically arranged in pairs. *Pseudomonas* was subdivided into a number of new genera, with *Burkholderia* and *Stenotrophomonas* being the most common human pathogens. Members of these three genera are found in the soil, decaying organic matter, and water, as well as in moist areas of the hospital such as sinks. These bacteria can use many organic compounds as a source of carbon and nitrogen, so they can survive and replicate in environments where nutrients are minimal. The bacteria, particularly *Pseudomonas*, produce an impressive array of virulence factors, and all are resistant to the most commonly used antibiotics. It is not surprising that these bacteria are particularly important opportunistic pathogens in hospitalized patients. In this chapter, I will focus on the most commonly isolated species of each genus: *P. aeruginosa*, *Burkholderia cepacia*, and *S. maltophilia*.

The genus *Pseudomonas* consists of more than 250 species, and a number of these will be encountered in the hospital environment. Likewise, there are a number of species closely related to *B. cepacia* (frequently these are

Opportunistic Pathogens of Plants, Animals, and Humans	
Bacteria	**Historical Derivation**
P. aeruginosa	*Pseudo*, false; *monas*, unit (refers to the Gram stain appearance of pairs of organisms that resemble a single cell); *aeruginosa*, full of copper rust or green (refers to the green color of colonies of this species due to production of blue and yellow pigments)
B. cepacia	*Burkholderia*, named after the microbiologist Burkholder; *cepacia*, like an onion (original strains isolated from rotten onions)
S. maltophilia	*Steno*, narrow; *trophos*, one who feeds; *monas*, unit (refers to the fact that these narrow bacteria require few substrates for growth); *malto*, malt; *philia*, friend (friend of malt [good growth with malt])

referred to as the *B. cepacia* complex), as well as one species, *Burkholderia pseudomallei*, that is a significant cause of **respiratory infections** ranging from asymptomatic colonization to cavitary disease resembling tuberculosis (**melioidosis**). The virulence of *B. pseudomallei* is well recognized, and this organism has been classified as a "select agent" for the risk of its use as an agent of bioterrorism. In contrast to *Pseudomonas* and *Burkholderia*, *S. maltophilia* is the only species in this genus of medical importance.

PSEUDOMONAS AERUGINOSA

This is the most common nonfermentative gram-negative rod responsible for opportunistic infections in hospitalized patients. *P. aeruginosa* produces a variety of adhesins, toxins, and tissue-destroying enzymes, so it is amazing not that these organisms produce disease, but that infections are not more common in the hospital. The explanation for this is that infection is defined by three factors: the organism's

virulence factors, a susceptible host (e.g., immunocompromised patients), and opportunity for exposure.

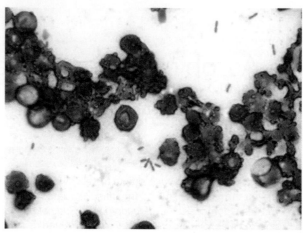

Pseudomonas aeruginosa in positive blood culture. Short gram-negative rods typically arranged in pairs.

PSEUDOMONAS AERUGINOSA	
Properties	• Bacterial surface components (i.e., pili, flagella, lipopolysaccharide, mucoid alginate capsule) bind to host cells • Alginate **capsule** protects from phagocytosis and antibiotic killing • **Exotoxin A** disrupts host protein synthesis (similar to the diphtheria toxin) • Pigments (pyocyanin, pyoverdin) produce toxic forms of oxygen, stimulate cytokine release, and regulate toxin secretion • Elastase, phospholipase, and extracellular toxins mediate tissue destruction and inhibit neutrophil function • Innate and acquired **antibiotic resistance** make treatment difficult
Epidemiology	• Ubiquitous in nature and in moist environmental hospital sites (e.g., flowers, sinks, toilets, mechanical ventilation, dialysis equipment) • No seasonal incidence of disease • Can transiently colonize the respiratory and gastrointestinal tracts of hospitalized patients, particularly those treated with broad-spectrum antibiotics, exposed to respiratory therapy equipment, or hospitalized for extended periods • Patients at high risk of developing infections include neutropenic or immunocompromised patients, cystic fibrosis patients, and burn patients
Clinical Disease	• **Pulmonary infection**: ranges from mild irritation of the bronchi (**tracheobronchitis**) to necrosis of the lung parenchyma (**necrotizing bronchopneumonia**) • **Primary skin infections**: opportunistic infections of existing wounds (e.g., burns) to localized infections of hair follicles (e.g., associated with immersion in contaminated waters such as hot tubs) • **Urinary tract infections**: opportunistic infections in patients with indwelling urinary catheters and following exposure to broad-spectrum antibiotics that select these antibiotic-resistant bacteria • **Ear infections**: can range from mild irritation of the external ear ("**swimmer's ear**") to invasive destruction of cranial bones adjacent to the infected ear ("**malignant otitis**") • **Eye infections**: opportunistic infections of mildly damaged corneas; can be very aggressive with complete loss of vision • **Bacteremia**: dissemination of bacteria from primary infection in other organs and tissues; can be characterized by necrotic skin lesions (**ecthyma gangrenosum**)

PSEUDOMONAS AERUGINOSA—cont'd	
Diagnosis	• Grows rapidly on common laboratory media and Gram stain morphology is characteristic • Identified by colonial characteristics (β-hemolysis on blood agar, green pigment, grapelike odor) and simple biochemical tests (positive oxidase reaction, oxidative utilization of carbohydrates)
Treatment, Control, and Prevention	• Treatment consists primarily of antibiotic combinations (e.g., aminoglycoside combined with active β-lactam antibiotic); monotherapy is generally ineffective; resistance to multiple antibiotics is common • Hospital infection control efforts should concentrate on preventing contamination of sterile medical equipment and nosocomial transmission; unnecessary use of broad-spectrum antibiotics can select for resistant organisms • No vaccine is available for high-risk patients

BURKHOLDERIA CEPACIA

B. cepacia is a complex of a number of closely related species that colonize and produce disease in a select group of patients: those with cystic fibrosis, chronic granulomatous disease (CGD; a primary immunodeficiency in which white blood cells have defective intracellular microbial killing) or indwelling urinary or vascular catheters.

In contrast to *P. aeruginosa*, *B. cepacia* has relatively few virulence factors, and infections can generally be treated with trimethoprim-sulfamethoxazole (TMP-SMX; a drug to which *Pseudomonas* is uniformly resistant). For this reason, it is important to differentiate between infections caused by *Pseudomonas* and *Burkholderia*.

BURKHOLDERIA CEPACIA	
Properties	• Relatively low level of virulence
Epidemiology	• Present in moist areas of hospital environment • Colonizes patients with increased susceptibility to infections
Clinical Disease	• **Pulmonary infections**: most worrisome infections are in patients with chronic granulomatous disease or cystic fibrosis, in whom infections can progress to cause significant destruction of pulmonary tissues • **Opportunistic infections**: urinary tract infections in catheterized patients; bacteremia in immunocompromised patients with contaminated intravascular catheters
Diagnosis	• Grows readily on common laboratory media • Can be classified in the *B. cepacia* complex by biochemical testing, but species identification requires gene sequencing or mass spectroscopy
Treatment, Control, and Prevention	• Generally susceptible to the sulfa drug, trimethoprim-sulfamethoxazole; may be susceptible *in vitro* to piperacillin, broad-spectrum cephalosporins, and ciprofloxacin, but the clinical response is poor • Avoid exposure of at-risk patients, and carefully monitor colonized patients for progression of the disease • No vaccine is available

STENOTROPHOMONAS MALTOPHILIA

Much like *B. cepacia*, *S. maltophilia* is an opportunistic

pathogen of immunocompromised patients, and the drug of choice for treating infections is TMP-SMX.

STENOTROPHOMONAS MALTOPHILIA

Properties	• Primary virulence property is antibiotic resistance
Epidemiology	• Present in moist areas of hospital • Immunocompromised patients receiving broad-spectrum antibiotics, particularly carbapenems, are at the greatest risk of disease • Infections traced to contaminated intravenous catheters, disinfectant solutions, mechanical ventilation equipment, and ice machines
Clinical Disease	• **Opportunistic infections**: a variety of infections (most commonly bacteremia and pneumonia) in immunocompromised patients
Diagnosis	• Grows readily on common laboratory media • Can be identified by biochemical tests or mass spectroscopy
Treatment, Control, and Prevention	• Generally susceptible to the sulfa drug, trimethoprim-sulfamethoxazole; uniformly resistant to carbapenem antibiotics • Avoid exposure of at-risk patients and carefully monitor colonized patients for progression of the disease • No vaccine is available

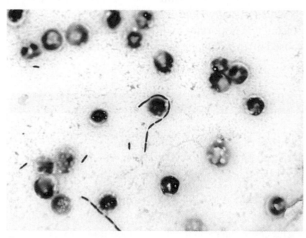

Stenotrophomonas maltophilia in positive blood culture. Like *Pseudomonas* and *Burkholderia*, *Stenotrophomonas* is typically arranged in pairs or occasionally short chains.

CLINICAL CASES (REFER TO SECTION VI)

Upper Respiratory Tract Infections
• *Pseudomonas* ear infection

Lower Respiratory Tract Infections
• *Pseudomonas* pulmonary infection
• *Burkholderia* pulmonary infection

Skin and Soft Tissue Infections
• *Pseudomonas* folliculitis

Sepsis and Cardiovascular Infections
• *Stenotrophomonas* sepsis in a neutropenic patient

Miscellaneous Infections
• *Pseudomonas* eye infection

SUPPLEMENTAL READING

1. Breidenstein E, Fuente-Nunez C, Hancock R. *Pseudomonas aeruginosa*: all roads lead to resistance. *Trends Microbiol.* 2011;19(5):419–426.
2. Sfeir M. *Burkholderia cepacia* complex infections: more complex than the bacterium name suggests. *J Infect.* 2018;77(3):166–179.
3. Brooke JS. *Stenotrophomonas maltophilia*: an emerging global opportunistic pathogen. *Clin Microbiol Rev.* 2012;25(1):2–41.

Anaerobic Bacteria

Anaerobic bacteria are the predominant population of microbes in humans, outnumbering aerobic bacteria by 10-fold to 1000-fold in different anatomic sites. These organisms play an important role in maintaining human health by taking part in metabolic functions, such as digestion of food, stimulation of innate and regulatory immunity, and prevention of colonization with unwanted pathogens. The majority of infections with anaerobic bacteria are **endogenous**, resulting from the transfer of the organisms from their normal residence on the skin or mucosal surfaces to normally sterile sites such as deep tissues and fluids (e.g., pleural fluid and peritoneal fluid). As might be expected, these endogenous infections are characteristically **polymicrobial** with a mixture of aerobic and anaerobic bacteria. The exceptions to this are infections caused by members of the genera *Clostridium* and *Clostridioides*, collectively referred to as clostridia. These bacteria are spore-forming organisms (the anaerobic counterpart to the aerobic spore-former, *Bacillus*). Because of their ability to form spores, clostridia are found in soil and other environmental sites and typically cause monomicrobic exogenous infections. The best-known clostridia are **Clostridium tetani** (cause of **tetanus**), **Clostridium botulinum** (cause of **botulism**), **Clostridium perfringens** (cause of **gas gangrene**), and **Clostridioides difficile** (cause of **antibiotic-associated diarrheal disease**). Each of these pathogens has well-characterized virulence mechanisms and is fully capable of causing significant disease. In contrast, most other anaerobes are relatively avirulent and produce disease most effectively in a complex of different organisms. One exception to this is **Bacteroides fragilis**, which has a number of important virulence

Anaerobic Bacteria

Bacteria	Historical Derivation
Clostridium	*closter*, a spindle
Clostridium tetani	*tetani*, related to tension (disease caused by this organism is characterized by muscle spasms)

Continued

Anaerobic Bacteria—cont'd

Bacteria	Historical Derivation
Clostridium botulinum	botulus, sausage (the first outbreak caused by this organism was associated with contaminated sausage)
Clostridium perfringens	perfringens, breaking through (this organism is highly virulent and associated with invasive tissue necrosis)
Clostridioides difficile	difficile, difficult (refers to the extreme oxygen sensitivity of this organism making it difficult to grow)
Bacteroides	bacter, staff or rod; idus, shape (rod shaped)
Bacteroides fragilis	fragilis, fragile (organism was believed to be fragile or rapidly killed by oxygen exposure)

factors and, when present in a polymicrobial infection, is primarily responsible for the pathology.

A brief discussion of the other groups of anaerobic bacteria is appropriate. The **gram-positive cocci** consist of a number of genera that colonize the oral cavity, gastrointestinal tract, genitourinary tract, and skin. These bacteria are commonly present in polymicrobial infections and contribute to abscess formation and tissue destruction, but all can generally be treated with β-lactam antibiotics, such as penicillin. The anaerobic gram-positive rods are subdivided into spore-forming rods (*Clostridium*) and non-spore-forming rods. The most common non-spore-forming genera associated with disease are **Actinomyces** (actinomycosis, a chronic suppurative disease), **Lactobacillus** (endocarditis), and **Cutibacterium** (acne; also, a common contaminant of blood cultures). **Veillonella** is the most commonly isolated gram-negative cocci, but is rarely responsible for disease. The following is a summary of the most important anaerobic species.

CLOSTRIDIUM TETANI

C. tetani is ubiquitous, found in soil and transiently in the gastrointestinal tracts of many animals and humans. The vegetative (replicating) form of *C. tetani* is extremely susceptible to oxygen toxicity, but the spores can survive in nature for many years. Disease is mediated by a plasmid-encoded, heat-labile neurotoxin (**tetanospasmin**). Tetanospasmin is an A-B toxin that inactivates proteins that regulate the release of the inhibitory neurotransmitters glycine and gamma-aminobutyric acid. This leads to unregulated excitatory synaptic activity in the motor neurons, resulting in **spastic paralysis**. Because the binding is irreversible, recovery from disease is prolonged even with aggressive therapy.

CLOSTRIDIUM TETANI	
Properties	• **Tetanospasmin** interferes with the release of inhibitory neurotransmitters (glycine, gamma-aminobutyric acid)
Epidemiology	• Ubiquitous, spores found in most soils and can transiently colonize the gastrointestinal tract of humans and animals • Exposure to spores is common, but disease is uncommon except in developing countries where there is limited access to vaccine and medical care • Risk of disease is highest for people with inadequate vaccine-induced immunity • Disease is uncommon in the USA and other high-income regions, but almost 700,000 new cases occur annually (5–10% mortality) primarily in South Asia and sub-Saharan Africa; approximately half of the reported cases occur in children <5 years • Disease does not induce immunity
Clinical Disease	• **Generalized tetanus**: generalized musculature spasms and involvement of the autonomic nervous system in severe disease (e.g., cardiac arrhythmias, fluctuations in blood pressure, profound sweating, dehydration) • **Localized tetanus**: musculature spasms restricted to localized area of primary infection • **Neonatal tetanus**: neonatal infection primarily involving the umbilical stump; very high mortality

CLOSTRIDIUM TETANI—cont'd	
Diagnosis	• Diagnosis is based on clinical presentation and not laboratory tests (used to confirm clinical diagnosis) • Microscopy and culture are insensitive, and tetanus toxin and antibodies are not typically detected; culture of *C. tetani* is difficult because the organism rapidly dies after exposure to oxygen
Treatment, Control, and Prevention	• Treatment requires debridement, antibiotic therapy (penicillin, metronidazole), passive immunization with antitoxin globulin to bind free toxin, and vaccination with tetanus toxoid to stimulate immunity • Prevention through the use of vaccination, consisting of three doses of tetanus toxoid followed by booster doses every 10 years

CLOSTRIDIUM BOTULINUM

As with *C. tetani*, *C. botulinum* is commonly isolated from soil worldwide. Similar to tetanus toxin, *C. botulinum* produces a **heat-labile A-B toxin** that inactivates the proteins that regulate the release of acetylcholine, blocking neurotransmission at peripheral cholinergic synapses. Acetylcholine is required for the excitation of muscles; therefore, the resulting clinical presentation of botulism is **flaccid paralysis**. As with tetanus, recovery of function after botulism is prolonged because regeneration of the nerve endings is required. Seven antigenically distinct botulinum toxins (A to G) are described, with human disease associated with types A, B, E, and rarely F, so multiple bouts of botulism are theoretically possible.

CLOSTRIDIUM BOTULINUM	
Properties	• **Botulinum toxin** blocks neurotransmission at motor nerve synapses
Epidemiology	• *C. botulinum* spores are found in the soil worldwide • Classified as a "select agent" because of the concern that the spores can be used as a bioterrorism agent • Relatively few cases of botulism in the USA but prevalent in developing countries • Infant botulism more common than other forms in the USA, but has significantly decreased in frequency following the recommendation not to give infants honey, which can be contaminated with *C. botulinum* spores • Botulinum toxin is sensitive to heating but resistant to gastric acids
Clinical Disease	• **Food-borne botulism**: initial presentation of blurred vision, dry mouth, constipation, and abdominal pain; progresses to bilateral descending weakness of the peripheral muscles with flaccid paralysis • **Infant botulism**: initially nonspecific symptoms (e.g., constipation, weak cry, failure to thrive) that progresses to flaccid paralysis and respiratory arrest • **Wound botulism**: clinical presentation same as with food-borne disease, although the incubation period is longer and fewer gastrointestinal symptoms are reported • **Inhalation** botulism: rapid onset of symptoms (flaccid paralysis, pulmonary failure) and high mortality from inhalation exposure to botulinum toxin
Diagnosis	• Diagnosis is based on clinical presentation and not laboratory tests (confirmatory) • Culture of *C. botulinum* is difficult because the organism rapidly dies after exposure to oxygen • Food-borne botulism is confirmed if toxin activity is demonstrated in the implicated food or in the patient's serum, feces, or gastric fluid • Infant botulism is confirmed if toxin is detected in the infant's feces or serum or the organism is cultured from feces • Wound botulism is confirmed if toxin is detected in the patient's serum or wound or the organism is cultured from the wound

Continued

CLOSTRIDIUM BOTULINUM—cont'd

Treatment, Control, and Prevention	• Treatment involves the combination of administration of metronidazole or penicillin, trivalent botulinum antitoxin, and ventilatory support • Spore germination in foods is prevented by maintaining food at an acid pH, by high sugar content (e.g., fruit preserves), or by storing the foods at 4°C or colder • Toxin is heat labile and therefore can be destroyed by heating the food for 10 min at 60°C to 100°C • Infant botulism associated with ingestion of contaminated soil or consumption of contaminated foods (particularly honey)

CLOSTRIDIUM PERFRINGENS

C. perfringens has a characteristic Gram stain morphology of large rectangular gram-positive rods and rarely forms spores in clinical specimens. These characteristics are important because they differentiate this species from other clostridia and make recognition of cells in clinical specimens easy for an experienced microbiologist. The species also grows rapidly in culture, forming characteristic large spreading β-hemolytic colonies. The production of one or more **"lethal" toxins** by *C. perfringens* (alpha, beta, epsilon, and iota toxins) is used to subdivide isolates into five types (A through E). Type A strains (with all four lethal toxins) are most commonly associated with human diseases including soft-tissue infections, food poisoning, necrotizing enteritis, and septicemia.

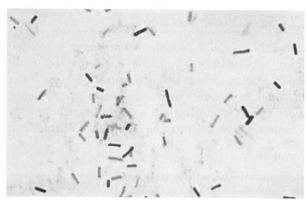

Gram stain of *Clostridium perfringens* in a wound specimen. Cells are uniformly rectangular in shape, may decolorize, and appear gram negative; spores are rarely observed with this species.

CLOSTRIDIUM PERFRINGENS

Properties	• Lethal toxins:
	  • **Alpha toxin** is a lecithinase that lyses erythrocytes, platelets, leukocytes, and endothelial cells; mediates massive hemolysis and tissue destruction characteristic of overwhelming disease
	  • **Beta toxin** is responsible for intestinal stasis, loss of mucosa with the formation of necrotic lesions, and progression to necrotizing enteritis
	  • **Epsilon toxin** increases vascular permeability of the gastrointestinal wall
	  • **Iota toxin** has necrotic activity and increases vascular permeability
	• Enterotoxin binds to receptors on the brush border membrane of the small intestine epithelium in the ileum and jejunum, leading to altered membrane permeability and loss of fluids and ions; acts as a superantigen, stimulating T-lymphocyte activity and massive release of cytokines

Epidemiology	• Ubiquitous; present in the soil, water, and intestinal tract of humans and animals • Type A strains are responsible for most human infections • Soft-tissue infections typically associated with bacterial contamination of wounds or localized trauma • Food poisoning associated with contaminated meat products (beef, poultry, gravy) held at temperatures between 5°C and 60°C, which allows the organisms to grow to large numbers

CLOSTRIDIUM PERFRINGENS—cont'd

Clinical Disease	• **Cellulitis**: localized edema and erythema with gas formation in the soft tissues; generally not painful • **Suppurative myositis**: accumulation of pus in the muscle planes, without muscle necrosis or systemic symptoms • **Myonecrosis**: painful, rapid destruction of muscle tissue with rapid systemic spread and high mortality • **Food poisoning**: rapid onset of abdominal cramps and watery diarrhea with no fever, nausea, or vomiting; short duration and self-limited • **Necrotizing enteritis**: acute, necrotizing destruction of jejunum with abdominal pain, vomiting, bloody diarrhea, and peritonitis
Diagnosis	• Reliably seen in Gram-stained tissues (large rectangular gram-positive rods) although spores will not be observed • Grows rapidly in culture as a large, spreading colony surrounded by a zone of β-hemolysis and an outer zone of partial hemolysis • Laboratories rarely culture stool specimens in suspected cases of food poisoning
Treatment, Control, and Prevention	• Rapid treatment is essential for serious infections • Severe infections require surgical debridement and high-dose penicillin therapy • Symptomatic treatment for food poisoning • Proper wound care and judicious use of prophylactic antibiotics will prevent most infections

CLOSTRIDIOIDES DIFFICILE

C. difficile is currently the most commonly encountered clostridial pathogen, responsible for antibiotic-associated gastrointestinal diseases ranging from self-limited diarrhea to life-threatening colitis. The disease is mediated by two toxins: an **enterotoxin** (toxin A) and a **cytotoxin** (toxin B). The enterotoxin is chemotactic for neutrophils, stimulating the infiltration of polymorphonuclear neutrophils into the ileum with the release of cytokines. The cytotoxin causes the destruction of the epithelial cytoskeleton. The cytotoxin alone is sufficient for producing the disease but not the enterotoxin. Highly virulent stains have been observed and were initially thought to be due to increased toxin production. More recent studies have discounted this explanation although it is widely cited. Disease is widespread in hospitals, particularly in patients treated with clindamycin, broad-spectrum β-lactam antibiotics, and other agents. It is now recognized that a significant proportion of infections recognized in the hospital were acquired in the community; that is, the patients are colonized with *C. difficile* at the time of hospitalization. In many cases, this is related to previous hospitalization in a health care facility.

CLOSTRIDIOIDES DIFFICILE

Properties	• **Enterotoxin (toxin A)** stimulates infiltration of neutrophils and release of cytokines • **Cytotoxin (toxin B)** causes the destruction of the intestinal epithelium
Epidemiology	• Colonizes the intestines of a small proportion of healthy individuals • Exposure to antibiotics is associated with depletion of the normal intestinal population of bacteria, overgrowth of *C. difficile*, and subsequent disease (endogenous infections) • Spores can be detected in hospital rooms of infected patients (particularly around beds and bathrooms); these can be an exogenous source of infection • Highly virulent stains periodically circulate in the hospital and community

Continued

CLOSTRIDIOIDES DIFFICILE — cont'd

Clinical Disease	• **Antibiotic-associated diarrhea**: acute diarrhea generally developing 5 to 10 days after initiation of antibiotic treatment (particularly clindamycin, penicillins, cephalosporins, fluoroquinolones); may be brief and self-limited or more protracted • **Pseudomembranous colitis**: most severe form of *C. difficile* disease with profuse diarrhea, abdominal cramping, and fever; whitish plaques (pseudomembranes) form over intact colonic tissue (seen on colonoscopy)
Diagnosis	• Diagnosis of *C. difficile* disease is by detection of the genes encoding the bacterial toxins or direct detection of the toxin in stool specimens • Use of culture is slow, and isolation of *C. difficile* must be further validated by demonstrating that the isolate produces toxin B, so culture is rarely done for routine diagnostic purposes • Immunoassays for toxins in stool specimens are insensitive and not reliable • Tests for detection of *C. difficile* cytoplasmic antigens (i.e., glutamine dehydrogenase) are sensitive but not specific, so should only be used as a screening assay • Nucleic acid amplification tests for the toxin genes are the most sensitive and specific diagnostic tests and are considered the test of choice for documenting *C. difficile* infection
Treatment, Control, and Prevention	• The implicated antibiotic should be discontinued • Treatment with fidaxomicin should be used in severe disease; vancomycin is an acceptable alternative; fecal transplants (repopulation of the bowel with the indigenous population of bacteria) has been used to treat recurrent disease • Relapse is common because antibiotics do not kill spores; a second course of therapy is usually successful, but multiple courses may be required • The hospital room should be carefully cleaned after the infected patient is discharged

BACTEROIDES FRAGILIS

B. fragilis is the most important member of a complex of closely related species (*B. fragilis* **group**). The bacteria are pleomorphic in size and shape and resemble a mixed population of gram-negative rods in a casually examined Gram stain. *B. fragilis* grows rapidly in culture and is stimulated by the presence of bile; both features serve the bacteria well *in vivo* because *B. fragilis* is found most commonly in the intestines. The most important structural feature of this species is an antiphagocytic **polysaccharide capsule** that stimulates abscess formation.

Bacteroides fragilis in positive blood culture. Cells are faintly staining pleomorphic gram-negative rods.

BACTEROIDES FRAGILIS

Properties	• Polysaccharide capsule is the primary virulence factor, responsible for abscesses characteristic of infections with *B. fragilis* • Fimbriae on the cell surface are responsible for adherence to host cells • Production of fatty acids (e.g., succinic acid) inhibits phagocytosis and intracellular killing • Catalase and superoxide dismutase protect the bacteria by inactivating hydrogen peroxide and super-oxide free radicals • Heat-labile toxin (*B. fragilis* toxin) stimulates chloride secretion and fluid loss in the small intestine and induces interleukin-8 secretion, which contributes to the inflammatory damage of the intestinal epithelium
Epidemiology	• Colonizes the gastrointestinal tract of animals and humans as a minor member of the microbiome; rare or absent from the oropharynx or genital tract of healthy individuals • Endogenous infections are most commonly polymicrobial, involving both aerobic and anaerobic bacteria
Clinical Disease	• **Intra-abdominal infections**: characterized by abscess formation and associated with leakage of bowel contents or dissemination by bacteremia • **Skin and soft-tissue infections**: associated with trauma and can progress from localized colonization to life-threatening **myonecrosis** • **Gynecologic infections**: include pelvic inflammatory disease, abscesses, endometritis, and surgical wound infections; abscess formation is characteristic of *B. fragilis* infections • **Gastroenteritis**: presents as self-limited watery diarrhea when caused by enterotoxin-producing *B. fragilis*; primarily in children younger than 5 years old
Diagnosis	• Characteristic Gram stain (pleomorphic gram-negative rods) from clinical specimens • Grows rapidly in cultures incubated anaerobically • Easily identified by biochemical tests, gene sequencing, or mass spectrometry laser desorption/ionization mass spectroscopy
Treatment, Control, and Prevention	• Resistant to penicillin and 25% of isolates are resistant to clindamycin; uniformly susceptible to metronidazole and most strains are susceptible to carbapenems and piperacillin-tazobactam • Prevention is difficult because infections are endogenous • No vaccine is available

CLINICAL CASES (REFER TO SECTION VI)

Gastrointestinal Tract Infections
• *Clostridium perfringens* food poisoning
• *Clostridium perfringens* gastroenteritis
• *Clostridioforme difficile* colitis

Genitourinary Tract Infections
• Pelvic actinomycosis

Central Nervous System Infections
• *Clostridium tetani* infection
• *Clostridium botulinum* infection
• Infant botulism

Skin and Soft-Tissue Infections
• *Bacteroides fragilis* necrotizing fasciitis

Sepsis and Cardiovascular Infections
• *Lactobacillus* endocarditis
• *Lactobacillus* bacteremia
• Shunt infection with *Propionibacterium* (*Cutibacterium*) acnes
• Contaminated blood culture with *Propionibacterium* (*Cutibacterium*)
• *Clostridium perfringens* sepsis
• *Clostridium septicum* sepsis with occult malignancy

SUPPLEMENTAL READING

1. Chatham-Stephens K, et al. Clinical features of foodborne and wound botulism: a systematic review of the literature, 1932–2015. *Clin Infect Dis.* 2018;66(Suppl):S11–S16.

2. Yan L, Thwaites C. Tetanus. *Lancet.* 2019;393:1657–1668.

3. Uzal F, et al. Towards and understanding of the role of *Clostridium perfringens* toxins in human and animal disease. *Future Microbiol.* 2014;9(3):361–377.

4. Finn E, Andersson FL, Madin-Warburton M. Burden of *Clostridioides difficile* infection (CDI)—a systematic review of the epidemiology of primary and recurrent CDI. *BMC Infect Dis.* 2021;21:456–467.

5. McDonald LC, Gerding D, Johnson S, et al. Clinical practice guidelines for *Clostridium difficile* infection in adults and children: 2017 update by IDSA and SHEA. *Clin Infect Dis.* 2018;66:987–994.

6. Wexler H. Bacteroides: the good, the bad, and the nitty-gritty. *Clin Microbiol Rev.* 2007;20(4):593–621.

Spiral-Shaped Bacteria

INTERESTING FACTS

- *Campylobacter jejuni* is the most common cause of bacterial gastroenteritis, responsible for an estimated 1.5 million illnesses every year in the USA.
- *Helicobacter pylori* is the most common cause of bacterial gastritis and peptic ulcer disease.
- *Treponema pallidum* is the most common cause of painless genital ulcers.
- Lyme disease caused by *Borrelia burgdorferi* is the most common arthropod-transmitted bacterial disease.

The bacteria discussed in this chapter are neither cocci nor rods; rather, they are spiral or helical shaped. Five organisms will be discussed in detail:

There are also related bacteria that should be briefly mentioned because they are important human pathogens, but will not be discussed further:

Spiral- or Helical-Shaped Bacteria

Bacteria	Historical Derivation
Campylobacter jejuni	*kampylos*, curved; *bacter*, rod; *jejuni*, of the jejunum (curved rod of the jejunum [site of disease])
Helicobacter pylori	*helix*, spiral; *bacter*, rod; *pylorus*, lower part of the stomach (spiral rod in the lower part of the stomach)
Treponema pallidum	*trepo*, turn; *nema*, a thread; *pallidum*, pale (refers to very thin, spiral rods that do not stain with traditional dyes)
Borrelia burgdorferi	named after A. Borrel and W. Burgdorfer
Leptospira species	*lepto*, thin; *spira*, a coil (refers to the thin coiled morphology of the bacteria)

Related Bacteria

Related Bacteria	Human Diseases
Campylobacter coli	Gastroenteritis
Campylobacter upsaliensis	Gastroenteritis
Campylobacter fetus	Vascular infections (e.g., septicemia, septic thrombophlebitis, endocarditis)
Helicobacter cinaedi	Gastroenteritis, proctocolitis
Helicobacter fennelliae	Gastroenteritis, proctocolitis
Borrelia afzelii	Lyme disease (in Europe and Asia)
Borrelia garinii	Lyme disease (in Europe and Asia)
Borrelia recurrentis	Epidemic (louse-borne) relapsing fever
Borrelia, many species	Endemic (tick-associated) relapsing fever

CAMPYLOBACTER JEJUNI

Campylobacters, primarily *C. jejuni* and *C. coli*, are the most common causes of **bacterial gastroenteritis** in both developed and developing countries. The role of these gram-negative bacteria in human disease was not recognized for many years because they are small (0.2–0.5 µm wide and 0.5–5.0 µm long) and grow best in reduced oxygen, increased carbon dioxide conditions and at 42°C. They were initially discovered when stool specimens were processed for viruses by filtration through 0.45-µm filters, allowing the thin bacteria to pass through the filters while eliminating the other enteric bacteria in the specimens.

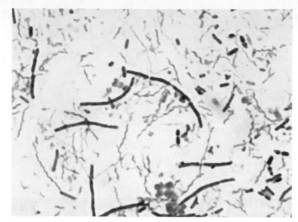

Campylobacter jejuni in stool specimen. *C. jejuni* is the thin, curved, gram-negative bacteria in the midst of larger gram-negative rods and gram-positive diplococci.

CAMPYLOBACTER JEJUNI	
Properties	• Polysaccharide capsule provides protection from phagocytosis • Lipopolysaccharide with endotoxin is absent in these gram-negative bacteria • Adhesins, cytotoxic enzymes, and enterotoxins are detected in *C. jejuni*, but specific role in disease is poorly defined • Cross-reactivity with host tissues responsible for autoimmune complications of *Campylobacter* infections (Guillain-Barré syndrome, reactive arthritis)
Epidemiology	• Zoonotic infection; improperly prepared **poultry** is a common source of human infections • Infections acquired by ingestion of contaminated food, unpasteurized milk, or contaminated water • Person-to-person spread is unusual • Dose required to establish disease is high because the organism is susceptible to gastric acids • Previous exposure provides partial immunity and results in less severe disease • Worldwide distribution with enteric infections seen throughout the year
Clinical Disease	• **Gastroenteritis**: damage to mucosal surfaces of jejunum, ileum, and colon; acute enteritis with diarrhea, fever, and severe abdominal pain; can mimic acute appendicitis, particularly in children and young adults • **Guillain-Barré syndrome**: well-recognized complication of *Campylobacter* infection; autoimmune disorder of the peripheral nervous system characterized by the development of symmetric weakness over several days, with recovery requiring months or longer • **Reactive arthritis**: complication of *Campylobacter* infection; characterized by joint pain and swelling involving the hands, ankles, and knees; persisting from 1 week to several months
Diagnosis	• Microscopic detection of thin "S-shaped" gram-negative rods in stool specimens is specific but insensitive • Commercial multiplex, nucleic acid amplification tests are highly sensitive and specific for enteric pathogens and particularly useful for the detection of *C. jejuni* and *C. coli* infections • Culture requires the use of specialized media incubated with reduced oxygen, increased carbon dioxide, and elevated temperatures; requires incubation for 2 or more days and is relatively insensitive unless fresh media are used • Detection of *Campylobacter* antigens in stool specimens is moderately sensitive and very specific compared with culture

CAMPYLOBACTER JEJUNI—cont'd

Treatment, Control, and Prevention	• For gastroenteritis, infection is self-limited and is managed by fluid and electrolyte replacement • Severe gastroenteritis and septicemia are treated with erythromycin or azithromycin; fluoroquinolone resistance is common • Gastroenteritis is prevented by proper preparation of food and consumption of pasteurized milk; preventing contamination of water supplies also controls infection • Experimental vaccines targeting the outer capsular polysaccharides are promising for the control of infections in animal reservoirs

HELICOBACTER PYLORI

Like *C. jejuni*, *H. pylori* is a relatively recently appreciated human pathogen. Helicobacters are similar in size and shape to campylobacters, and growth requires complex media supplemented with blood, serum, charcoal, starch or egg yolk, and microaerophilic conditions. *H. pylori* was initially associated with gastritis in 1983 and subsequently implicated as a cause of peptic ulcers, gastric adenocarcinomas, and gastric mucosa-associated lymphoid tissue lymphomas. Helicobacters are subdivided into species that primarily colonize the stomach (**gastric helicobacters**) and those that colonize the intestines (**enterohepatic helicobacters**). *H. pylori* is a gastric helicobacter.

HELICOBACTER PYLORI

Properties	• Initial colonization facilitated by blockage of acid production and neutralization of gastric acids with ammonia produced by bacterial **urease** activity • Actively motile, permitting migration through gastric mucosa to gastric epithelial cells where attachment is mediated by bacterial adhesin proteins • Localized tissue damage caused by urease byproducts, mucinase, phospholipases, and the activity of vacuolating cytotoxin A • Type VI secretion system injects bacterial proteins into epithelial cells, which interferes with normal cytoskeletal structure
Epidemiology	• Infections are common, particularly in people in a low socioeconomic class or developing nations, and colonization can be lifelong • **Humans** are the primary reservoir • Person-to-person spread is important (typically fecal-oral) • Ubiquitous and worldwide, with no seasonal incidence of disease • *H. pylori* responsible for >80% of peptic ulcer disease and 75% of noncardia (lower part of the stomach) gastric cancers
Clinical Disease	• **Gastritis**: inflammation of gastric mucosa, characterized by feeling of fullness, nausea, vomiting, and hypochlorhydria (decreased acid production); can progress to chronic disease • **Peptic ulcers**: development of ulcers, commonly at the junction between the corpus and antrum of the stomach or the proximal duodenum (duodenal ulcer) • **Gastric adenocarcinoma**: progression of chronic gastritis to stomach cancer • **Mucosa-associated lymphoid tissue B-cell lymphomas**
Diagnosis	• Microscopy: histologic examination of biopsied gastric antrum specimens is sensitive and specific • **Urease test** is relatively sensitive and highly specific; urea breath test is a noninvasive test • *H. pylori* antigen test is sensitive and specific; performed with stool specimens • Culture requires incubation in microaerophilic conditions; growth is slow; relatively insensitive unless multiple biopsies are cultured • Serology is useful for demonstrating exposure to *H. pylori* but not the disease

Continued

HELICOBACTER PYLORI—cont'd

Treatment, Control, and Prevention	• Multiple regimens have been evaluated for the treatment of *H. pylori* infections (Saleem and Howden reference). Combined therapy with a proton pump inhibitor (e.g., omeprazole), bismuth subcitrate, tetracycline, and metronidazole for 2 weeks has had a high success rate • Recommended to only treat symptomatic patients because prophylactic treatment of colonized individuals has not been useful and potentially has adverse effects, such as predisposing patients to adenocarcinomas of the lower esophagus • Human vaccines are not currently available

TREPONEMA PALLIDUM

T. pallidum is the organism responsible for the sexually transmitted disease **syphilis**. Although this disease has been recognized for centuries, diagnosis by traditional tests such as microscopy and culture is not useful because *T. pallidum* and related treponemes are small (0.1–0.2 μm × 6–20 μm) tightly coiled spirochetes that are too thin to be observed by light microscopy and *T. pallidum* has not been cultured in the laboratory. **Serology** remains the primary diagnostic test for syphilis, with **nontreponemal** tests (measurement of antibodies that develop against lipids released from damaged host cells during the early stages of disease) used for screening patients and **treponemal** tests (antibodies specifically directed against *T. pallidum*) used as confirmatory tests.

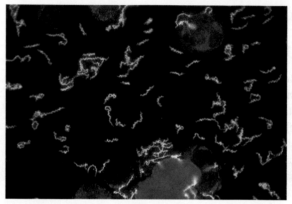

Treponema pallidum can be observed in an ulcer specimen using fluorescein-labeled antibodies for *T. pallidum* although this test is not widely available today.

TREPONEMA PALLIDUM

Properties	• Outer membrane proteins promote adherence to host cells • Hyaluronidase facilitates perivascular infiltration • Coating of fibronectin protects against phagocytosis • Tissue destruction primarily results from the host's immune response to infection
Epidemiology	• **Humans** are the only natural host • Venereal syphilis transmitted by sexual contact or congenitally from mother to fetus • Syphilis occurs worldwide with no seasonal incidence • Third most common sexually transmitted bacterial disease in the USA (after *Chlamydia* and *Neisseria gonorrhoeae* infections) • Patients with genital ulcers at increased risk of acquiring and transmitting HIV

Clinical Disease	• **Syphilis** develops in stages:
	  • **Primary disease: painless ulcer** or **chancre** at the site of infection with regional lymphadenopathy and bacteremia
	  • **Secondary syphilis:** flulike syndrome with generalized mucocutaneous rash and bacteremia
	  • **Late-stage syphilis:** diffuse chronic inflammation and destruction of any organ or tissue
	• **Neurosyphilis:** neurologic symptoms, primarily **meningitis**, can develop in the early or late stages of disease
	• **Congenital syphilis:** may result in fetal death; child born with multiorgan malformations; or latent disease that initially presents as rhinitis followed by a widespread desquamating maculopapular rash; teeth and bone malformation, blindness, deafness, and cardiovascular syphilis are common in untreated infants

TREPONEMA PALLIDUM—cont'd	
Diagnosis	• Darkfield or direct fluorescent antibody microscopy useful if mucosal ulcers are observed in primary or secondary stages of syphilis • **Serology** is very sensitive in the secondary and late stages of syphilis • Nucleic acid amplification tests have been developed but are not widely available
Treatment, Control, and Prevention	• Penicillin is drug of choice; doxycycline or tetracycline is administered if the patient is allergic to penicillin • Safe sex practices should be emphasized, and sexual partners of infected patients should be treated • No vaccine is available

BORRELIA BURGDORFERI

Borreliae are large spirochetes $(0.2–0.5\,\mu m \times 830\,\mu m)$ that stain best with aniline dyes (e.g., Giemsa or Wright stain). *B. burgdorferi* and related organisms are responsible for **Lyme disease**, named after Lyme, Connecticut, where the disease was first described. Typically, few organisms are present in the skin lesions or blood of the patients, and borreliae are microaerophilic with complex nutritional needs, so diagnosis is primarily by serology. **Serology** is relatively insensitive during the early stage of disease but is uniformly positive in the late stages of disease. False-positive tests can occur, so tests should only be performed in patients with the appropriate history and clinical presentation, a fact that is frequently overlooked and is responsible for many misdiagnosed patients.

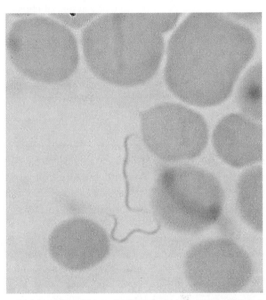

Giemsa stain of *Borrelia* spp. in the blood of a patient with endemic relapsing fever. Although *Borrelia burgdorferi* observed in tissues has the same appearance, it is rarely seen in clinical specimens.

BORRELIA BURGDORFERI	
Properties	• A number of *Borrelia* species responsible for Lyme disease with *B. burgdorferi* the most common in the USA • Outer surface antigens important for bacteria to evade host immune response
Epidemiology	• *B. burgdorferi* causes disease in the USA and Europe; *B. garinii* and *B. afzelii* cause disease in Europe and Asia • Transmitted by hard **ticks** from mice to humans; reservoir: mice, deer, and ticks • The most common tick-borne disease in the USA • Nymph stage of ticks responsible for more than 90% of human diseases so, although the ticks must feed for more than 2 days, they may not be noticed because of their small size • In the USA, 95% of Lyme disease cases are from two principle foci: Northeast and mid-Atlantic states (Maine to Virginia) and Upper Midwest states (Minnesota, Wisconsin) • Worldwide distribution • Seasonal incidence corresponds to feeding patterns of vectors; most cases of Lyme disease in the USA occur in late spring and early summer (feeding pattern of nymph stage of ticks); peak in June and July

Continued

BORRELIA BURGDORFERI—cont'd	

Clinical Disease	• **Lyme disease** develops in stages:
	  • **Early localized disease**: small macule or papule develops at the site of the tick bite and then enlarges to a lesion with a flat, red border and central clearing (**erythema migrans**)
	  • **Early disseminated disease**: hematogenous dissemination is characterized by systemic signs (severe fatigue, headache, fever, malaise), arthritis and arthralgia, myalgia, erythematous skin lesions, and cardiac and neurologic symptoms
	  • **Late-stage** manifestations include **arthritis** and **chronic skin involvement**

Diagnosis	• Microscopy and culture of limited value • Nucleic acid amplification tests are available for Lyme disease but are relatively insensitive due to few circulating bacteria • Serology is test of choice for Lyme disease
Treatment, Control, and Prevention	• For early localized or disseminated Lyme disease, treatment is with amoxicillin, doxycycline, or cefuroxime; late manifestations are treated with ceftriaxone • Reduced exposure to hard ticks through the use of insecticides, application of insect repellents to clothing, and wearing protective clothing that reduces exposure of skin to insects • Vaccines are not available

LEPTOSPIRA SPECIES

The taxonomy of this genus is a source of confusion in the literature. It is sufficient to recognize that a number of *Leptospira* species can cause the human disease **leptospirosis**. The organisms are very thin $(0.1\,\mu m \times 6\text{--}20\,\mu m)$, so brightfield microscopy is not useful. Additionally, they have complex nutritional requirements and grow slowly in culture, so diagnosis is based on serology.

LEPTOSPIRA SPECIES	
Properties	• Immune reactivity against *Leptospira* may be responsible for the clinical disease
Epidemiology	• US reservoirs: rodents (particularly rats), dogs, farm animals, and wild animals • **Humans: accidental end-stage host** • Organism can penetrate the skin through minor breaks in the epidermis • People are infected with leptospires through exposure to water contaminated with urine from an infected animal or handling of tissues from an infected animal • People at risk are those exposed to urine-contaminated streams, rivers, and standing water; occupational exposure to infected animals for farmers, meat handlers, and veterinarians • Infection is rare in the USA but has worldwide distribution • Disease is more common during warm months (recreational exposure)

Clinical Disease	• Most human infections are clinically unapparent and detected only through the demonstration of specific antibodies
	• Symptomatic infections (**leptospirosis**) develop in two stages:
	  • Initial phase is flulike symptoms with fever, muscle pain, chills, headache, vomiting, or diarrhea
	  • Second phase characterized by more severe disease with sudden onset of headache, myalgia, chills, abdominal pain
	• May present as **aseptic meningitis**
	• **Icteric form** of disease (**Weil disease**) is characterized by jaundice, vascular collapse, thrombocytopenia, hemorrhage, and hepatic and renal dysfunction

LEPTOSPIRA SPECIES—cont'd

Diagnosis	• Microscopy not useful because too few organisms are generally present in fluids or tissues • Culture: leptospires detected in blood or cerebrospinal fluid in the first 7 to 10 days of illness; and in urine after the 1st week • **Serology** using the microscopic agglutination test is relatively sensitive and specific but not widely available in resource-limited countries; enzyme-linked immunosorbent assay tests are less accurate but can be used to screen patients
Treatment, Control, and Prevention	• Treatment with penicillin or doxycycline • Doxycycline but not penicillin is used for prophylaxis • Herds and domestic pets should be vaccinated • Rats should be controlled

CLINICAL CASES

Gastrointestinal Tract Infections
• *Campylobacter jejuni* enteritis and Guillain-Barre syndrome
• *Helicobacter pylori* peptic ulcers

Genitourinary Tract Infections
• *Treponema pallidum* syphilis

Central Nervous System Infections
• *Treponema pallidum* neurosyphilis

Skin and Soft-Tissue Infections
• Congenital syphilis
• Lyme disease in Lyme CT
• Outbreak of tick-borne relapsing fever

Sepsis and Cardiovascular Infections
• *Campylobacter fetus* septicemia

Miscellaneous Infections
• *Leptospirosis* in triathlon participants

SUPPLEMENTAL READING

1. Silva J, Leite D, Fernandes M, et al. *Campylobacter* spp. as a foodborne pathogen: a review. *Front Microbiol.* 2011. https://doi.org/10.3389/fmicb.2011.00200.

2. Garza-Gonzalez E, Perez-Perez G, Maldonado-Garza H, Bosques-Padilla F. A review of *Helicobacter pylori* diagnosis, treatment, and methods to detect eradication. *World J Gastroenterol.* 2014;20(6):1438–1449.

3. Wang Y-K, Kuo F-C, Liu C-J, et al. Diagnosis of *Helicobacter pylori* infection: current options and development. *World J Gastroenterol.* 2015;21(40):11221–11235.

4. Saleem N, Howden C. Update on the management of *Helicobacter pylori* infection. *Curr Treat Options Gastro.* 2020. https://doi.org/10.1007/s11938-020-00300-3.

5. Radolf J, Deka R, Anand A, et al. *Treponema pallidum*, the syphilis spirochete: making a living as a stealth pathogen. *Nat Rev Microbiol.* 2016;14:744–759.

6. Steere A, Strle F, Wormser G, et al. Lyme borreliosis. *Nat Rev.* 2017. https://doi.org/10.1038/nrdp.2016.90.

7. Levett P. Leptospirosis. *Clin Microbiol Rev.* 2001;14(2):296–326.

Intracellular Bacteria

The bacteria discussed in this chapter are obligate aerobic intracellular organisms with a gram-negative cell wall structure. Beyond these features, they are taxonomically unrelated and classified into five separate families:

- Rickettsiaceae: *Rickettsia* and *Orientia*
- Ehrlichiaceae: *Ehrlichia*
- Anaplasmataceae: *Anaplasma*
- Coxiellaceae: *Coxiella*
- Chlamydiaceae: *Chlamydia*

Four Species of Intracellular Bacteria of Interest	
Bacteria	**Historical Derivation**
Rickettsia rickettsii	*Rickettsia*, named after Howard Ricketts who implicated the wood tick as the vector of Rocky Mountain spotted fever
Ehrlichia chaffeensis	*Ehrlichia*, named after the German microbiologist Paul Ehrlich; *chaffeensis*, bacteria first isolated in a soldier at Fort Chaffee, Arkansas
Coxiella burnetii	*Coxiella burnetii*, named after Herald Cox and F.M. Burnet who isolated the bacterium from ticks in Montana and patients in Australia, respectively
Chlamydia trachomatis	*Chlamydis*, a cloak; *trachomatis*, of trachoma or rough (disease characterized by rough granulations on the conjunctival surfaces that lead to chronic inflammation and blindness)

There are a number of related bacteria that should be mentioned because they are important human pathogens:

Other Intracellular Pathogens

Pathogens	Human Diseases
Rickettsia akari	Rickettsial pox: spotted fever transmitted by infected mites in urban areas such as New York
Rickettsia prowazekii	Typhus (three forms: epidemic, recrudescent, sporadic)
Rickettsia typhi	Endemic or murine typhus
Orientia tsutsugamushi	Scrub typhus: transmitted by mites ("chiggers")
Anaplasma phagocytophilum	Human granulocytic anaplasmosis
Chlamydia psittaci	Psittacosis (parrot fever): asymptomatic colonization to severe bronchopneumonia
Chlamydia pneumoniae	Asymptomatic or mild disease to severe atypical pneumonia

RICKETTSIA RICKETTSII

The genus *Rickettsia* is subdivided into two groups of diseases:

- **The spotted fever** group: many species of *Rickettsia* in the spotted fever group are associated with the human disease, although *R. rickettsii* and *R. akari* are the most important. *R. prowazekii* is the etiologic agent of **epidemic or louse-borne typhus**, with **humans as the principal reservoir** and the human body louse as the vector. Recrudescent disease can occur years after the initial infection.
- **The typhus** group: *R. typhi* is responsible for **endemic or murine typhus**, with rodents as the primary reservoir and the rat flea and cat flea as the principal vectors.

Members of the family Rickettsiaceae are small and grow only in the cytoplasm of eukaryotic cells. Although they have a gram-negative cell wall, they stain poorly with the Gram stain. The following is a summary of *R. rickettsii*:

RICKETTSIA RICKETTSII

Properties	- Outer membrane protein A on the surface of bacteria is responsible for attachment to endothelial cells; after penetration into the cell, *R. rickettsii* is released from the phagosome and multiplies in the cell - Endothelial cell damage related to bacterial replication resulting in vasculitis
Epidemiology	- *R. rickettsii* is the most common rickettsial pathogen in the USA - Hard ticks (e.g., dog tick, wood tick) are the primary reservoirs and vectors - Transmission requires prolonged contact - Distribution in the Western Hemisphere; in the USA, primarily in North Carolina, Oklahoma, Arkansas, Tennessee, and Missouri - Disease is most common from April to September
Clinical Disease	- **Rocky Mountain spotted fever** develops an average of 7 days after the tick bite; onset heralded by high fever and headache, associated with malaise, myalgias, nausea, vomiting, abdominal pain, and diarrhea; macular rash develops after 3 days, evolving to petechial form - Complications include neurologic manifestations, pulmonary and renal failure, and cardiac abnormalities

Continued

RICKETTSIA RICKETTSII—cont'd

Diagnosis	• Serology (e.g., microimmunofluorescence tests) is most commonly used • Gram stain and culture are of no value; staining of infected tissues with fluorescein-labeled antibodies is useful but generally available only in reference laboratories • Nucleic acid amplification tests are insensitive
Treatment, Control, and Prevention	• Doxycycline is the drug of choice • Should avoid tick-infected areas, wear protective clothing, and use effective insecticides • Should remove attached ticks immediately • No vaccine is available

EHRLICHIA CHAFFEENSIS

Ehrlichia and *Anaplasma* (formerly classified in the genus *Ehrlichia*) are small intracellular bacteria that parasitize blood cells (e.g., granulocytes, monocytes, erythrocytes, and platelets) and produce very similar diseases. Three species are important human pathogens: *E. chaffeensis* (infects monocytes), *Ehrlichia ewingii* (infects granulocytes), and *A. phagocytophilum* (infects granulocytes). In contrast to *Rickettsia*, these bacteria remain in the phagosome and prevent fusion with lysosomes. The masses of replicating bacteria in the phagosome (called **morulae**) can be detected by staining infected cells with Giemsa or Wright stains. *E. chaffeensis* is a model for infections with these organisms.

EHRLICHIA CHAFFEENSIS

Properties	• Replicates in infected cells and is protected from the host's immune response • Initiates host inflammatory response that contributes to pathology
Epidemiology	• Infections found predominantly in Midwestern USA (Missouri, Arkansas, Oklahoma) and the coastal Atlantic states (Maryland, Virginia, New Jersey, New York) • White-tailed deer is the primary reservoir, and the Lone Star tick is the vector • Humans are accidental hosts and not the natural hosts • Infects blood monocytes and mononuclear phagocytes in tissues and organs
Clinical Disease	• **Human monocytic ehrlichiosis**: 1 to 2 weeks after the tick bite, patients develop high fever, headache, malaise, and myalgias; late-onset rash develops in less than half of the patients; leucopenia, thrombocytopenia, and elevated serum transaminases develop in the majority of the patients and recovery is prolonged
Diagnosis	• Diagnosis primarily based on history and clinical presentation • Microscopy is of limited value; bacteria stain poorly with Gram stain, and Giemsa-stained intracytoplasmic inclusions are detected only early in the infection • Bacteria are not cultured • Nucleic acid amplification tests are useful but not widely available • Serology is useful but antibodies develop slowly (3–6 weeks after initial presentation)
Treatment, Control, and Prevention	• Doxycycline is the drug of choice; rifampin is an acceptable alternative • Prevention involves avoidance of tick-infested areas, use of protective clothing and insect repellents, and prompt removal of embedded ticks • Vaccine is not available

COXIELLA BURNETII

C. burnetii is a gram-negative bacterium that stains weakly with the Gram stain, grows intracellularly in eukaryotic cells, and causes the disease **Q (query) fever**, so named because the causal organism was not identified in the original Australian outbreak. Two structural forms of the bacterium develop: small cell variants that are stable in the environment and large cell variants that are the metabolically active, replicating form.

The small cell variants can also undergo phase variation (**phase I** and **phase II**). Small cell variants attach to macrophages and monocytes and are internalized in a phagocytic vacuole. If phase II variants are internalized, then the vacuole will fuse with lysosomes resulting in bacterial death. This is avoided if phase I variants are internalized. The disease is mostly asymptomatic, but symptomatic disease can present acutely and persist into chronic infections. The following is a summary of *C. burnetii*:

COXIELLA BURNETII	
Properties	• Replicating bacteria are protected in their intracellular location • Chronic infections develop if persistent intracellular survival occurs; mediated by overproduction of interleukin-10 that interferes with phagosome-lysosome fusion
Epidemiology	• There are many reservoirs including mammals, birds, and ticks • Most human infections are associated with contact with infected cattle, sheep, goats, dogs, and cats • Bacteria in high concentrations in the placenta; the soil becomes contaminated with dried placentas left on the ground after parturition, feces, and urine • The disease is mostly acquired through inhalation of aerosolized bacteria; possible exposure from consumption of contaminated milk; ticks are not an important vector for the human disease • Worldwide distribution • No seasonal incidence
Clinical Disease	• Most human infections are **asymptomatic** or mild, with exposure confirmed by serology • **Q fever**: symptomatic infections present with nonspecific flulike symptoms with an abrupt onset, high fever, fatigue, headache, and myalgias. More severe disease progresses to include hepatitis or pneumonia • **Chronic Q fever**: can develop months to years after the initial exposure, with **subacute endocarditis** as the most common presentation
Diagnosis	• Microscopy is not useful, and culture is rarely performed • Serology is the test of choice with detection of the antibody response to phase I and phase II antigens; antibodies against phase II detected in acute disease; antibodies against both phase I and II antigens develop in chronic disease • Nucleic acid amplification tests are not sensitive and not widely available
Treatment, Control, and Prevention	• Doxycycline is the drug of choice for acute infections; hydroxychloroquine combined with doxycycline is used to treat chronic infections • Phase I antigen vaccine is protective and safe if administered in a single dose before the animal or human has been exposed to *Coxiella*; not available in the USA

CHLAMYDIA TRACHOMATIS

Members of the family Chlamydiaceae are obligate intracellular parasites that have a unique developmental cycle, forming metabolically inactive infectious forms (**elementary bodies**, EBs) and metabolically active, replicating forms (**reticulate bodies**, RBs). EBs are extremely stable in the environment. EBs bind to receptors on the surface of host cells, are internalized, prevent fusion of phagosomes with lysosomes, and convert to replicating RBs. After about 24 h of replication, RBs are reorganized into EBs, the host cell ruptures, and infectious EBs are released. The following is a summary of *C. trachomatis*:

CHLAMYDIA TRACHOMATIS	
Properties	• Receptors for elementary bodies are restricted to nonciliated columnar, cuboidal, and transitional epithelial cells • Intracellular survival because bacteria prevent fusion of phagosome with lysosomes
Epidemiology	• **Most common sexually transmitted bacteria in the USA** • Leading cause of preventable **blindness** worldwide • Ocular trachoma presents primarily in North and sub-Saharan Africa, the Middle East, South Asia, and South America • Lymphogranuloma venereum prevalent in Africa, Asia, and South America
Clinical Disease	• **Trachoma**: chronic inflammatory granulomatous process of the eye surface, leading to corneal ulcerations, scarring, pannus formation, and blindness • **Adult inclusion conjunctivitis**: acute process with mucopurulent discharge, dermatitis, and corneal infiltrates; corneal vascularization occurs in chronic disease • **Neonatal conjunctivitis**: acute process characterized by a mucopurulent discharge • **Infant pneumonia**: after a 2- to 3-week incubation period, the infant develops rhinitis, followed by bronchitis with a characteristic dry cough • **Urogenital infections**: an acute process involving the genitourinary tract with characteristic mucopurulent discharge; asymptomatic infections are common in women • **Lymphogranuloma venereum**: a **painless ulcer** develops at the site of infection that spontaneously heals, followed by inflammation and swelling of lymph nodes draining the area; then a progression to systemic symptoms
Diagnosis	• Culture is highly specific but relatively insensitive and not widely available • Antigen tests are insensitive • Nucleic acid amplification tests are the most sensitive and specific tests are currently available
Treatment, Control, and Prevention	• Ocular and genital infections are treated with azithromycin or doxycycline • Newborn conjunctivitis and pneumonia treated with erythromycin • Lymphogranuloma venereum treated with doxycycline or erythromycin • Safe sex practices and prompt treatment of the patient and sexual partners help control infections • Vaccine not available

CLINICAL CASES (REFER TO SECTION VI)

Lower Respiratory Tract Infections
- *Chlamydia trachomatis* pneumonia in newborn infants
- Psittacosis in a previously healthy man

Genitourinary Tract Infections
- *Chlamydia trachomatis* Reiter syndrome and pelvic inflammatory disease
- *Chlamydia trachomatis* lymphogranuloma venereum

Skin and Soft-Tissue Infections
- Rocky mountain spotted fever
- Rickettsial pox in New York City

- Human granulocytic anaplasmosis
- *Rickettsia prowazekii* epidemic typhus
- *Rickettsia typhi* murine typhus
- *Orientia* scrub typhus

Sepsis and Cardiovascular Infections
- Human monocytic ehrlichiosis
- *Coxiella burnetii* endocarditis

Miscellaneous Infections
- *Chlamydia trachomatis* trachoma

SUPPLEMENTAL READING

1. Blanton L. The rickettsioses: a practical update. *Infect Dis Clin North Am.* 2019;33(1):213–229.
2. Madison-Antenucci S, Kramer L, Gebhardt L, Kauffman E. Emerging tick-borne diseases. *Clin Microbiol Rev.* 2020;33(2):e00083–18. https://doi.org/10.1128/CMR.00083-18.
3. Ismail N, McBride J. Tick-borne emerging infections: ehrlichiosis and anaplasmosis. *Clin Lab Med.* 2017;37(2):317–340.
4. Eldin C, Melenotte C, Mediannikov O, et al. From Q fever to *Coxiella burnetii* infection: a paradigm change. *Clin Microbiol Rev.* 2017;30(1):115–190.
5. Elwell C, Mirrashidi K, Engel J. *Chlamydia* cell biology and pathogenesis. *Nat Rev Microbiol.* 2016;14(6):385–400.

12

Introduction to Viruses

OVERVIEW

Viruses are the simplest and, generally, smallest microbe. They are obligate intracellular parasites, dependent on their host cell for survival and replication. In many ways, these are the most efficient microbes, carrying the minimum amount of genetic information as DNA or RNA (but not both), possessing a simple protein shell (called capsid), and in some cases surrounded by a membranous envelope. Their life cycle consists of finding the right host cell (defined by specific receptors for the different viruses), penetrating the cell, and then either remaining dormant in the cell by integrating into the host DNA or taking over the host metabolic machinery for direct viral replication. After a period when many viral particles have been produced, the particles can either be slowly released from the host cell (to preserve the cell integrity and survival) or essentially explode from the cell in search of new cellular targets.

The replication and pathology of most viral infections are restricted to specific host cell types (e.g., cells of the hematopoietic system, respiratory tract, gastrointestinal tract, central nervous system, liver, etc.); therefore, virology is best understood by focusing on the viruses that infect specific target cells or organs. This is in contrast to bacteria where a single species can infect many tissues (consider infections caused by *Staphylococcus aureus*), or a bacterial infection at a specific site can be caused by many bacteria (consider all the bacteria that can cause pneumonia). Therefore, for the presentations in the virology chapters, the focus will be on the viruses associated with specific diseases. This section is not a comprehensive review of all viruses of medical importance. Rather, the focus is on the viruses that will be encountered most commonly in medical practice.

CLASSIFICATION

The classification of viruses has traditionally been done based on their structural properties:
- Presence of DNA or RNA
- Presence of nucleic acids in a single strand or double strand
- Shape of the protein shell (icosahedral, spherical, other)
- Presence or absence of an envelope
- Overall size

The following is a list of the 7 DNA and 14 RNA virus families organized by their structural properties and examples of some of the important human pathogens.

DNA and RNA Virus Families		
Structure[a]	Family	Most Important Members
DNA Viruses		
DS, brick-shaped, envelope	Poxviridae	Smallpox (Variola) virus Vaccinia virus Monkeypox Molluscum contagiosum

Continued

DNA and RNA Virus Families—cont'd

Structure[a]	Family	Most Important Members
DS, icosahedral, envelope	Herpesviridae	Herpes simplex virus 1, 2 (HSV-1, HSV-2)
		Varicella-zoster virus (VZV)
		Epstein-Barr virus (EBV)
		Cytomegalovirus (CMV)
		Human herpesvirus 6, 7, 8 (HHV-6, HHV-7, HHV-8)
DS, spherical, envelope	Hepadnaviridae	Hepatitis B virus (HBV)
DS, icosahedral, no envelope	Adenoviridae	Adenovirus
	Papillomaviridae	Human papillomavirus
	Polyomaviridae	JC virus
		BK virus
SS, icosahedral, no envelope	Parvoviridae	Parvovirus B19
RNA Viruses		
DS, icosahedral, no envelope	Reoviridae	Rotavirus
SS, bullet-shaped, no envelope	Rhabdoviridae	Rabies virus
SS, filamentous, envelope	Filoviridae	Ebola virus
		Marburg virus
SS, icosahedral, no envelope	Picornaviridae	Rhinovirus
		Poliovirus
		Echovirus
		Parechovirus
		Enterovirus
		Coxsackievirus
		Hepatitis A virus
SS, icosahedral, envelope	Caliciviridae	Norovirus
		Sapovirus
	Togaviridae	Rubella virus
		Equine encephalitis viruses
		Chikungunya virus
SS, spherical, envelope	Orthomyxoviridae	Influenza virus
	Paramyxoviridae	Parainfluenza virus
		Measles virus
		Mumps virus
		Hendra virus
		Nipah virus
	Pneumoviridae	Human metapneumovirus
		Respiratory syncytial virus (RSV)
	Coronaviridae	Human coronavirus (229E, NL63, OC43, HKU1)
		SARS-CoV-1[b]
		SARS-CoV-2[b]
		MERS-CoV[b]
	Arenaviridae	Lassa virus
		Lymphocytic choriomeningitis virus
	Hantaviridae	Hantaan virus
	Retroviridae	Human immunodeficiency virus (HIV)
		Primate T-lymphotropic virus
	Flaviviridae	Dengue virus
		Yellow fever virus
		West Nile virus
		Zika virus
		Hepatitis C virus

[a]DS, double-strand nucleic acids; SS, single-strand nucleic acids.
[b]SARS-CoV, severe acute respiratory syndrome coronavirus; MERS-CoV, Middle East respiratory syndrome coronavirus.

ROLE IN DISEASE

The clinical presentation of viral infections can be complex. For example, a primary respiratory pathogen could initially present with a diffuse rash and progress to later complications such as meningitis or encephalitis. The following is a summary of important presentations for many viral infections.

Viruses Responsible for Cutaneous Manifestations

Virus	Macules/Papules	Vesicles	Petechiae	Virus	Macules/Papules	Vesicles	Petechiae
DNA Viruses				**RNA Viruses**			
Herpes viruses				Flaviviridae			
• HSV		X		• Dengue virus	X		X
• VZV		X		• West Nile virus	X		
• CMV	X		X (congenital)	• Yellow fever virus	X		
• EBV	X		X	• Zika virus	X		
• HHV-6, HHV-7, HHV-8	X			Arenaviridae			
Poxviruses				• Lassa virus			
• Variola		X		• Lymphochoriomeningitis virus	X		
• Vaccinia		X		Hantaviridae			
• Monkeypox	X			• Hantaan virus			X
• Molluscum contagiosum virus	X			Filoviridae			
Other DNA viruses				• Ebola virus			X
• Adenovirus	X		X	• Marburg virus			X
• Human papillomavirus	X			Picornaviridae			
• Parvovirus B19	X			• Coxsackievirus	X	X	X
• HBV	X			• Echovirus	X	X	X
				Other RNA viruses			
				• HIV	X		
				• Rubella virus	X	X	X
				• Rubeola virus	X		

Viruses Responsible for Respiratory Infections

Virus	Rhinorrhea	Pharyngitis	Laryngitis	Croup	Bronchitis	Pneumonia
Rhinovirus	X	X	X		X	
Influenza virus	X	X	X	X	X	X
Paramyxoviruses						
• Parainfluenza virus	X	X	X	X	X	X
• RSV	X	X	X	X	X	X
• Human metapneumovirus	X	X	X		X	X
• Measles virus					X	X
Coronavirus	X	X	X		X	X
HIV		X				
Adenovirus	X	X	X	X	X	X

Viruses Responsible for Respiratory Infections—cont'd

Virus	Rhinorrhea	Pharyngitis	Laryngitis	Croup	Bronchitis	Pneumonia
Herpesviruses						
• HSV		X				X
• CMV		X				X
• EBV		X				

Viruses Responsible for Meningitis and Encephalitis

Virus	Meningitis	Encephalitis
Herpesviruses[a]	X	X (common)
Adenovirus	X	
Enteroviruses[b]	X (common)	X
Arboviruses[c]	X	X (common)
Paramyxoviruses		
• Parainfluenza virus	X	X
• Mumps virus	X	X (uncommon)
• Measles virus		X
Rubella virus		X
Arenaviruses		
• Lymphochorio-meningitis virus	X	X
• Lassa virus		X
Rabies virus		X
HIV	X	X

[a]Primarily HSV-2; other members include HSV-1, CMV, EBV, and VZV.
[b]Include echovirus, coxsackievirus, and (now rare) poliovirus.
[c]"Arboviruses" is a historic term still used commonly to refer to the many viruses transmitted by arthropods (primarily mosquitos); these include eastern equine encephalitis virus, western equine encephalitis virus, La Crosse virus, California encephalitis virus, Venezuelan equine encephalitis virus, St. Louis encephalitis virus, Murray Valley encephalitis virus, Japanese encephalitis virus, Hendra virus, Chikungunya virus, West Nile virus, and many others of restricted geographic regions.

Viruses Responsible for Pericarditis and Myocarditis

Virus	Pericarditis	Myocarditis
Herpesviruses	X	
Adenovirus	X	X
HBV	X	
Enteroviruses	X (common)	X
Influenza viruses	X	X
Mumps virus	X	X
Measles virus		X
Rubella virus		X
Lymphochoriomen-ingitis virus	X	
Arboviruses		X

Gastrointestinal symptoms can be a prominent presentation of many viral infections, but the gastrointestinal tract is the primary site of replication for the following viruses:

- Norovirus (most common)
- Rotavirus
- Sapovirus
- Adenovirus
- Astrovirus

It is well recognized that human immunodeficiency virus (HIV) is transmitted by sexual contact, but genital lesions are not observed. In contrast, three sexually transmitted viruses characteristically produce genital lesions:

- Herpes simplex virus types 1 and 2
- Human papillomavirus
- Molluscum contagiosum virus

Although a number of viruses produce hepatitis, five viruses are primary pathogens of the liver: hepatitis A, B, C, D, and E virus (HAV, HBV, HCV, HDV, and HEV). These will be discussed in a later chapter.

Infection of the eye, particularly keratitis, is observed with the adenovirus and the herpes simplex virus. Less commonly involved are other members of the herpes virus group and enteroviruses.

ANTIVIRAL AGENTS

In contrast to antibacterial agents, where relatively few new antibiotics have been introduced in recent years, there has been a proliferation of antivirals with more than 50 agents currently available. More than half of these are for the treatment of infections caused by three viruses: HIV and hepatitis B and C viruses. Many antivirals have also been developed to treat respiratory infections and herpesvirus group infections. The antivirals listed in this section are in current use, recognizing that other antivirals are in development and some will be introduced to the market within the next few years.

The spectrum of antiviral agents for the treatment of HIV infections is impressive, as well as bewildering. Any discussion here will most likely be rapidly outdated. Rather than a comprehensive summary, I will present the mode of action and some specific examples. The student should recognize that these antivirals are administered in carefully considered combinations.

Antiviral Agents for HIV Infections

Mode of Action	Antivirals
Nucleoside and nucleotide reverse transcriptase inhibitors	Zidovudine, didanosine, stavudine, lamivudine, abacavir, tenofovir, emtricitabine
Non-nucleoside reverse transcriptase inhibitors	Nevirapine, delavirdine, efavirenz, etravirine, rilpivirine
Protease inhibitors	Saquinavir, ritonavir, indinavir, nelfinavir, fosamprenavir
Viral entry inhibitors	Enfuvirtide, maraviroc
Integrase strand inhibitors	Raltegravir, dolutegravir

Antiviral Agents for Hepatitis Virus Infections

Antivirals	Mode of Action	Viral Targets
Adefovir	Analog of adenosine monophosphate; inhibitor of viral DNA polymerases and reverse transcriptase	HBV; also HIV, poxviruses, and herpesviruses
Entecavir	Deoxyguanosine analog; inhibits DNA polymerase and reverse transcriptase	HBV
Lamivudine	Analog of dideoxy-thiacytidine; inhibits DNA synthesis	HBV; also HIV
Tenofovir	Adenosine 5′-monophosphate analog; inhibits DNA polymerase and reverse transcriptase	HBV
Boceprevir	Inhibitor of NS3/NS4A protease	Hepatitis C virus
Telaprevir	Inhibitor of NS3/NS4A protease	Hepatitis C virus
Simeprevir	Inhibitor of NS3/NS4A protease	Hepatitis C virus
Sofosbuvir	Uridine nucleoside polymerase inhibitor	Hepatitis C virus

Antiviral Agents for Respiratory Infections

Antivirals	Mode of Action	Viral Targets
Amantadine, Rimantadine	Tricyclic amines; inhibit viral uncoating and assembly	Influenza A virus
Oseltamivir, Zanamivir, Peramivir	Sialic acid analog; inhibitor of neuraminidase and prevents viral release from infected cells	Influenza A and B viruses
Ribavirin	Guanosine analog; inhibits viral replication	RSV, as well as hepatitis C and E viruses
Remdesivir	Premature termination of RNA transcription	SARS-CoV-2
Ritonavir-nirmatrelvir	Inhibitor of essential viral proteases	SARS-CoV-2

Antiviral Agents for Herpesvirus Infections

Antivirals	Mode of Action	Viral Targets
Acyclovir Valacyclovir	Deoxyguanosine analog; inhibitors of viral DNA polymerase; inhibits DNA synthesis; valacyclovir converted to acyclovir	HSV-1, HSV-2, VZV
Penciclovir Famciclovir	Acyclic guanosine analog; inhibits DNA synthesis; famciclovir converted to penciclovir	HSV-1, HSV-2, VZV
Ganciclovir Valganciclovir	Deoxyguanosine analog; inhibits DNA synthesis; valganciclovir converted to ganciclovir	CMV
Foscarnet	Pyrophosphate analog; inhibits DNA polymerase and HIV reverse transcriptase	All herpesviruses, as well as HIV
Cidofovir	Deoxycytidine monophosphate analog; inhibits DNA synthesis	All herpesviruses, as well as papillomavirus, polyomaviruses, poxviruses, and some adenoviruses
Trifluridine	Pyrimidine nucleoside; inhibits DNA synthesis	Topical treatment of HSV keratitis

Human Immunodeficiency Viruses

Since the first infections by HIV were recognized in 1981, knowledge of the biology and pathology of these viruses has increased at an exponential rate. We have moved from fear of the unknown to the reality that scientific knowledge and countless hours of investigations have brought us to the conversion of an untreatable infection to chronic, manageable disease and to the belief that we will see preventive vaccines and therapeutic cures in the future. Despite this optimism, HIV and AIDS pose a daunting medical challenge. The World Health Organization estimates that in 2020, 37 million people were living with HIV, 1.5 million acquired their infection in 2020, and there were almost 700,000 AIDS-related deaths. Although these statistics show a significant improvement over the last decade, the morbidity and mortality associated with this virus are sobering. The highest incidences of the disease are in the poorest countries of the world in sub-Saharan Africa and in south, southeast, and eastern Asian countries. AIDS-related morbidity and mortality in these regions are further complicated by the high co-prevalence of malnutrition and infectious diseases such as hepatitis B and C, malaria, and tuberculosis. The reality is that a great deal of human suffering will occur before our dreams of conquering this disease are realized.

To provide a focus for this chapter, it is important to know the members of the Retroviridae family of viruses and an understanding of what will be discussed:

Retroviridae Family of Viruses

Virus	Disease
Lentivirus	
• Human immunodeficiency virus 1 (HIV-1)	Acquired immunodeficiency syndrome (AIDS)
• Human immunodeficiency virus 2 (HIV-2)	Acquired immunodeficiency syndrome (AIDS)
Delta retrovirus	
• Human T-cell lymphotropic virus 1 (HTLV-1)	Adult T-cell leukemia/lymphoma; tropical spastic paraparesis
• Human T-cell lymphotropic virus 2 (HTLV-2)	Atypical hairy cell leukemia

Additional delta retroviruses have been described but are not conclusively associated with human disease. HIV-2 causes a disease similar to HIV-1 but is geographically restricted to west Africa, progresses more slowly, and is less transmissible. The focus of this chapter will be restricted to HIV-1.

HUMAN IMMUNODEFICIENCY VIRUS 1 (HIV-1)

HIV-1 is subdivided into four groups (M, N, O, and P) based on the origin of the parent virus. Group M is responsible for the global spread of HIV-1, while the other groups have remained restricted to western Africa. Group M is subdivided further into nine subtypes with:

- Subtype B being predominant in western Europe, the Americas, and Australia
- Subtype C being predominant in Africa and India

The methods for transmission of HIV-1 are well known: genital contact with infectious body fluids such as semen, vaginal secretions, and blood; contact with contaminated blood or tissues; and infant exposure to an infected mother. Risk factors for transmission include unprotected sex, sexual exposure to multiple partners, sexual exposure to genital ulcers (e.g., due to syphilis or herpes simplex virus), men who have sex with men, intravenous drug abuse, and transfusion with unscreened blood products. The likelihood of transmission is directly related to the viral concentration in the infectious fluids or tissues, so the risk is highest when contact is with an individual with active, advanced disease.

Following exposure to HIV, the virus binds and penetrates CD4 T lymphocytes and other cells with the appropriate receptors. This is followed by rapid viral replication that induces inflammatory cytokines and chemokines. Viral replication is balanced by HIV-specific CD8 T-cell killing of the infected cells, thus depleting the CD4 T-cell population with resulting compromised T-cell immune response. Innate immunity mediated by natural killer cells is also important for containing the infection. Although viral exposure can progress to unrelenting immune suppression and associated complications, most infections are characterized by an extended period of latency where slow viral replication can occur; most infected cells remain dormant, only to reactivate months or years later.

The central role of the CD4 T cells is the initiation and regulation of innate and immune responses. Activated cells initiate immune responses by the release of cytokines required for the activation of epithelial cells, neutrophils,

macrophages, other T cells, B cells, and natural killer cells. Initially, this is manifested by increased susceptibility to infections with fungi (e.g., *Candida*, *Cryptococcus*, *Histoplasma*, *Pneumocystis*, and *Microsporidia*) and bacteria. Further depletion of immune responsiveness is associated with opportunistic infections with intracellular bacteria (e.g., mycobacteria and nocardia), parasites (e.g., *Toxoplasma*, *Cryptosporidium*, and *Cystoisospora*), and viruses (e.g., herpesvirus group and JC polyomavirus), as well as some viral related neoplasms (e.g., Epstein-Barr virus lymphoma and human herpesvirus 8 Kaposi sarcoma). These opportunistic infections and malignancies are the hallmark of AIDS and the primary contributor to AIDS-related mortality.

Laboratory diagnosis of HIV infections is complex with many different approaches in use. Rapid point-of-care immunoassays are widely used as screening tests for the assessment of patients with active infections. Generally, the tests are simple to use, test for antibody response to multiple viral antigens, and provide results within 30 min. The disadvantage of these tests is relatively poor sensitivity, particularly when used shortly following exposure to HIV. Laboratory-based immunoassays are also available, with significantly better analytic performance. The most recently designed tests detect both immunoglobulin M and immunoglobulin G antibodies to recombinant HIV antigens as well as expression of the HIV p24 antigen. Although these tests are an improvement over the point-of-care tests, they are unreliable for the detection of early infections. For this purpose, the detection of viral RNA by nucleic acid amplification tests is used to screen blood products or to assess the quantity of viral particles in the blood of an infected patient (for staging disease or monitoring response to therapy).

Therapy has made remarkable progress since the first antivirals were developed, providing a more manageable drug regimen, less toxicity, and better therapeutic outcomes. More than 25 drugs or combinations of drugs currently exist. Although treatment options are rapidly changing, current practice is the use of two nucleoside reverse transcriptase inhibitors with a non-nucleoside reverse transcriptase inhibitor, protease inhibitor, or integrase inhibitor. Prophylactic treatment of pregnant women and individuals exposed to contaminated blood (e.g., needlestick) is recommended. The use of vaginal microbicides to prevent male-to-female acquisition has not been demonstrated to be effective. Likewise, prophylactic use of antiviral for individuals engaged in high-risk activities is not recommended. An HIV vaccine is not currently available. The following is a summary of HIV:

HUMAN IMMUNODEFICIENCY VIRUS

Properties	• Enveloped RNA virus • Primary target for HIV is activated **CD4 T lymphocytes**; entry into the cell is via binding to the CD4 receptor and then binding to the CCR5 or CXCR4 coreceptor; other susceptible cells include resting CD4 T cells, monocytes, macrophages, and dendritic cells, as well as astrocytes (responsible for neurologic disorders) and renal epithelial cells (resulting neuropathy)
Epidemiology	• Worldwide distribution with the greatest prevalence in the poorest countries • Transmission via direct contact with contaminated fluids (e.g., blood, semen, vaginal fluid) and tissues • Recognition of HIV infection frequently occurs with the development of opportunistic bacterial, fungal, viral, or parasitic infections
Clinical Disease	• Acute disease develops 2–4 weeks after infections, presenting with flu-like symptoms or as infectious mononucleosis; aseptic meningitis may develop within the first 3 months; symptoms subside within 2–3 weeks although the virus continues to replicate with resultant CD4 cell death • When the CD4 T cells fall below 500 cells/µL and the viral concentration (viral load) is > 75,000 copies/mL, the onset of the more severe disease occurs with weight loss and diarrhea (HIV wasting syndrome) and opportunistic infections, malignancies, and dementia • Opportunistic infections include oral candidiasis (thrush), *Pneumocystis* pneumonia, *Cryptococcus* meningitis, cerebral toxoplasmosis, tuberculosis, diarrheal disease (caused by mycobacteria, *Salmonella*, *Shigella*, *Campylobacter*, *Cryptosporidia*, and other agents)
Diagnosis	• Initial screening of patients can be performed by point-of-care immunoassays or more sensitive laboratory-based immunoassays • Detection of viral RNA by nucleic acid amplification tests is the most sensitive method for screening blood products, assessment of the stage of infection, or monitoring response to antiviral therapy
Treatment, Control, and Prevention	• Antiviral treatment of HIV infections is rapidly evolving with the use of multiple agents to inhibit viral reverse transcriptase, protease, and integrase; refer to Infectious Diseases Society of America and World Health Organization treatment guidelines for current recommendations • Prevention of disease is by avoidance of high-risk activities • Prophylaxis with antiviral agents after the first trimester recommended for HIV-infected pregnant women; antiviral prophylaxis recommended for accidental exposure to HIV-contaminated blood • No HIV vaccine currently exists although clinical trials of candidate vaccine are underway

CLINICAL CASES

Lower Respiratory Tract Infections
• First Report of AIDS in Los Angeles

Central Nervous System Infections
• Cryptococcal Brain Abscess in HIV Patients
• Epstein-Barr Virus (EBV) Lymphoma in HIV Patients

Skin and Soft-Tissue Infections
• Kaposi's sarcoma in HIV patients
• *Mycobacterium* and *Pneumocystis* Lymphadenitis

Miscellaneous Infections
• Disseminated *Mycobacterium avium intracellulare* (MAI) infection in HIV patients

SUPPLEMENTAL READING

1. Kanters S, et al. Comparative efficacy and safety of first-line antiretroviral therapy for the treatment of HIV infection: a systematic review and network meta-analysis. *Lancet HIV.* 2016;3(11):e510–e520.
2. Hassan A, et al. Defining HIV-1 transmission clusters based on sequence data. *AIDS.* 2017;31(9):1211–1222.
3. Patel P, et al. Estimating per-act HIV transmission risk: a systematic review. *AIDS.* 2014;28(10):1509–1519.

Human Herpesviruses

The herpesvirus group is an important collection of eight human pathogens:

Eight Human Pathogens of Human Herpesviruses

| Virus | INFECTIONS IN: | |
	Immunocompetent Persons	Immunocompromised Persons
Herpes simplex virus, type 1 (HSV-1)	Gingivostomatitis*	Gingivostomatitis
	Keratoconjunctivitis	Keratoconjunctivitis
	Cutaneous herpes	Cutaneous herpes
	Genital herpes	Disseminated infection
Herpes simplex virus, type 2 (HSV-2)	Genital herpes*	Genital herpes
	Cutaneous herpes	Cutaneous herpes
	Gingivostomatitis	
	Encephalitis*	
	Neonatal herpes	Disseminated infection
Varicella-zoster virus (VZV)	Chickenpox (varicella)*	Disseminated infection
	Herpes zoster (shingles)*	
Cytomegalovirus (CMV)	Mononucleosis	Hepatitis
	Hepatitis	Retinitis
	Congenital disease*	Disseminated infection
Epstein-Barr virus (EBV)	Mononucleosis*	Lymphoproliferative syndromes*
	Hepatitis	Oral hairy leukoplakia
	Encephalitis	

Eight Human Pathogens of Human Herpesviruses—cont'd

Virus	INFECTIONS IN:	
	Immunocompetent Persons	Immunocompromised Persons
Human herpesvirus 6 (HHV-6)	Exanthem subitum* Childhood febrile seizures Encephalitis	Fever and rash Encephalitis Bone marrow suppression
HHV-7	Exanthem subitum Childhood febrile seizures Encephalitis	Encephalitis
HHV-8	Febrile exanthema	Kaposi sarcoma* Castleman disease Primary effusion lymphoma

* Virus is the most common cause.

The human herpesviruses (HHVs) are divided into three subfamilies:

- Alpha herpesviruses: herpes simplex virus 1 and 2 (HSV-1, HSV-2), VZV; latent infections established in neurons of sensory ganglia
- Beta herpesviruses: CMV, HHV-6, HHV-7; latent infections established in mononuclear cells
- Gamma herpesviruses: EBV, HHV-8; latent infections established in lymphoid cells

The ability to establish latent infections means that recurrent diseases can occur when natural immunity wanes, during times of immunosuppression, or under conditions such as stress or hormonal changes. Most infections with these viruses are asymptomatic or mild with the exception of VZV (chickenpox) and HHV-6 (fever and rash). In the following section, HSV-1, HSV-2, VZV, CMV, and EBV are discussed in detail.

HERPES SIMPLEX VIRUS, TYPES 1 AND 2

HSV-1 and HSV-2 are ubiquitous viruses transmitted person to person by contact with infectious secretions.

Herpes Simplex Virus, Types 1 and 2

Virus	Disease
HSV-1	Most common cause of viral orofacial lesions ("cold sores")
HSV-1	Most common cause of corneal blindness in the USA
HSV-1	Most common cause of acute viral encephalitis in the USA
HSV-2	Most common cause of painful genital ulcers

Infections include mucocutaneous lesions, involvement of the central nervous system, and disseminated infections, particularly in immunocompromised patients. The viruses establish lifelong latent infections with periodic asymptomatic and symptomatic episodes of virus production. These viruses are particularly important causes of some specific diseases.

The following is a summary of HSV-1 and HSV-2:

HERPES SIMPLEX VIRUS, TYPES 1 AND 2

Properties	
	• Enveloped DNA viruses
	• Infection initiated in abraded skin or mucosal surfaces; replication in epithelial cells precedes infection of sensory or autonomic nerve endings, followed by migration of the virus to nerve cell bodies in ganglia where latency is established
	• Reactivation of virus replication can be caused by a number of stimuli (e.g., heat, cold, stress) and can be characterized as either asymptomatic or symptomatic (i.e., presence of vesicular lesions) shedding of virus

HERPES SIMPLEX VIRUS, TYPES 1 AND 2—cont'd

Epidemiology	• Worldwide distribution; HSV-1 typically acquired earlier in life than HSV-2; HSV-2 generally acquired when sexual activity is initiated • Both viruses are inactivated rapidly in the environment so infection requires close contact • HSV-1 is the most common cause of orofacial lesions (**"cold sores"**) and acute **viral encephalitis** in the USA; HSV-2 is the most common cause of **genital ulcers**; both viruses overlap in sites of clinical disease
Clinical Disease	• **Orofacial infections** present most commonly as gingivostomatitis and pharyngitis; lesions may be present on the palate, gingiva, tongue, lip, and adjacent areas of the face; symptomatic reactivated disease typically with vesicular lesions at the edge of the lips (**herpes labialis**); recurrent lesions more frequent with HSV-1 • Primary **genital infections** characterized by up to 2 weeks of symptoms with painful ulcerative lesions and viral shedding; mucoid discharge and dysuria may be present; recurrent lesions more frequent with HSV-2 • **Eye infections**: HSV infection of the eye is the most frequent cause of **corneal blindness** in the USA • **Encephalitis**: HSV-1 infection is the most common cause of acute, viral encephalitis in the USA • **Disseminated disease**: complication of immunosuppression
Diagnosis	• HSV-1 and HSV-2 can be readily detected by culture of cutaneous lesions or corneal scrapings; nucleic acid amplification test (NAAT) of these specimens available for rapid diagnosis • NAAT is the test of choice for CNS or disseminated diseases • Serologic response to infections can be measured but does not distinguish between active primary infections and past or recurrent disease
Treatment, Control, and Prevention	• Acyclovir, valacyclovir, or famciclovir is used for mucocutaneous and disseminated infections; encephalitis is treated with acyclovir; topical acyclovir is used to treat herpes keratitis; foscarnet or cidofovir is used to treat acyclovir-resistant strains • Antivirals manage the symptoms of herpesvirus infection but do not eliminate carriage • Prevention of disease is difficult because infected patients may be shedding the virus asymptomatically; condom use is partially protective • No vaccine is currently available

VARICELLA-ZOSTER VIRUS

VZV is responsible for two distinct diseases: the primary infection is **varicella** or **chickenpox** and the recurrent infection is **zoster** or **shingles**. Chickenpox is characterized by a generalized maculopapular or vesicular rash and is generally a benign disease except in immunocompromised patients. Zoster is a disease where a painful vesicular rash develops along the nerve track where the virus reactivates. This can also present as a disseminated disease in an immunocompromised patient.

VARICELLA-ZOSTER VIRUS

Properties	• Enveloped DNA virus • Initial replication in the upper respiratory tract, followed by lymphatic spread to the reticuloendothelial system, viremia, and widespread infection of epithelial cells in the epidermis • Epithelial cells degenerate with viral replication, forming fluid-filled vesicles
Epidemiology	• Worldwide distribution with humans only host • Person-to-person spread primarily by the respiratory route; the virus is not stable in the environment, so close contact is required for transmission • Chickenpox is primarily a disease of school-aged children, except in populations where vaccination of children is widely used

VARICELLA-ZOSTER VIRUS—cont'd

Clinical Disease	• **Chickenpox**: rash, low-grade fever, and malaise develops following a 2-week incubation period; the rash develops over a 3- to 5-day period and is characterized as maculopapular and vesicular lesions with an erythematous base in different stages of development; the lesions resolve over a 1- to 2-week period; disease is generally benign and self-limited, although a more prolonged and severe rash occurs in immunocompromised patients and complications (**acute cerebellar ataxia, encephalitis**, or **pneumonia**) may occur and are associated with significant morbidity and mortality • **Zoster**: characterized by the development of vesicular lesion along a dermatome, with thoracic and lumbar dermatomes most commonly involved; if the fifth cranial nerve is involved, **herpes zoster ophthalmicus** can develop and threaten vision; onset of disease is identified by pain along the dermatome followed by the development of the lesion over a 3- to 5-day period; relief may take as long as 1 month; infections in immunocompromised patients (particularly HIV patients) may involve more chronic development of lesions
Diagnosis	• Clinical diagnosis is confirmed by culture (infrequently done), microscopy (specific stain is the Tzanck smear), detection of infected cells in lesions by immunofluorescent microscopy, or NAAT (test of choice because it is rapid, sensitive, and specific)
Treatment, Control, and Prevention	• Treatment is symptomatic and with the antiviral **acyclovir**; valacyclovir and famciclovir can also be used to treat zoster • Varicella-zoster immune globulin can be used as a prophylaxis in high-risk patients • Two doses of a live, attenuated **vaccine** are recommended for children for the prevention of vaccinia, and a high-titer attenuated vaccine is recommended for adults over the age of 50 to prevent zoster; inactivated vaccines are under evaluation for immunocompromised patients

CYTOMEGALOVIRUS

CMV is a ubiquitous virus that causes a wide spectrum of clinical diseases. The following are some of the most noteworthy.

Following the initial infection with CMV, which can frequently be asymptomatic or present with mild non-specific symptoms, latency is established in a variety of cells including polymorphonuclear cells, T lymphocytes, endothelial cells, renal epithelial cells, and the salivary glands. It is not surprising that this virus is a significant cause of complications following immunosuppression for transplantation or by disease.

Cytomegalovirus

Population	Disease
Unborn child	Congenital CMV syndrome
Healthy teenager	Infectious mononucleosis syndrome
Solid organ transplant patient	Disseminated infection with associated organ rejection
Bone marrow transplant patient	CMV pneumonia
HIV AIDS patient	CMV retinitis

CYTOMEGALOVIRUS

Properties	• Enveloped DNA virus; genetic variability similar to that seen with RNA viruses • Largest herpesvirus (genome 236 kb, encodes 164 proteins) compared with VZV (125 kb), HSV-1 and HSV-2 (155 kb), and EBV (172 kb)
Epidemiology	• Worldwide distribution • Asymptomatic primary infections are common in healthy individuals • Twenty percent of cases of infectious mononucleosis are caused by CMV

CYTOMEGALOVIRUS—cont'd

Clinical Disease	• **Infectious mononucleosis**: characterized with fever, lymphadenopathy, and lymphocytosis (lymphocytes >50% of peripheral white blood cells); pharyngitis less common than with EBV infections; symptoms persist for 1 month or longer; **Guillain-Barré syndrome** (progressive inflammatory polyneuropathy with muscle weakness and distal sensory loss) is a well-recognized complication of CMV mononucleosis • **Congenital CMV**: generally asymptomatic if the mother is immune; fulminant disease for the child of a nonimmune mother with multiorgan involvement including CNS with microcephaly, chorioretinitis, and cerebral calcification; death *in utero* or soon after birth; surviving infants with significant defects including mental retardation, retinitis, and hearing disorders • **CMV pneumonia**: interstitial pneumonia following infectious mononucleosis is typically mild and self-limited; in contrast, in bone marrow transplant patients, this is rapidly progressive and associated with high mortality despite aggressive treatment • **CMV retinitis**: CMV is a common opportunistic infection in patients with advanced HIV infections, and retinitis is the most common manifestation
Diagnosis	• Culture of CMV in epithelial cells can be done, but replication is slow and not practical for diagnostic purposes • Detection of CMV protein pp65 (protein in the outer layer beneath the envelope) by immunofluorescent staining of neutrophils in peripheral blood was widely used but has more recently been replaced by NAAT • Quantitative assessment of blood-borne CMV is useful for monitoring transplant patients (rising titers are an early indicator of disease)
Treatment, Control, and Prevention	• Antivirals used for treating CMV infections include ganciclovir, foscarnet (used to treat ganciclovir-resistant CMV), and cidofovir (not associated with ganciclovir or foscarnet resistance) • Ganciclovir and valganciclovir are used for CMV prophylaxis for high-risk immunocompromised patients • No vaccine is currently available

EPSTEIN-BARR VIRUS

EBV is the most common cause of infectious mononucleosis and is associated with a number of malignant diseases.

EPSTEIN-BARR VIRUS

Properties	• Enveloped DNA virus • Initial replication of the virus in oral epithelial cells with subsequent spread to B lymphocytes; replication of viral DNA (but not intact virus particles) is synchronized with host cell DNA replication, and limited gene products are produced in the infected cell (markers for identifying these cells)
Epidemiology	• Worldwide distribution with most infections occurring early in life • Asymptomatic infections occur most commonly in the very young • Person-to-person transmission through oral secretions (kissing, sharing utensils); close contact required for transmission • Virus can be cultured from the oral secretions of 10%–20% of healthy adults and a higher proportion of immunocompromised patients

EPSTEIN-BARR VIRUS—cont'd

Clinical Disease	• **Infectious mononucleosis**: acute infections characterized by pharyngitis, fever, fatigue, lymph-adenopathy, and leukocytosis, with monocytes and atypical lymphocytes observed in peripheral blood; symptoms typically resolve within 1 month • **Burkitt lymphoma**: undifferentiated B-cell lymphoma of the jaw that is observed in Central Africa • **Lymphoproliferative disease**: uncontrolled proliferation of infected B lymphocytes observed in immunocompromised patients (solid organ and bone marrow transplants) • **Nasopharyngeal carcinoma**: proliferation of EBV-infected epithelial cells in nasopharynx; disease in South Chinese and Alaskan Inuit Eskimo populations • **Central nervous system lymphoma**: EBV lymphoma in the brains of HIV AIDS patients and stem cell transplant patients
Diagnosis	• Diagnosis of infectious mononucleosis is based on clinical presentation and the presence of **heterophile antibodies** (positive reaction: ability to agglutinate sheep erythrocytes as absorption of serum with guinea pig kidney cells) • Diagnosis of infections is also performed by measuring the antibody response to structural proteins (viral capsid antigens), nonstructural proteins expressed early in the lytic cycle (early antigens), and nuclear proteins expressed in latently infected cells (EBV nuclear antigens) • Diagnosis now commonly performed with NAAT
Treatment, Control, and Prevention	• Treatment of infectious mononucleosis is supportive • Acyclovir and ganciclovir are active against replicating EBV; however, most disease manifestations are the result of the immune response to EBV-infected cells, so antiviral agents will be ineffective • No vaccine is currently available

HUMAN HERPESVIRUSES 6, 7, AND 8

HHV-6 is responsible for infantile fevers (frequently associated with **febrile seizures**) and a common pediatric disease, **exanthema subitum** or **roseola infantum** (also called the sixth disease). This is a disease that presents with a high fever after a 1-week incubation period, persisting for 3 to 4 days. At the time of defervescence, a maculopapular rash will develop and spread from the trunk to the extremities. This will last for up to 2 days. HHV-7 is also associated with infantile fevers and exanthema subitum, although less commonly than HHV-6. HHV-8 is responsible for **Kaposi sarcoma**, typically manifested as cutaneous plaques or nodules in immunocompromised patients (e.g., highly advanced HIV disease).

CLINICAL CASES (REFER TO SECTION VI)

Upper Respiratory Tract Infections
• HSV-1 Gingivostomatitis

Lower Respiratory Tract Infections
• CMV pneumonia post-bone marrow transplant

Genitourinary Tract Infections
• Genital HSV infection in patients with diabetes mellitus

Central Nervous System Infections
• Aseptic meningitis complicating acute HSV-2 proctitis
• Congenital Cytomegalovirus infection
• Epstein-Barr Virus (EBV) lymphoma in HIV patients

Skin and Soft-Tissue Infections
• Neonatal HSV infection
• Concurrent presentation of Varicella and Zoster
• Human Herpesvirus 6 (HHV-6) Exanthem Subitum
• Kaposi's sarcoma in HIV patients

Miscellaneous Infections
• EBV infectious mononucleosis associated with agranulocytosis

SUPPLEMENTAL READING

1. Whitley RJ, Roizman B. Herpes simplex virus infections. *Lancet.* 2001;357:1513–1518.
2. Arvin AM. Varicella-zoster virus. *Clin Microbiol Rev.* 1996;9:361–381.
3. Freer G, Pistello M. Varicella-zoster virus infection: natural history, clinical manifestations, immunity and current and future vaccination strategies. *New Microbiol.* 2018;41:95–105.
4. Nowalk A, Green M. Epstein-Barr virus. *Microbiol Spectr.* 2016. https://doi.org/10.1128/microbiolspec.DMIH2-0011-2015.
5. Caserta MT, Hall CB. Human herpesvirus 6. *Annu Rev Med.* 1993;44:377–383.
6. Lebbe C, Frances C. Human herpesvirus 8. *Cancer Treat Res.* 2009;146:169–188.

Respiratory Viruses

Several viruses produce upper and/or lower respiratory tract infections, ranging from the "common cold" to life-threatening overwhelming pneumonia. The significance of these viruses has been reinforced by the global medical and economic impact of the current SARS-CoV-2 pandemic and is rivaled by the influenza virus pandemic 100 years ago. This chapter focuses on six RNA virus groups to illustrate the range of respiratory infections produced by viruses. Many infections caused by these viruses occur during the cold months of the year and frequently produce symptoms indistinguishable from each other. This is generally not a problem because neither antiviral treatment nor vaccines are available for most of these pathogens. There are two notable exceptions. Seasonal vaccines are available to prevent or attenuate influenza virus infections, and effective antiviral treatments have been developed. Additionally, vaccines were introduced within one year after the start of the SARS-CoV-2 pandemic and, to date, have proven effective in limiting the spread and severity of COVID-19.

Historically, most viral respiratory infections were documented by viral cultures or serology (measuring the patient's immune response to specific viruses). Neither procedure was widely used for routine diagnostics. However, this has changed in recent years with the commercial introduction of highly multiplex nucleic acid amplification tests (NAATs) where 20 or more respiratory pathogens can be tested simultaneously. This has rapidly expanded our diagnostic skills and appreciation for the prevalence of these pathogens.

RHINOVIRUSES

Although most rhinovirus infections are not severe and complications are rare, the prevalence of infections and duration of symptoms result in prolonged periods of feeling miserable (and coughing and sneezing are not welcomed by anyone). The following is a summary of key facts about rhinoviruses.

RHINOVIRUSES

Properties	• Nonenveloped RNA viruses; more than 100 serotypes described
	• Symptoms caused by infection of respiratory ciliated epithelial cells, stimulates cellular inflammatory response with the expression of cytokines and chemokines
Epidemiology	• Worldwide distribution, with infections in both children and adults
	• Infections occur throughout the year but typically peak in the fall and spring, with decreased activity during the winter and summer months
	• Transmission most common with large droplets (cough, sneeze) where hands are contaminated and then transferred to the nose or eyes
	• Transmission most efficient when symptoms are most severe (high virus concentration in respiratory secretions)
	• Multiple serotypes and short-lived immunity make recurrent disease inevitable
Clinical Disease	• Primarily an upper respiratory tract infection
	• Initiated with sore, "scratchy" throat followed closely by rhinorrhea and nasal obstruction; cough, sneezing, headache, and low-grade fever (particularly in children) also develop
	• Symptoms can persist for 1 week or more
Diagnosis	• Definitive diagnosis cannot be made based on clinical parameters
	• Virus can be grown in culture, but this is rarely performed
	• Antigen tests have been replaced in recent years by nucleic acid amplification tests (NAATs)
Treatment, Control, and Prevention	• No specific antiviral therapy is available
	• Vaccines are not available

CORONAVIRUSES

Human coronaviruses primarily cause respiratory infections. Four strains of coronaviruses are responsible for "cold-like" symptoms: 229E, NL63, OC43, and HKU1. I see no intrinsic value in remembering these names. What is important is to recognize that coronaviruses are common, circulate through populations annually during the cold months, and are easily spread by contact with infectious respiratory secretions present in the air or on environmental surfaces. The three highly pathogenic coronaviruses (SARS-CoV-1, MERS-CoV, and SARS-CoV-2) share many of these same attributes. In 2002 a new coronavirus strain emerged in China that rapidly spread in the region and then to Hong Kong, Vietnam, and Singapore. Focal outbreaks were also reported in other countries by travelers from the endemic region who became ill when they returned home. The virus was named **SARS-CoV** (Severe Acute Respiratory Syndrome—Coronavirus). Two facts about this virus are critical: person-to-person spread occurred readily, including among the healthcare workers exposed to the patients, and the disease was responsible for a high overall mortality rate (10%), particularly for patients with underlying pulmonary disease and in the elderly. The outbreak ended 18 months later, but in 2012, a new coronavirus infection erupted in the Middle East, again associated with a high mortality rate (35%). This strain, **MERS-CoV**, has spread from the initial focus in the Kingdom of Saudi Arabia through the Middle East and to other countries via travelers. In contrast with the SARS-CoV-1 strain, this coronavirus is only intermittently spread person to person; however, the strain continues to circulate in the Middle East primarily because individuals in the region frequently come into contact with camels, the reservoir host for this virus. Unfortunately, we must view our experiences with SARS-CoV-1 and MERS-CoV as a prelude to what we are confronted with today. In December 2019, the first reports of new coronavirus infections in Wuhan, China, were published. The virus spread globally very rapidly, with little success in controlling the infections. This was different from the experience with SARS-CoV-1 and MERS-CoV but maybe more similar to the common cold coronaviruses. This new coronavirus, SARS-CoV-2, caused more serious infections with a high incidence of morbidity and mortality particularly in the elderly or those with underlying medical conditions. Finally, like many RNA viruses, we now see mutant variants of the virus that are even more highly contagious and able to at least partially evade immunity developed to the original virus strain (by either natural infection or vaccination). At the time of this writing, SARS-CoV-2 has infected more than 620 million people, is responsible for almost seven million deaths, continues to spread globally, and will likely be with us for many years to come. It should be noted that global efforts to develop diagnostics and vaccines literally within months of the onset of infections are unparalleled in the history of infectious diseases. Despite these efforts, infections continue at an unprecedented rate. It is interesting that the three highly virulent coronaviruses are related to bat coronavirus strains. It is also a bit frightening that similar coronaviruses are circulating in the bat population, so it is likely that other virulent strains may be introduced in the human population in the future.

CORONAVIRUSES	
Properties	• Enveloped RNA virus • Replicate in ciliated and nonciliated epithelial cells of the nasopharynx • Stimulates production of cytokines and chemokines resulting in cold symptoms; hyperproduction of this inflammatory response is responsible for the pathology with SARS-CoV-1, MERS-CoV, and SARS-CoV-2
Epidemiology	• Responsible for about 15% of common colds; infections in pediatric and adult patients primarily in winter and spring • Common cold coronaviruses with worldwide distribution; SARS-CoV-1 and MERS-CoV with more restricted geographic distribution (the former initially in China, the latter in the Kingdom of Saudi Arabia); SARS-CoV-1 with global spread
Clinical Disease	• Infections with the common cold coronaviruses have a 2-day incubation period, with peak symptoms 3 to 4 days after exposure: symptoms similar to rhinovirus infections (sore throat, rhinorrhea, cough, headache) • SARS-CoV-1 and SARS-CoV-2 not typically associated with cold-like symptoms; typically present with fever, headache, myalgia, and followed by a nonproductive cough; progression to severe pulmonary disease most likely in older adults and patients with underlying disease (e.g., diabetes, cardiac disease, hepatitis, chronic pulmonary disease) • MERS-CoV infections may be restricted to mild upper respiratory tract symptoms, but more likely progresses to respiratory and multiorgan failure
Diagnosis	• Although the viruses can be grown with some difficulty in culture, this is rarely done except in public health laboratories • Diagnosis most commonly by NAATs or in the case of SARS-CoV-2 by point-of-care rapid immunoassays
Treatment, Control, and Prevention	• Remdesivir and ritonavir-nirmatrelvir used to treat SARS-CoV-2 infections • Vaccines are only available for SARS-CoV-2 • Rigorous infection control practices used to control infections with SARS-CoV-1 and MERS-CoV; the use of masks, social distancing, hand hygiene, and vaccines have been demonstrated to reduce the spread of SARS-CoV-2, but the effectiveness is limited by irregular adoption of these practices and the evolution of more infectious variant viruses

INFLUENZA VIRUSES

These are the oldest recognized respiratory viruses producing epidemic disease every few years. The structural properties of these viruses are important to understand. The genetic information is encoded in single-stranded RNA. Single-stranded nucleic acids (as with the other respiratory viruses discussed in this chapter) are more susceptible to mutations during replication, so gene products such as the surface proteins (in the case of influenza these would be hemagglutinin [H] and neuraminidase [N]) can be altered. This can create a previously unrecognized virus (new virus: little or no immunity). The influenza viruses have the RNA arranged in discrete segments, so if a cell is infected with two different influenza viruses, rearrangement can occur creating a unique third virus.

This is the reason novel viruses can be created every few years and produce epidemics. A worldwide pandemic can occur if the virus is both unique and highly infectious, and if the strain is highly virulent, a pandemic associated with high mortality can occur. There are three distinct influenza groups: A, B, and C. Influenza A and B viruses are responsible for epidemic disease, with influenza A causing more severe disease; and influenza C virus causes milder upper respiratory infections. The circulating strain of the influenza virus is identified by its type and surface proteins, such as A (H3N2). Influenza A strains circulate in bird populations ("avian flu"), so the opportunity for a new strain to emerge is great. Sometimes these strains will also circulate in pig populations ("swine flu") further increasing their genetic uniqueness and virulence. The following is a summary of these viruses.

INFLUENZA VIRUSES	
Properties	• Enveloped RNA viruses with genome divided into eight segments • Three types of influenza viruses: A, B, and C; A and B associated with epidemics; A is the most virulent • Strains identified by their surface proteins: hemagglutinin (H), neuraminidase (N) • Virus infects ciliated columnar epithelial cells of the trachea and bronchials
Epidemiology	• Worldwide distribution with infections primarily in the cold months • Person-to-person spread either by the airborne route (sneezing, coughing) or by contact with infectious particles on contaminated surfaces (hand to nose) • Severity of disease determined by the virulence of the virus strain and immunity to the circulating strain
Clinical Disease	• After a 1- to 2-day incubation period, onset is acute with fever, chills, myalgias, and headache, as well as cough, chest pain, and nasal discharge; symptoms may last 1 week or longer • Complications include primary viral pneumonia or secondary bacterial pneumonia (most commonly with *Staphylococcus aureus* and *Streptococcus pneumoniae*)
Diagnosis	• Viral culture has generally been replaced with immunoassays or NAATs • Specific diagnosis is important for guiding antiviral therapy
Treatment, Control, and Prevention	• Treatment and prophylaxis of influenza A and B infections with neuraminidase inhibitors zanamivir, oseltamivir, or peramivir; must be initiated early in infection • Previously, influenza A but not B was treated with amantadine or rimantadine, but resistance is now widespread • Multiplex vaccines widely used to control disease; however, if the circulating strain is not included in the vaccine, it will be ineffective • Vaccine effectiveness is limited, with many recipients infected but protected against severe disease

PARAMYXOVIRIDAE

Paramyxoviridae is an important family of respiratory pathogens in both children and adults. Three members are discussed below: parainfluenza virus, respiratory syncytial virus (RSV), and human metapneumovirus (HMV). Two other members of this family, measles virus and mumps virus, can also present with respiratory symptoms.

PARAINFLUENZA VIRUSES (PIV)

Parainfluenza viruses are the most important cause of **croup** in children and a significant cause of severe lower respiratory tract viral disease in immunocompromised patients.

PARAINFLUENZA VIRUSES

Properties	• Enveloped RNA virus with four major human serotypes: parainfluenza virus-1 (PIV-1), PIV-2, PIV-3, and PIV-4 • Preferentially infect ciliated epithelial cells of the upper and lower respiratory tract
Epidemiology	• Worldwide distribution with infections in both children and adults • Person-to-person spread by exposure to respiratory droplets or contact with contaminated surfaces • PIV-1 and PIV-2 cause seasonal outbreaks in the fall; PIV-3 and PIV-4 cause outbreaks in spring
Clinical Disease	• Most pediatric infections are limited to upper respiratory tract with cold symptoms developing about 1 day after exposure to the virus and persisting for a week or more; involvement of the sinuses and middle ear occurs in up to half of the children infected • PIV-1 and PIV-2 associated with laryngotracheobronchitis (**croup**) with the initial development of fever, rhinorrhea, and pharyngitis, and then progressing to barking cough associated with stridor and difficulty in breathing; the PIV-1 disease is generally more severe than the PIV-2 disease • PIV-3 disease is more commonly associated with pneumonia and bronchiolitis in children, and PIV-4 primarily causes mild upper respiratory infections • PIV infections in adults are generally asymptomatic or mild upper respiratory infections, except in immunocompromised patients where severe lower respiratory tract disease can develop and is associated with high mortality
Diagnosis	• Although PIV can be grown in culture, most clinical diagnoses are by NAATs
Treatment, Control, and Prevention	• No specific antiviral treatment • Croup is managed symptomatically with glucocorticoids and nebulized epinephrine • Vaccine is not available

RESPIRATORY SYNCYTIAL VIRUS (RSV)

RSV infections are most severe in infants and young children and responsible for the majority of bronchial infections (**bronchiolitis**), as many as half of the hospitalizations due to **pneumonia**, and the majority of middle ear infections (**otitis media**). Mild disease is widespread in adults, but severe complications can occur in high-risk patients, particularly those with underlying pulmonary disease.

RESPIRATORY SYNCYTIAL VIRUS

Properties	• Enveloped RNA virus; two major antigenic groups (A and B) with multiple subgroups; both groups can circulate in the population simultaneously • RSV infects the ciliated columnar epithelial cells of the lower airways as well as pneumocytes in the lungs
Epidemiology	• Worldwide distribution with infections in both children and adults • Person-to-person spread by exposure to respiratory droplets or contact with contaminated surfaces • Infections occur annually from late fall through early spring; may extend throughout the year in warmer climates • Initial infections in early years of life, followed by milder recurrent infections throughout life

Continued

RESPIRATORY SYNCYTIAL VIRUS—cont'd	
Clinical Disease	• Infection in infants primarily involves the lower respiratory tract, presenting after a 2- to 5-day incubation period as bronchiolitis; pneumonia can develop but croup occurs less commonly • RSV infections in children and adults present initially as an upper respiratory tract infection with nasal congestion and cough • Otitis media is associated with pediatric disease, and co-infections with bacterial pathogens are responsible for more severe otitis • Adult disease is primarily mild, although severe lower respiratory disease is well recognized in the elderly, immunocompromised adults, and those with underlying cardiopulmonary disease (chronic obstructive pulmonary disease, congestive heart failure)
Diagnosis	• Although RSV can be grown in culture, most clinical diagnoses are by NAATs • Virus shedding in adult patients, even with severe disease, is quantitatively lower than in infants, which makes diagnosis more challenging
Treatment, Control, and Prevention	• Mild infections are treated symptomatically • Bronchiolitis is generally managed with bronchodilators and corticosteroids • Ribavirin is approved for the treatment of hospitalized infants with lower respiratory tract disease, although benefits have not been consistently demonstrated for this population or for older children or adults with RSV infections • Vaccine is not available

HUMAN METAPNEUMOVIRUS (HMV)

HMV was recently discovered, although serologic evidence demonstrates this virus was widely disseminated in the population and is an important human pathogen.

HUMAN METAPNEUMOVIRUS	
Properties	• Enveloped RNA virus closely related to RSV • Two genotypes with multiple subgroups; genetic diversity observed with two surface glycoproteins, resulting in a number of novel circulating strains of virus • Immunity to HMV is incomplete and reinfections occur throughout life • Infection of bronchial epithelial cells results in a prolonged inflammatory response
Epidemiology	• Worldwide distribution with infections most common in winter and spring in temperate climates, as with RSV and influenza virus • Primary infections by 5 years of age • Severity of HMV infections related to co-infections with RSV or *S. pneumoniae*
Clinical Disease	• Diseases range from mild upper respiratory infections to bronchitis and severe pneumonia • Infections in children characterized by fever, cough, wheezing, and rhinorrhea; conjunctivitis, pharyngitis, laryngitis, and otitis may occur; involvement of the bronchial airways and lungs may develop • Adult disease is similar to that in children, with lower respiratory complications more common in patients with underlying respiratory disease or immunosuppression
Diagnosis	• Although HMV can be grown in culture, most clinical diagnoses are by NAATs
Treatment, Control, and Prevention	• No specific antiviral treatment • Vaccine is not available

ADENOVIRUS

Although most respiratory infections are caused by RNA viruses, the nonenveloped DNA virus, adenovirus, has been associated with respiratory infections in children, including cold-like symptoms, an exudative pharyngitis indistinguishable from group A streptococcal infection, a pertussis-like syndrome, and pneumonia. Outbreaks of upper respiratory tract disease progressing to more severe lower respiratory tract involvement have been reported in military recruits.

CLINICAL CASES (REFER TO SECTION VI)

Lower Respiratory Tract Infections

- Previously healthy patients with SARS-CoV-1 infection
- MERS-CoV infection in visitors to Saudi Arabia
- Reinfection in a patient with SARS-CoV-2
- H5N1 avian influenza infection
- Outbreak of parainfluenza virus (PIV) in neonatal intensive care unit
- Respiratory syncytial virus (RSV) infection in elderly immunocompetent patients
- Adenovirus 14 pneumonia in military recruits

SUPPLEMENTAL READING

1. Moriyama M, et al. Seasonality of respiratory viral infections. *Annu Rev Virol.* 2020;7(1):83–101.
2. Chafekar A, Fielding B. MERS-CoV: understanding the latest human coronavirus threat. *Viruses.* 2018;10(2):93. https://doi.org/10.3390/v10020093.
3. Liu YC, et al. COVID-19: the first documented coronavirus pandemic in history. *Biomed J.* 2020;43(4):328–333.
4. Rabaan AA, et al. SARS-CoV-2, SARS-CoV, and MERS-CoV: a comparative overview. *Infez Med.* 2020;28(2):174–184.
5. Labella AM, Merel SE. Influenza. *Med Clin North Am.* 2013;97(4):621–645.
6. Griffiths C, et al. Respiratory syncytial virus: infection, detection, and new options for prevention and treatment. *Clin Microbiol Rev.* 2017;30(1):277–319.
7. Radke JR, Cook JL. Human adenovirus infections: update and consideration of mechanisms of viral persistence. *Curr Opin Infect Dis.* 2018;31(3):252–256.
8. Huang HS, et al. Multiplex PCR system for the rapid diagnosis of respiratory virus infection: systematic review and meta-analysis. *Clin Microbiol Infect.* 2018;24(10):1055–1063.

Hepatitis Viruses

A number of viruses can infect the liver (e.g., herpesvirus group, adenoviruses, paramyxovirus group, and enteroviruses), but five viruses are responsible for primary infections:

Virus	Genus	Nucleic Acid	Exposure
Hepatitis A virus (HAV)	Hepatovirus (*hepa*, liver)	RNA	Fecal-oral
Hepatitis B virus (HBV)	Orthohepadnavirus (*hepa* DNA virus)	DNA	Sexual, blood
Hepatitis C virus (HCV)	Hepacivirus (*hepa* C virus)	RNA	Blood
Hepatitis D virus (HDV)	Delta virus (*delta*, D virus)	RNA	Sexual, blood
Hepatitis E virus (HEV)	Hepevirus (*hep* E virus)	RNA	Fecal-oral

The viruses can present with acute symptoms of hepatitis ranging from mild disease to fulminant, rapidly fatal disease. Additionally, HBV, HCV, and hepatitis D virus (HDV) are the most common causes of chronic hepatitis

worldwide, increasing the risk of cirrhosis and hepatocellular carcinoma. The enteric hepatitis viruses (HAV and hepatitis E virus [HEV]) are not associated with chronic disease, with the exception of HEV infections in immunosuppressed patients. The clinical presentation of acute disease can be indistinguishable for the hepatitis viruses, with the majority of infections resulting in asymptomatic or mild disease. Progression to fulminant disease is primarily observed with HBV and HCV, with HAV progressing less often. Chronic infections are most troublesome because the infected patients serve as a reservoir for viral transmission and this population is at risk of long-term hepatic complications. The following is a summary of the five hepatitis viruses:

	HAV	HBV	HCV	HDV	HEV
Acute disease	+	+	+	+	+[a]
Fulminant disease	–	+	+	–	–
Chronic disease	–	+	+[a]	+	–
Antiviral treatment available	–	+	+	–	+
Vaccine available	+	+	–	–	+[b]

[a]Most common cause.
[b]Currently only licensed for China.

The following are summaries of each pathogen.

HEPATITIS A VIRUS

HAV is a member of the Picornavirus family (*pico*, small RNA virus) and related to rhinovirus (cause of common cold), echovirus and coxsackievirus (causes of viral meningitis), and poliovirus (cause of paralytic disease). HAV causes acute, self-limited infections and is not responsible for chronic liver disease.

HEPATITIS A VIRUS	
Properties	• Nonenveloped RNA virus; three genotypes are responsible for human infections • In the absence of an envelope, these viruses are resistant to heat, organic solvents, and detergents; they are inactivated by bleach and quaternary ammonium compounds • Infects hepatocytes; pathology believed to be related to cellular immune response, while humoral immunity limits cell-to-cell spread
Epidemiology	• Worldwide distribution, although vaccine programs have reduced the risk of transmission • Fecal-oral transmission; the highest concentration of virus in stools during the 2 weeks before jaundice develops; although stool concentrations decrease after jaundice develops, viruses are in stool specimens for as long as 6 months (particularly in infants) • Virus can remain stable and infectious in the environment for prolonged periods
Clinical Disease	• Asymptomatic disease more common in young children than in older children and adults • Onset of symptomatic disease with dark urine (bilirubinuria) with development of pale stools and jaundice a few days later; hepatomegaly and elevated liver enzymes; about half of the patients will experience itching due to cholestasis; resolution of symptoms typically within 1 month
Diagnosis	• Majority of patients have elevated anti-HAV immunoglobulin M antibodies at the time symptoms develop • Immunoassay for HAV antigens or nucleic acid amplification test (NAATs) also useful
Treatment, Control, and Prevention	• No specific antiviral treatment • Inactivated **HAV vaccines** have effectively controlled this infection; should be administered to children at 1 year of age • Immunoglobulins were administered following exposure but now have been replaced with the HAV vaccine • Transmission is difficult to control because peak shedding of virus is before symptoms develop, and shedding can occur for months after symptoms disappear

HEPATITIS B AND D VIRUSES

HBV is the only DNA virus that primarily infects hepatic cells. Hepatitis D virus (delta virus or HDV) is a defective RNA virus that requires the envelope of HBV for viral assembly. Infections with HBV range from asymptomatic to icteric, including both fulminant acute disease and chronic progressive disease.

HEPATITIS B AND D VIRUSES	
Properties	• Replication of HBV is distinguished by the production of large quantities of defective particles without viral DNA but with viral surface antigen (HBsAg) expressed on the surface; this antigen is highly immunogenic • Two other viral antigens of importance: core antigen (HBcAg) that forms the protein shell around the viral DNA, and soluble "e" antigen (HBeAg) that is secreted from infected cells; antibody response to the antigens are important markers for infection • HDV expresses a protein antigen (HDAg) that is an important marker for infection • Pathology in acute and chronic disease related to host cellular and humoral immune response to infection

Continued

HEPATITIS B AND D VIRUSES—cont'd

Epidemiology	• Worldwide distribution; vaccination programs have modified prevalence • HDV found only in patients with HBV infections • Transmission by contact with blood (very high concentrations of virus) or sexual contact; virus not found in urine or stool • The highest incidence of chronic disease in Africa, the Middle East, Southeast Asia, China, northern Canada, and Greenland • Populations at risk include intravenous drug abusers, male homosexuals, and HIV-infected individuals • Risk of chronic disease greatest with infants
Clinical Disease	• Incubation period of 1 to 4 months before symptoms develop • Acute disease may be subclinical or initiated with flulike symptoms; jaundice is uncommon in infants, more common in older children and most common in adults; jaundice and elevation of liver enzymes (serum aminotransferases) typically resolve by 4 months; persistence of elevated enzymes indicative of chronic disease • Fulminant hepatitis occurs in <1% of HBV-infected patients, but is more common in patients co-infected with HDV • Chronic hepatitis is defined as persistence of HBsAg for more than 6 months; patients are at significant risk of cirrhosis, liver failure, hepatocarcinoma, and death • Co-infection with HDV or HCV increases the risk of adverse outcomes
Diagnosis	• Diagnosis of HBV infection is by detection of HBsAg, HBcAg, and HBeAg and the host antibody response to these proteins (see below) • Presence of HDAg is indicative of co-infection with HDV
Treatment, Control, and Prevention	• Management of acute HBV infection is supportive • Acute fulminant disease treated with lamivudine or entecavir • Active chronic disease treated with entecavir, lamivudine, or tenofovir • Widespread use of recombinant **vaccine** expressing HBsAg provides long-lasting immunity following three doses (at 0, 1–2, and 6–12 months) or two doses (at 11–15 years and 6 months later) • Postexposure immunization recommended for nonimmune individuals

Serologic diagnosis of HBV infection and disease:

Test	Acute HBV Disease	Active Chronic HBV Disease	Inactive Chronic HBV Disease
HBsAg	+	+	+
Anti-HBs	–	–	–
HBeAg	+	+/–	–
Anti-HBe	–	+/–	+
HBcAg	+	+	+
Anti-HBc	+	–	–
Alanine aminotransferase	Elevated	Elevated	Normal

HEPATITIS C VIRUS

HCV is a member of the Flaviviridae family (*flavi*, yellow), which includes yellow fever virus (jaundice is a prominent feature of this disease), dengue virus (hemorrhagic fever), and a number of arthropod-transmitted viruses responsible for encephalitis including West Nile virus, St. Louis encephalitis virus, Japanese encephalitis virus, and Murray Valley encephalitis virus. HCV is the **most common cause of chronic hepatitis** worldwide.

HEPATITIS C VIRUS

Properties	• Small enveloped RNA virus; six genotypes and significant strain differences
Epidemiology	• Worldwide distribution with the highest prevalence in northern Africa, the Middle East, Southeast Asia, and China • Transmission by exposure to contaminated blood through intravenous drug abuse or unsafe medical practices; through sexual contact is uncommon • Virus detected within days of exposure and remains elevated for the first 2 to 3 months of infection; low-level viremia can be detected intermittently in persistent infections • HCV is the leading cause of chronic hepatitis
Clinical Disease	• Acute infections are typically asymptomatic; if symptoms are present, they are indistinguishable from other acute hepatitis virus infections • Development of fulminant disease is determined by virus genotype, host factors, and co-infection with other hepatitis viruses (e.g., HAV) • Chronic disease is associated with long-term persistence of virus production, development of cirrhosis and metabolic disorders, and hepatocellular carcinoma
Diagnosis	• Patients are initially screened for antibodies to HCV; confirmation of active disease is by detection of viral RNA with NAATs
Treatment, Control, and Prevention	• Treatment of HCV infections is rapidly evolving; please refer to the Infectious Disease Society of America and American Association for the Study of Liver Diseases guidelines • Prevention by reduced exposure to contaminated blood • Anti-HCV vaccines are not available because of the rapid development of strain variations

HEPATITIS E VIRUS

HEV is an enteric RNA virus that causes acute, self-limited hepatitis in immunocompetent individuals and chronic disease in immunocompromised patients. Although HEV infections are uncommon in developed countries, this is the most common cause of **acute hepatitis** in developing countries with poor sanitary controls.

HEPATITIS E VIRUS

Properties	• Nonenveloped RNA virus stable on environmental surfaces and resistant to many disinfectants (similar to HAV) • Four genotypes with many subtypes
Epidemiology	• Worldwide distribution with the highest prevalence in India, China, and northern Africa • Transmission through the fecal-oral route; most commonly from ingestion of fecal-contaminated water or foods; person-to-person transmission is uncommon because of low levels of virus in stools (in contrast with HAV) • Outbreaks common in developing countries but not in developed countries • Prevalence of infection more common in older children and adults than in infants (in contrast to HAV)
Clinical Disease	• Acute disease indistinguishable from other forms of acute viral hepatitis • HEV infection of pregnant women associated with a high risk of fulminant disease and mortality • HEV genotype 3 has been associated with chronic hepatitis in immunocompromised patients (solid organ transplants, stem cell transplants, HIV infections)
Diagnosis	• Serology is used, but NAATs are more sensitive and specific
Treatment, Control, and Prevention	• Acute HEV infections managed with supportive care • Fulminant disease can be managed with ribavirin, but this is contraindicated in pregnant women, so an alternative is needed • Ribavirin used in immunosuppressed patients with chronic HEV infections • Recombinant **vaccine** currently available in China • Prevention by implementation of appropriate sanitary conditions to prevent fecal contamination of water supplies

CLINICAL CASES (REFER TO SECTION VI)

Miscellaneous Infections
- Severe Hepatitis A virus infection in a family
- Hepatitis B virus infection in an immunized man
- Hepatitis C virus infection in a previously healthy woman

SUPPLEMENTAL READING

1. Shin EC, Jeong SH. Natural history, clinical manifestations, and pathogenesis of Hepatitis A. *Cold Spring Harbor Perspect Med.* 2018;8(9), a031708.
2. Nguyen MH, et al. Hepatitis B virus: advances in prevention, diagnosis, and therapy. *Clin Microbiol Rev.* 2020;33(2). e00046-19.
3. Applegate TL, et al. Hepatitis C virus diagnosis and the Holy Grail. *Infect Dis Clinic North Am.* 2018;32(2):425–445.

Gastrointestinal Viruses

Five viruses are responsible for primary gastrointestinal disease:
- Rotavirus
- Norovirus
- Sapovirus
- Astrovirus
- Adenovirus

Of these viruses, **rotavirus and norovirus are the most common**, with the other viruses being less prevalent. Before rotavirus was detected in the mid-1970s, no virus had been demonstrated to cause gastroenteritis. The role of these viruses was not appreciated because most of them could not be grown *in vitro* in cell cultures. Early diagnosis required observation of viral particles in stool specimens by electron microscopy.

This problem has been overcome, first by the use of immunoassays to detect viral antigens and then more recently by detecting viral nucleic acids using nucleic acid amplification tests (NAATs, e.g., polymerase chain reaction [PCR]).

ROTAVIRUS

Rotavirus was the first virus demonstrated to cause human gastrointestinal disease by observing large numbers of viral particles in the stool of symptomatic children. Despite the recognition of the importance of this virus and the introduction of vaccines to control the spread of the pathogen, rotaviruses are still the **most common cause of viral diarrhea** in most countries.

ROTAVIRUS

Properties	• Nonenveloped RNA virus that binds to cell surface carbohydrates of epithelial cells of the small intestinal villi • Absence of envelope renders these viruses stable in the environment • Mucosal damage leads to malabsorption and **secretory diarrhea**
Epidemiology	• Exposure is worldwide with most children infected by age 2 or 3 years • Severe disease most common in children between 6 months and 2 years of age • Most common cause of severe, dehydrating viral diarrhea in children in all countries; mortality highest in developing countries where vaccines are not widely utilized • Multiple strains can circulate in a community simultaneously • Reinfections with milder disease due to partial immunity occur throughout life • Major route of person-to-person spread is the fecal-oral route
Clinical Disease	• Asymptomatic infections can occur, particularly in previously exposed individuals • Following a 1- to 3-day incubation period, onset of disease is characterized by **vomiting** and **fever** lasting 2 to 3 days, progressing to profuse **watery diarrhea** that can last up to 1 week • Severe dehydration and electrolyte abnormalities can occur due to the watery diarrhea
Diagnosis	• Clinical diagnosis is confirmed by detection of viral antigens in stool specimens by immunoassays (generally positive for the first week or longer after onset); more recently, nucleic acid amplification tests (NAATs) by polymerase chain reaction have come into widespread use
Treatment, Control, and Prevention	• Therapy is supportive with maintenance of hydration; no antivirals are currently available • Live, attenuated **rotavirus vaccines** are available and associated with a significant decrease in symptomatic disease

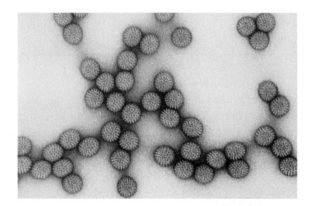

NOROVIRUS AND SAPOVIRUS

Two members of the Caliciviridae family, norovirus and sapovirus, are important enteric pathogens. A number of genetic variants of both viruses exist, so reinfection and disease can occur, particularly with norovirus. Because norovirus is far more common than sapovirus and the clinical disease is similar, the following comments refer to norovirus.

NOROVIRUS

Properties	• Nonenveloped RNA virus that is relatively heat- and acid-stable • Produces damage to the microvilli of the small intestine
Epidemiology	• Worldwide distribution • Major viral enteric pathogen in both children and adults • **Most common cause of outbreaks of viral gastroenteritis**, e.g., cruise ships, schools, hospitals, long-care facilities • Commonly responsible for sporadic disease • Exposure occurs throughout life • Major route of person-to-person spread is the fecal-oral route, although food-borne disease can also occur

NOROVIRUS—cont'd	
Clinical Disease	• Following a 1- to 2-day incubation period, the initial symptoms include **abdominal cramping** and nausea, followed by **vomiting** and **nonbloody diarrhea** • Symptoms generally resolve after 2 to 3 days
Diagnosis	• Virus is present in the stool of symptomatic patients for 2 to 3 days, although elderly patients and immunocompromised patients may shed the virus for weeks to months • Virus cannot be cultured • Immunoassays to detect viral antigens in stool are widely used, although NAATs are more sensitive and are considered the test of choice
Treatment, Control, and Prevention	• No specific antiviral therapy is available • Symptomatic treatment including fluid replacement is generally sufficient • Vaccines are not currently available • Use of bleach to clean potentially contaminated surfaces such as in health care institutions, schools, or cruise ships can help control outbreaks

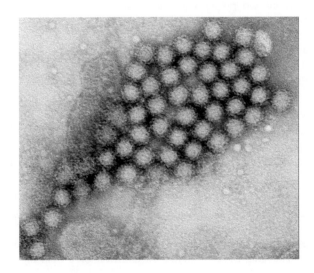

ASTROVIRUS

Astroviruses were initially detected in stool specimens by electron microscopy.

ASTROVIRUS	
Properties	• Nonenveloped RNA virus • Multiple genotypes are recognized
Epidemiology	• Worldwide distribution • Disease most common in young children but can occur in adults • Transmission by the fecal-oral route
Clinical Disease	• Incubation period is 3–4 days • Symptomatic disease is characterized by **diarrhea**, **headache**, malaise, and nausea; vomiting less prominent, and dehydration not as severe as with rotavirus; symptoms persist for less than 5 days
Diagnosis	• Diagnosis by immunoassay or more recently NAATs
Treatment, Control, and Prevention	• Illness is self-limited and treatment is supportive • Antivirals are not available

ADENOVIRUS

Adenovirus is the only DNA virus responsible for gastrointestinal diseases. Although many serotypes have been described, types 40 and 41 are the most commonly associated with diarrheal disease.

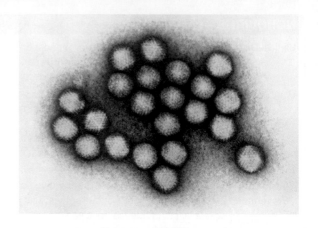

ADENOVIRUS	
Properties	• Nonenveloped DNA virus
Epidemiology	• Adenovirus exposure is common and worldwide, with most initial exposures during childhood and re-exposure throughout life • Enteric adenovirus types 40 and 41 associated with infantile diarrhea • Outbreak-related adult disease can occur
Clinical Disease	• Majority of infections are subclinical • Acute infantile disease presents as **watery diarrhea** that lasts 8–12 days, accompanied by fever and **vomiting**
Diagnosis	• The enteric viruses cannot be cultured • Diagnosis by immunoassay or, more commonly, by NAATs
Treatment, Control, and Prevention	• No approved antiviral treatment is available • Vaccines for the enteric adenovirus are not available

CLINICAL CASES (REFER TO SECTION VI)

Gastrointestinal Infections
• Severe rotavirus infection in an infant
• Outbreak of acute rotavirus infection
• Norovirus outbreak in children
• Norovirus transmission on cruise ships
• Adenovirus gastroenteritis in an immunocompromised child

SUPPLEMENTAL READING

1. Sadiq A, et al. Rotavirus: genetics, pathogenesis, and vaccine advances. *Rev Med Virol.* 2018;28, e2003.

2. Robilotti E, Deresinski S, Pinsky BA. Norovirus. *Clin Microbiol Rev.* 2015;28:134–164.

3. Becker-Dreps S, Gonzalez F, Bucardo F. Sapovirus: an emerging cause of childhood diarrhea. *Curr Opin Infect Dis.* 2020;33:388–397.

4. Johnson C, et al. Astrovirus pathogenesis. *Virus.* 2017;9:22.

5. Lee B, Damon C, Platts-Mills J. Pediatric acute gastroenteritis associated with adenovirus 40/41 in low-income and middle-income countries. *Curr Opin Infect Dis.* 2020;33:398–403.

Human Papillomavirus

In 2011, Peyton Rous discovered a tumor-inducing virus in chicken, and in 1964, Howard Temin proposed a theory of virus-induced oncology. Both investigators received the Nobel Prize for their pioneering work. Despite this work, the association of viruses with human cancer is relatively recent. In the 1960s, it was demonstrated that a herpesvirus, Epstein-Barr virus (EBV), was responsible for Burkitt's lymphoma. This was the first of seven viruses associated with human cancers. These seven viruses are:

Viruses	Associated Malignancies
Epstein-Barr virus (EBV)	Burkitt's lymphoma, nasopharyngeal carcinoma
Human herpesvirus-8 (HHV-8)	Kaposi's sarcoma, primary infusion lymphoma
Hepatitis B virus (HBV)	Hepatocellular carcinoma
Hepatitis C virus (HCV)	Hepatocellular carcinoma
Human adult T-cell leukemia virus type 1 (HTLV-1)	T-cell leukemia
Merkel cell polyomavirus	Merkel cell sarcoma
Human papillomavirus (HPV)	Carcinomas of the cervix, vulva, vagina, penis, anus, and oropharynx

The virus of interest in this chapter is the human papillomavirus (HPV), a virus with circular DNA surrounded by a nonenveloped, round shell. DNA sequencing has identified more than 100 genotypes of HPV that can be subdivided into viruses that infect and replicate in the squamous epithelial cells of the skin (producing **warts**) and mucous membranes (producing **genital, anal**, and **oropharyngeal cancers**). HPV is the most common sexually transmitted pathogen, and it is estimated that as many as 80% of unvaccinated, sexually active men and women are infected during their lifetime. Two HPV types (6 and 11) are responsible for more than 90% of the genital warts and, although more than 40 HPV types have been implicated in cancers, HPV types 16 and 18 are responsible for more than 70% of cervical cancers and five additional HPV types are responsible for 10%–20% of the cancers. The currently available multivalent vaccine is effective in preventing infection and disease with these nine HPV types.

HUMAN PAPILLOMAVIRUS

Properties	• Nonenveloped, DNA virus, 50–55 nm in diameter • More than 100 genotypes identified by DNA sequencing, tissue tropism, and associated with oncogenesis • Infects squamous epithelial cells of the skin and mucous membranes
Epidemiology	• Most common sexually transmitted pathogen • More than 80% of sexually active men and women will acquire infection during their lifetime, with lifelong persistence of the virus • HPV is present in virtually all cervical carcinomas
Clinical Diseases	• Infections are **asymptomatic** at the time of exposure, with pathology observed months to more than a year later • HPV types that infect the skin can produce **warts**, a benign self-limited proliferation of the infected cells • High-risk HPV types, including types 16 and 18, are associated with intraepithelial **cervical cancer**, progressing from mild to moderate neoplasia to severe neoplasia, occurring over a period of 1–4 years • HPV responsible for **penile, anal,** and **laryngeal carcinoma**
Diagnosis	• **NAAT tests** for most high-risk HPV types are the most sensitive diagnostic test for cervical infections • Pap smears historically used for diagnosis of cervical dysplasia, but the test is insensitive and nonspecific; replaced with automated liquid-based cytology in high-resource countries • Cytological examination of other implicated tissues (e.g., anal, oral) currently approved, although NAAT tests in research laboratories have proven highly effective
Treatment, Control, and Prevention	• Precancerous and cancerous treatment include surgery, radiotherapy, chemotherapy • Vaccination with multivalent vaccine highly effective in preventing infection and disease; recommended first dose for all 11- or 12-year-olds followed by a second dose 6–12 months later; the multivalent vaccine followed by two booster doses recommended for 15- to 27-year olds; currently, vaccination of older adults is considered less effective because most have prior exposure to HPV • Routine screening with a combination of liquid-based cytology and NAAT used for early detection of disease

CLINICAL CASES (REFER TO SECTION VI)

Upper Respiratory Tract Infections
• HPV-associated nasopharyngeal carcinoma

Genitourinary Tract Infections
• Invasive cervical carcinoma missed by colposcopy
• HPV type 16 penile cancer

SUPPLEMENTAL READING

1. White MK, Pagano JS, Khalili K. Viruses and human cancers: a long road of discovery of molecular paradigms. *Clin Microbiol Rev.* 2014;27(3):463–481.

2. Brianti P, De Flammineis E, Mercuri SR. Review of HPV-related diseases and cancers. *New Microbiol.* 2017;40(2):80–85.

3. Gravitt PE, Winer RL. Natural history of HPV infection across the lifespan: role of viral latency. *Viruses.* 2017;9(10):267. https://doi.org/10.3390/v9100267.

4. Wang R, et al. Human papillomavirus vaccine against cervical cancer: opportunity and challenge. *Cancer Lett.* 2020;471:88–102.

19

Introduction to Fungi

OVERVIEW

Fungi are more complex than bacteria and viruses. These are eukaryotic organisms that share a well-defined nucleus, mitochondria, Golgi bodies, and endoplasmic reticulum. They are distinguished from other eukaryotic organisms by a rigid cell wall composed of **chitin** and **glucan** and a cell membrane in which **ergosterol** is substituted for cholesterol as the major sterol component. These unique structural properties are exploited both for diagnosis and as targets for antifungal treatment.

As with the word of caution in the Introduction of the Bacteriology Section, the student should not be intimidated by the lists of fungi, diseases, and antifungal agents found in this chapter. Rather, I felt it was important to provide a structure to organize the information presented in this section, and I encourage students to return to this chapter as they master the information in the other chapters on fungi.

CLASSIFICATION

Fungi are classified in their own separate kingdom, Kingdom Fungi, and exist either as unicellular organisms (**yeasts**) that can replicate asexually or as multicellular filamentous organisms (**molds**) that replicate both sexually and asexually. Although most fungi exist in only one of the two forms, some clinically important fungi can assume either morphology (**dimorphic fungi**). A few other morphologic features are important for the student

to understand. Fundamentally, the multicellular molds consist of filaments called **hyphae** with budding forms or **spores**. Molds have been historically identified by the size, shape, and color of these structures. The hyphae can be subdivided into a string of individual compartments or cells separated by walls (**septum**) and are either pigmented (**dematiaceous mold**) or nonpigmented (**hyaline mold**). Thus, the molds can be subdivided into three groups: nonseptate (generally nonpigmented) molds; septate, dematiaceous molds; and septate, hyaline molds. Although this may be a bit confusing, it has a practical application in classifying some of the fungal diseases, as will be seen in the subsequent chapters.

The taxonomy of fungi is complex and, frankly, beyond the interest of most students and physicians. It is suffice to say that the asexual form of molds (**anamorph**) and the sexual form of molds (**teleomorph**) have different morphologies and have historically had different names. For the purpose of this textbook, only the commonly recognized names (primarily the anamorph names) will be used.

In contrast with the chapters on bacteria and the later chapters on parasites, this section of the textbook has been organized based on the clinical presentation of disease: cutaneous and subcutaneous fungi, systemic dimorphic fungi, and opportunistic fungi. The following table is a list of the most common diseases and associated genera of fungi in each group. It should be recognized that this is not an exhaustive list; rather, these are the fungi that a physician is likely to see.

Superficial, Cutaneous, and Subcutaneous Fungi	Dimorphic Fungi	Opportunistic Fungi
Pityriasis versicolor • *Malassezia furfur* Dermatophytoses • *Microsporum* spp. • *Trichophyton* spp. • *Epidermophyton floccosum* Onychomycosis • *Candida* spp. • *Aspergillus* spp. • *Trichosporon* spp. • *Geotrichum* spp. Mycotic keratitis • *Fusarium* spp. • *Aspergillus* spp. • *Candida* spp. Lymphocutaneous sporotrichosis • *Sporothrix schenckii*	Blastomycosis • *Blastomyces dermatitidis* Histoplasmosis • *Histoplasma capsulatum* Coccidioidomycosis • *Coccidioides immitis* • *Coccidioides posadasii* Penicilliosis • *Talaromyces (Penicillium) marneffei* Paracoccidioidomycosis • *Paracoccidioides brasiliensis*	Candidiasis • *Candida albicans* • *Candida glabrata* • *Candida aurus* • *Candida*, other spp. Cryptococcosis • *Cryptococcus neoformans* • *Cryptococcus gattii* Trichosporonosis • *Trichosporon* spp. Aspergillus • *Aspergillus fumigatus* • *Aspergillus*, other spp. Mucormycosis • *Rhizopus* spp. • *Mucor* spp. Hyalohyphomycosis • *Acremonium* spp. • *Fusarium* spp. • *Paecilomyces* spp. • *Scedosporium* spp. Phaeohyphomycosis • *Alternaria* spp. • *Bipolaris* spp. • *Curvularia* spp. Pneumocystosis • *Pneumocystis jiroveci* Microsporidiosis

ROLE IN DISEASE

This section is a summary of the fungi associated with human disease. Again, I have restricted this to the most common fungal pathogens, recognizing that many of the molds are opportunistic pathogens that can cause disease in immunocompromised patients. Additionally, some fungi are restricted to residents of tropical areas of the world and would primarily be treated by physicians living in those communities. For those physicians, a more comprehensive book on tropical medicine would be appropriate.

	FUNGAL PATHOGEN		
Infection Site	Yeast and Yeast Like	Mold	Dimorphic Fungi
Blood	*Candida* *Cryptococcus* *Trichosporon* *Malassezia* *Rhodotorula*	*Fusarium* *Talaromyces*	*Blastomyces* *Histoplasma*

Infection Site	FUGAL PATHOGEN		
	Yeast and Yeast Like	Mold	Dimorphic Fungi
Bone marrow		Talaromyces	Histoplasma
Central nervous system	Cryptococcus	Scedosporium	Coccidioides
	Candida	Mucormycetes	Histoplasma
Bone and joint	Candida	Sporothrix	Histoplasma
		Fusarium	Blastomyces
		Aspergillus	Coccidioides
		Talaromyces	
Eye	Candida	Fusarium	
	Cryptococcus	Aspergillus	
		Mucormycetes	
Urogenital system	Candida		
	Cryptococcus		
	Trichosporon		
Respiratory tract	Cryptococcus	Aspergillus	Blastomyces
		Mucormycetes	Histoplasma
	Pneumocystis	Fusarium	Coccidioides
		Scedosporium	
Skin and mucous membranes	Candida	Trichophyton	
		Microsporum	
	Cryptococcus	Epidermophyton	
	Trichosporon	Aspergillus	
		Mucormycetes	
		Fusarium	
		Dematiaceous molds	
		Sporothrix	
Multiple systemic sites	Candida	Hyaline molds	
	Cryptococcus	Dematiaceous molds	
	Trichosporon		

ANTIFUNGAL AGENTS

Management of fungal infections is complex because patients typically require prolonged treatment with a limited number of available drugs, many of which are toxic. Despite this, progress has been made in recent years with the development of new antifungals and less toxic alternatives to older agents. This table is a list of the most commonly used antifungals for specific clinical indications. No effort has been made here to indicate the treatment of choice for specific diseases. That will be done in the following chapters.

Drug Class	Examples	Clinical Indications
Polyene	Amphotericin B	Candidiasis, cryptococcosis, aspergillosis, mucormycosis, dimorphic fungal infections
	Lipid-associated amphotericin B	
	Nystatin	Candidiasis (oral, topical)
Imidazole	Ketoconazole	Dermatophytosis (topical)
	Clotrimazole	Candidiasis (oral), dermatophytosis (topical)
	Miconazole	Dermatophytosis (topical)
Triazole	Itraconazole	Blastomycosis, coccidioidomycosis, paracoccidioidomycosis, histoplasmosis, sporotrichosis, dermatophytosis (topical), onychomycosis
	Fluconazole	Candidiasis, cryptococcal meningitis, coccidioidomycosis, onychomycosis
	Voriconazole	Candidiasis, aspergillosis, fusariosis, pseudallescheriasis
	Posaconazole	Candidiasis (oral pharyngeal)
Flucytosine	Flucytosine	Candidiasis, cryptococcosis, chromoblastomycosis
Echinocandin	Caspofungin	Candidiasis, aspergillosis
	Anidulafungin	Candidiasis
	Micafungin	Candidiasis
Sulfonamide	Trimethoprim-sulfamethoxazole	Pneumocystis
Aromatic diamidine	Pentamidine	Pneumocystis

20

Cutaneous and Subcutaneous Fungi

INTERESTING FACTS

- Ringworm is caused by fungi (dermatophytes) and not parasitic worms, and the cutaneous disease caused by dermatophytes does not resemble any parasitic infection.
- *Microsporum canis* is a common dermatophyte in cats that can be spread among cats and dogs, with humans as an accidental host.
- *Sporothrix* is a dimorphic fungus found in sphagnum moss, organic-rich soil, and rotting vegetation; infection is caused when the fungus is introduced into the subcutaneous tissues of nursery workers, farm laborers, gardeners, and others working with soil through cuts in the skin produced by thorns from roses, barberry bushes, and the like.
- *Sporothrix* produces painless, nonhealing ulcers on the skin surface.

There are a large number of fungi that are responsible for cutaneous and subcutaneous diseases. Rather than offering a comprehensive presentation of all diseases and pathogens, I want to focus on just a few clinical conditions: infections of the outermost layers of the skin caused by the dermatophytes (**dermatophytosis**), a specific subset of infections of the nails (**onychomycosis**), eye infections (**fungal keratitis**), and subcutaneous infections caused by *Sporothrix* (**lymphocutaneous sporotrichosis**). I will briefly mention other related fungal diseases as appropriate.

There are three primary genera of fungi responsible for infections of the keratinized outer layers of the skin, hair, and nails, as well as a number of minor genera—well, minor if you are not infected with these fungi. These minor fungi, their disease, and their presentation are listed below.

Fungus	Disease	Presentation
Malassezia furfur	Tinea versicolor	Hypopigmented or hyperpigmented macules on the upper trunk, arms, chest, shoulders, face, and neck
Hortaea werneckii	Tinea nigra	Solitary, irregular, brown to black macule usually on the palms or soles (resembles a melanoma in appearance)
Trichosporon spp.	White piedra	White to brown swelling along the shaft of hairs of the groin and axillae
Piedraia hortae	Black piedra	Small, dark nodules surrounding the shaft of scalp hairs

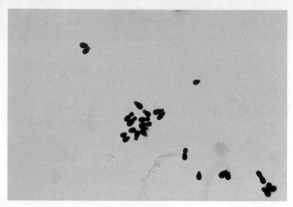

Gram stain of *Malassezia furfur* in skin scraping.

DERMATOPHYTOSIS

The three genera responsible for most cutaneous fungal infections are *Trichophyton*, *Epidermophyton*, and *Microsporum*. All dermatophytes have the common ability to invade the skin, hair, or nails (not all species invade all these sites) and break down the outermost keratin layer. The fungi are grouped into the anatomic site where infection occurs:

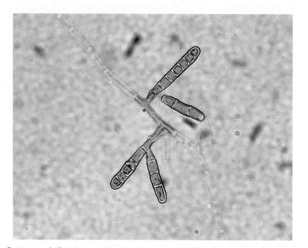

Culture of *Epidermophyton floccosum* showing smooth-walled macroconidia and absence of microconidia.

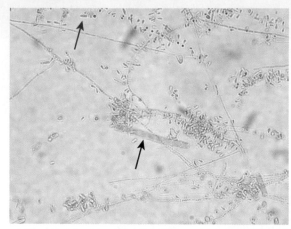

Culture of *Trichophyton rubrum*, showing multicelled macroconidia (*black arrow*) and microconidia (*red arrow*).

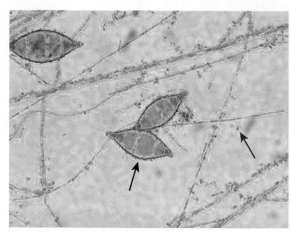

Culture of *Microsporum canis* showing rough-walled macroconidia (*black arrow*) and microconidia (*red arrow*).

Disease	Anatomic Site	Examples
Tinea capitis	Scalp, eyebrows, eyelashes	*Trichophyton tonsurans*
Tinea barbae	Beard	*Trichophyton rubrum, Trichophyton verrucosum*
Tinea corporis	Smooth or glabrous skin	*T. rubrum, Microsporum canis*
Tinea cruris	Groin	*T. rubrum, Epidermophyton floccosum*

Disease	Anatomic Site	Examples
Tinea pedis	Foot	*T. rubrum*
Tinea unguium	Nails	*T. rubrum*

Many species of dermatophytes are restricted to specific geographic areas of the world. Because the individual species may have very unique presentations, it is important to know the most common dermatophytes that you might encounter and their clinical presentation. White et al have presented a good summary of these species.

Epidemiology	• Dermatophytes classified into three categories based on natural habitat: geophilic, zoophilic, and anthropophilic
	  • Geophilic: live in soil and are an occasional pathogen of animals and humans
	  • Zoophilic: infect animals and some species can be transmitted to humans
	  • Anthropophilic: infect humans and may be transmitted person to person
	• Infections occur worldwide, especially in tropical and subtropical regions

Clinical Disease	• The clinical presentation is a function of the fungus, site of infection, and immune response of the host • Classic presentation on the skin is the development of a ring of inflammation "**ringworm**"; papules, pustules, or vesicles may develop • **Nail infections** are typically chronic with the nails becoming thickened, discolored, raised, friable, and deformed
Diagnosis	• Demonstration of fungal hyphae by direct microscopy of skin, hair, or nail samples • Isolation of the organism in culture • Hair infections with some species can be diagnosed by a fluorescent yellow-green appearance when exposed to a Wood's light (long wave ultraviolet light)
Treatment, Control, and Prevention	• Localized infections that do not involve hair or nails may be treated effectively with topical antifungal agents (imadazoles) • All other infections require oral therapy (griseofulvin, itraconazole, fluconazole)

One additional comment should be made about nail infections. In addition to dermatophytes, there are a number of bacteria, as well as the yeast *Candida*, that can infect nails. Because treatment may differ for the specific pathogen, it is important to make the diagnosis by culture. One caution is that damaged nail beds may be superficially colonized with fungi that are not responsible for the primary infection, so it is important to recover the fungus from multiple cultures or demonstrate the fungus specifically invading the nail tissues.

FUNGAL KERATITIS

This is a specific fungal infection that deserves mention. Fungal keratitis (infection of the cornea) is far less common than bacterial or viral infections, but threatens vision unless specifically diagnosed and treated. Although a number of molds can cause keratitis, the most common are *Fusarium* and *Aspergillus*. These and other molds are most commonly introduced following trauma to the eye. The yeast most commonly associated with keratitis is *Candida*. This yeast is acquired from the patient's normal population of organisms, and *Candida* infections are associated with prolonged ulceration, recent eye surgery, or corticosteroid use.

LYMPHOCUTANEOUS SPOROTRICHOSIS

Sporothrix schenckii is responsible for this lymphocutaneous disease that is characterized by the development of a skin ulcer at the primary site of inoculation of the fungus found in the soil and then the development of subsequent ulcers along the lymphatics that drain the initial lesion. This is a dimorphic fungus, existing as yeast cells in the infected patient and a mold form in nature and when grown in laboratory culture. It is discussed in this chapter rather than in the following chapter because the skin lesions are the primary presentation of the disease. The clinical picture will develop slowly and can mimic infections caused by other organisms (e.g., mycobacteria and *Nocardia*), so a specific diagnosis is important for the proper treatment of the patient.

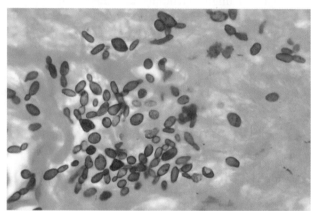 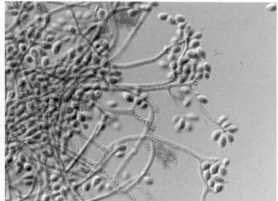

Sporothrix schenckii. (Left) Yeast cells in tissue biopsy; (Right) mold form in culture.

LYMPHOCUTANEOUS SPOROTRICHOSIS	
Epidemiology	• Worldwide distribution, especially in tropical and subtropical regions; present in North, Central, and South America • Infections associated with exposure to soil and plants, particularly organic-rich soils • Trauma such as a minor cut while gardening (e.g., on rose thorn) is a common method for subcutaneous inoculation of the fungus
Clinical Disease	• **Lymphocutaneous disease** presents as an indolent papulonodular lesion that can ulcerate; secondary nodules and ulcerative lesions develop along the lymphatics draining the primary inoculation site • **Disseminated infections** can occur in the bones, lungs, and central nervous system although this is not common
Diagnosis	• Demonstration of the yeast form of the fungus in lesions is frequently difficult (relatively few organisms may be present), but the culture of the lesions will be positive • Dimorphic fungus with cigar-shaped yeast cells in the lesions when observed and classic mold in the laboratory culture at 25–30°C; the mold has very thin hyphae and budding spores that resemble a flower ("flowerette"; a reminder of the source of the organism and association with gardening)
Treatment, Control, and Prevention	• Itraconazole is the treatment of choice for the lymphocutaneous disease, with 3–6 months of treatment required • Disseminated disease may be treated with more prolonged itraconazole or the use of amphotericin B followed by itraconazole

OTHER SUBCUTANEOUS INFECTIONS

Finally, as with cutaneous infections, there is a large collection of other fungi that cause subcutaneous infections. Most of these are observed in tropical areas and may be uncommonly seen outside the endemic regions.

Still, it is important to be aware of these pathogens. Diagnosis is by observation of the fungus in the involved tissues and isolation in culture. Because these are slowly progressive infections, treatment must be provided for months or years.

Disease	Examples of Pathogens	Comments
Eumycotic mycetoma	*Phaeoacremonium, Curvularia, Fusarium*; many other molds	Slowly developing infection particularly on lower limbs; characterized by chronic inflammation and fibrosis with progressive disfigurement
Chromoblastomycosis	*Fonsecaea, Cladosporium, Exophiala*; many other pigmented (dematiaceous) molds	As with mycetoma, chronically progressive infection of lower limbs or exposed skin; characterized by "cauliflower-like" growth with satellite lesions; disfiguring; with secondary lesions and infections
Subcutaneous mucormycosis	*Conidiobolus, Basidiobolus* (nonseptate molds)	Subcutaneous introduction of the fungus to the face or skin (shoulder, pelvis, thighs) that develops into a large subcutaneous mass
Subcutaneous phaeohyphomycosis	*Exophilia, Alternaria, Curvularia*; other dematiaceous molds	Usually single inflammatory cyst on the feet or legs; less commonly on the hands or other body surfaces; grows slowly over months to years

CLINICAL CASES (REFER TO SECTION VI)

Skin and Soft-Tissue Infections
- *Tinea versicolor* in an immunocompetent woman
- Dermatophytosis in an immunocompromised man
- *Tinea capitis* in an adult woman
- *Candida keratitis* following cataract surgery
- Sporotrichosis in a fisherman

SUPPLEMENTAL READING

1. White TC, et al. Fungi on the skin: dermatophytes and *Malassezia. Cold Spring Harb Perspect Med.* 2014;4(8), e019802.
2. Malmoudi, et al. Fungal keratitis: an overview of clinical and laboratory aspects. *Mycoses.* 2018;61(12):916–930.
3. de Lima Barros MB, de Almeida Paes R, Schubach AO. *Sporothrix schenckii* and sporotrichosis. *Clin Microbiol Rev.* 2011;24(4):633–654.

21

Systemic Dimorphic Fungi

The fungi discussed in this chapter are associated with disseminated or systemic disease and characteristically exist in two morphologies: most commonly in a **yeast form** in human tissues (*Coccidioides* is the exception) and a multicellular **mold form** in nature. Disease with these fungi is initiated by exposure to the infectious mold form; specifically, spores of the molds are inhaled, followed by the development of mild to severe respiratory disease. Dissemination may occur to characteristic body sites (e.g., central nervous system [CNS], skin, bone marrow). Thus, knowledge of the prevalent dimorphic fungi in specific geographic areas and the most common clinical presentation allows a rapid narrowing of the differential diagnosis. Three dimorphic fungi will be discussed in this chapter:

Dimorphic Fungus	Historic Perspective
Blastomyces dermatitidis	Blastomyces was first described by Thomas Gilchrist who named the fungus *B. dermatitidis*, recognizing the dermal presentation. The French biologist Philippe Van Tieghem recognized the disseminated form and named the disease **blastomycosis**. The disease is also referred to as **Gilchrist disease** after Thomas Gilchrist
Coccidioides immitis, Coccidioides posadasii	The first case of **coccidioidomycosis** was described by Alejandro Posadas (1892) in an Argentinean patient who had disseminated disease. The organism *C. immitis* and associated disease were first described by Rixford and Gilchrist (1896) from a patient observed in California. *C. immitis* infections are localized in California and *C. posadasii* is responsible for the majority of infections outside California.
Histoplasma capsulatum	**Histoplasmosis** was first described by Samuel Darling (1905), who reported the disease in a fatal case from Martinique. The name is derived from the observation that the yeast form of the fungus is found in the cytoplasm of reticuloendothelial cells. The disease is also referred to as **Darling disease**

Two additional dimorphic fungi deserve brief mention: *Paracoccidioides brasiliensis* and *Talaromyces (Penicillium) marneffei*. *P. brasiliensis* was originally described by Adolfo Lutz in 1908 in a Brazilian patient. In 1930, the current name was selected because the mold resembles *Coccidioides* and the majority of cases had been described in Brazil. Although the fungus resembles *Coccidioides*, disease is more like that caused by *Blastomyces*, hence the common name **South American Blastomycosis**. Disease is endemic throughout Latin America in areas with high humidity, rich vegetation, and moderate temperatures. **Paracoccidioidomycosis** may be subclinical, progressive with acute or chronic pulmonary disease, or disseminated disease involving the skin, lymph nodes, liver, spleen, CNS, and bones.

T. marneffei is an important cause of morbidity and mortality in HIV-infected and other immunosuppressed patients in Southeast Asia. The fungus was originally isolated in rats from Vietnam in 1952. It was believed to be a *Penicillium* species and was named in honor of Hubert Marneffe, Director of the Pasteur Institute in Indochina. It was renamed *T. marneffei* in 2015; however, the disease is still referred to as **penicilliosis**. Disease presents with fever, cough, and pulmonary infiltrates, and can progress to disseminated disease characterized by organomegaly, skin lesions, and hematologic disorders.

BLASTOMYCES DERMATITIDIS

B. dermatitidis is responsible for the disease **blastomycosis**. It is a dimorphic fungus that grows as a filamentous mold in moist, organic-rich soil and as yeast cells in patients. Animals, particularly dogs, are also susceptible to disease with this organism.

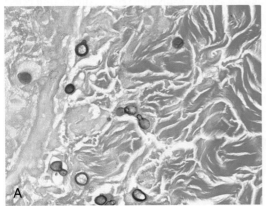 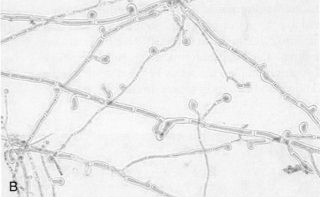

Blastomyces dermatitidis. (A) Yeast cells in biopsy tissue; (B) mold phase in culture with spores described as "lollipops" (infectious form found in nature).

BLASTOMYCES DERMATITIDIS	
Epidemiology	• Endemic in southeastern and south-central states, especially bordering the Ohio and Mississippi river basins; Midwest states and Canadian provinces bordering the Great Lakes; and an area of New York and Canada along the St Lawrence River • Outbreaks of infections have been associated with occupational or recreational contact with soil and decaying organic matter • Infection is acquired by inhalation of infectious spores • Person-to-person spread does not occur
Clinical Disease	• Exposure may result in asymptomatic, transient colonization, or disease • Disease is initiated with the development of **pneumonia** and may progress to dissemination to the **skin and subcutaneous tissues** (most common) as well as to bones, prostate, central nervous system, or other organs • Severity of disease is influenced by the magnitude of exposure and immune status of the patient

Continued

BLASTOMYCES DERMATITIDIS—cont'd

Diagnosis	• Microscopic detection of characteristic yeast cells (typically large, single cells or pairs of cells with a thick wall) in tissue or draining skin lesions • Antigen detection in urine may be useful for diagnosis but is rarely performed • Antibody detection is not useful • Grows as a mold form (room temperature; 2–4 weeks) or yeast form (37°C; 3–5 days) in culture
Treatment, Control, and Prevention	• Itraconazole is the drug of choice for mild to moderate pulmonary or non-CNS disease • Amphotericin B followed by itraconazole is the treatment for severe infection • Prevention and control of infections are not feasible because this fungus is endemic in the environment • Care should be taken in handling laboratory cultures

COCCIDIOIDES IMMITIS AND COCCIDIOIDES POSADASII

C. immitis and *C. posadasii* are responsible for the disease **coccidioidomycosis**. The species are indistinguishable in appearance or pathogenicity, differentiated only by molecular methods. In contrast to the other dimorphic fungi, *Coccidioides* forms a spherule containing endospores in human tissues. A key to diagnosis is the detection of these "bags of spores" in clinical specimens.

The mold form of the fungus also has a characteristic morphology. Instead of forming spores along the sides or end of hyphae (mycelia), the growing mycelia are subdivided by septae (walls) into cells. Alternating cells will disintegrate, leaving mature barrel-shaped cells called **arthroconidia**. These arthroconidia are infectious spores and are extremely resilient to harsh environmental conditions (typically this fungus is found in dry, hot climates). The spores can be carried hundreds of miles in wind currents to cause disease in distant populations.

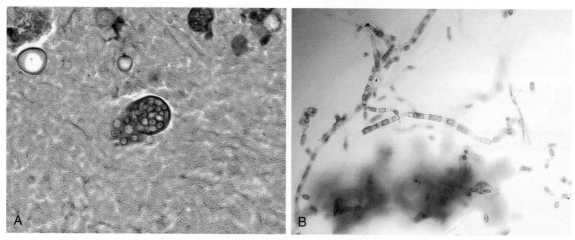

Coccidioides immitis. (A) Spherule observed in sputum; (B) mold phase in culture (infectious form found in nature).

COCCIDIOIDES IMMITIS AND COCCIDIOIDES POSADASII	
Epidemiology	• Endemic to US southwest desert, northern Mexico, scattered areas of Central and South America • Spores can survive in nature for an extended period; germinate and grow as molds following rain; then be disseminated in the wind during a windy, dry period • Exposure and asymptomatic or mild infection are very common in endemic areas • Infection caused by inhalation of infectious spores (arthroconidia) • Risk of disseminated disease highest in certain ethnic groups (Filipino, African American, Native American, Hispanic), women in the third trimester of pregnancy, individuals with cellular immune deficiency, persons at extremes of age • Person-to-person spread does not occur • Laboratory infections with exposure to the mold form of this organism are not uncommon, so care must be exercised
Clinical Disease	• Infections can be asymptomatic or progress to disease • **Pneumonia** is the most common clinical disease • Extrapulmonary dissemination is most commonly to the skin, joints and bones, and **central nervous system** (meningitis)
Diagnosis	• Histopathologic examination of tissues for endosporulating spherules • Spherules can also be observed in sputa or wound drainage • The mold form grows rapidly in culture and can be detected as soon as 1–2 days; caution is needed because sporulation can occur within a day or two, so the mold form is highly infectious • Serology may be useful for diagnosis or prognostic evaluation
Treatment, Control, and Prevention	• Most patients with primary infections do not require treatment • Those with severe disease or risk factors for progressive disease should be treated with amphotericin B followed by an oral azole as maintenance therapy • Azoles are used for chronic cavitary pulmonary disease or nonmeningeal disseminated disease • Meningeal coccidioidomycosis is treated with fluconazole, with other azoles as secondary choices • With the exception of careful handling of laboratory cultures, prevention and control of exposure are not feasible because the fungus is endemic in the regions

HISTOPLASMA CAPSULATUM

Histoplasmosis is caused by two variants of *H. capsulatum*: *H. capsulatum* var. *capsulatum* is responsible for pulmonary and disseminated disease in the eastern half of the USA and most of Latin America, and *H. capsulatum* var. *duboisii* causes predominantly skin and bone lesions in tropical areas of Africa. The mold forms of the fungi are indistinguishable, but the variants are separated by the different morphology of the yeast cells. The yeast forms of both variants are only observed as intracellular pathogens.

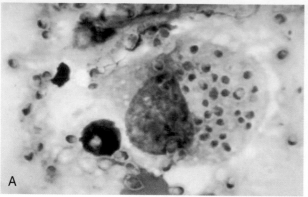 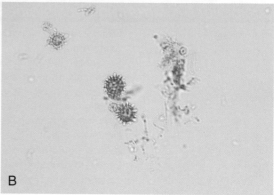

Histoplasma capsulatum. (A) Giemsa stain of intracellular yeast forms; (B) infectious mold form found in nature.

HISTOPLASMA CAPSULATUM	
Epidemiology	<ul><li>*H. capsulatum* var. *capsulatum* is localized to Ohio and Mississippi river valleys and throughout Mexico and Central and South America</li><li>*H. capsulatum* var. *duboisii* is confined to tropical Africa (e.g., Gabon, Uganda, Kenya)</li><li>Found in soil with high nitrogen content such as areas contaminated with bird or bat droppings</li><li>Outbreaks of disease associated with exposure to bird roosts, caves, and decaying buildings or urban renewal projects involving excavation and demolition</li><li>Infection acquired by inhalation of infectious spores</li><li>Person-to-person spread does not occur</li><li>Immunocompromised patients and children are most susceptible to symptomatic disease</li><li>Reactivation of disease and dissemination common among immunosuppressed individuals (e.g., AIDS patients)</li></ul>
Clinical Disease	<ul><li>Severity of symptoms and course of disease depend on the extent of exposure and immune status of the infected individual</li><li>Most infections are asymptomatic or mild, self-limited flulike disease</li><li>Acute **pulmonary disease** caused by *H. capsulatum* var. *capsulatum* is characterized by high fever, headache, nonproductive cough, and chest pain; symptoms most commonly resolve within 10 days but can progress to disseminated disease, involving multiple organ systems</li><li>Pulmonary disease is rare in African histoplasmosis caused by *H. capsulatum* var *duboisii*; disease is characterized by regional lymphadenopathy with **lesions of skin and bone**; a more fulminant progressive disease can occur in AIDS patients</li></ul>
Diagnosis	<ul><li>Direct microscopy and culture of respiratory material confirm the diagnosis of histoplasmosis</li><li>Serology is useful for all but AIDS patients</li><li>Detection of *Histoplasma* antigen in urine or serum is useful for extrapulmonary disease</li></ul>
Treatment, Control, and Prevention	<ul><li>Mild or moderate pulmonary histoplasmosis can be treated symptomatically or with itraconazole</li><li>Moderate to severe disease is treated with amphotericin B followed by itraconazole</li><li>Exposure in endemic areas is difficult to avoid, but areas where birds may have roosted should be avoided, particularly for immunocompromised patients</li><li>Care should be exercised in handling laboratory cultures</li></ul>

CLINICAL CASES

Lower Respiratory Tract Infections
- Histoplasmosis
- Coccidioidomycosis

Central Nervous System Infections
- Central nervous system blastomycosis

Skin and Soft-Tissue Infections
- *Talaromyces marneffei* infection in an HIV/AIDS patient
- *Paracoccidioides brasiliensis* infection in a Brazilian man
- Disseminated histoplasmosis in an HIV/AIDS patient
- Cutaneous blastomycosis

SUPPLEMENTAL READING

1. Castillo CG, Kauffman CA, Miceli MH. Blastomycosis. *Infect Dis Clin North Am.* 2016;30(1):247–264.
2. Marques SA. Paracoccidioidomycosis. *Clin Dermatol.* 2012;30(6):610–615.
3. Stockamp NW, Thompson GR. Coccidioidomycosis. *Infect Dis Clin North Am.* 2016;30(1):229–246.
4. Wheat LJ, et al. Histoplasmosis. *Infect Dis Clin North Am.* 2016;30(1):207–227.
5. Limper AH, et al. Fungal infections in HIV/AIDS. *Lancet Infect Dis.* 2017;17(11):e334–e343.

Opportunistic Fungi

There are many examples of opportunistic fungi but this chapter will be restricted to examples of the most commonly encountered human pathogens. Most of the opportunistic fungi are filamentous molds commonly found in the environment and produce disease in humans following inhalation of spores or following trauma (**exogenous infections**). In general, infections are primarily restricted to individuals with a compromised immune system or some other underlying disease (e.g., diabetes). There are three important exceptions to the rule that opportunistic fungi are molds. *Cryptococcus* is a yeast that exists in nature and is acquired by inhalation of the yeast cells and not spores. *Candida* is a yeast that colonizes humans and produces **endogenous infections**; that is, the yeast moves from normally colonized mucosal surfaces to the blood or other normally sterile sites. *Pneumocystis*, formerly classified as a parasite, is another yeast-like fungus that colonizes humans but produces disease in immunocompromised patients.

The three genera of fungi that will be the focus of this chapter are *Candida*, *Cryptococcus*, and *Aspergillus*. Other fungi of interest will be mentioned briefly at the end of the chapter.

CANDIDA ALBICANS AND RELATED SPECIES

More than 20 species of *Candida* have been associated with human disease, but most infections are caused by relatively few species.

Candida Speciess	Most Common Diseases
Candida albicans	Mucosal infections (thrush, vaginitis), cutaneous and nail infections, cardiovascular infections (fungemia, endocarditis, intravenous line-related or intravenous drug abuse-related sepsis), deep tissue infections
Candida glabrata	Urinary tract infections; many other less common infections
Candida auris	Skin colonization; catheter-related sepsis
Candida parapsilosis	Catheter-related fungemia, particularly in children receiving lipid-rich hyperalimentation
Candida tropicalis	Fungemia in patients with hematologic malignancies
Candida krusei	Fungemia

Candida species are the most common cause of all fungal diseases, infecting healthy individuals (e.g., cutaneous and nail infections, vaginitis, and urinary tract infections) as well as life-threatening infections in immunocompromised patients. Diagnosis is generally not a problem because these yeasts will grow in 1 to 3 days in culture and identification can be easily accomplished for the most common species. One potential diagnostic problem is relatively few yeasts circulate in the blood of patients with disseminated infections, so documentation of fungemia may be difficult. Therapeutic management of infected patients has been complicated in recent years by the increased observation of azole resistance in certain *Candida* species (e.g., **Candida auris, Candida krusei, and Candida glabrata**). The following is a summary of *Candida* species:

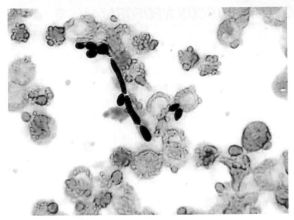

Candida albicans in blood culture.

CANDIDA ALBICANS AND RELATED SPECIES

Epidemiology	• Opportunistic yeasts • Most infections caused by *C. albicans* • Colonize humans and other warm-blooded animals • Primary site of colonization is gastrointestinal tract, although present in mouth, vagina, and on warm, moist skin surfaces; *C. glabrata* common colonizer on genitourinary tract; *C. auris* most commonly found colonizing the skin • Most infections are endogenous • Risk factors for blood infections with *Candida* include hematologic malignancies and neutropenia, HIV infections, contaminated intravascular line, prior exposure to broad-spectrum antibacterials, recent abdominal surgery or trauma, prematurity in infants, elderly patients • Use of azoles for antifungal prophylaxis in hematologic malignancy patients and recipients of stem cell transplantation increase the risk for infections caused by *C. auris*, *C. glabrata*, and *C. krusei*
Clinical Disease	• Cause infections ranging from superficial mucosal and cutaneous disease to hematogenously disseminated, often fatal, infections
Diagnosis	• Observation of yeasts by microscopy and culture • Use of antigen tests to detect fungal antigens or nucleic acid amplification tests to detect presence of *Candida* in normally sterile specimens • Care must be used to interpret microscopy and culture because *Candida* normally colonizes the skin and mucosal surfaces; abnormal predominance of yeast in body sites is consistent with disease
Treatment, Control, Prevention	• Mucosal and cutaneous infections can be treated with itraconazole, fluconazole, miconazole, and many other agents; invasive infections, particularly in immunocompromised patients, must be treated more aggressively using azoles, echinocandins, or amphotericin B • *C. auris*, *C. glabrata*, and *C. krusei* have decreased susceptibility to azoles (e.g., fluconazole) so treatment with an echinocandin (e.g., anidulafungin, caspofungin, micafungin) or amphotericin B may be required • Antifungal prophylaxis for high-risk patients has reduced the incidence of disease

CRYPTOCOCCUS NEOFORMANS

Cryptococci are spherical yeasts that are surrounded by a large, prominent **polysaccharide capsule** (an important diagnostic feature). *C. neoformans* is found worldwide in soil, particularly soil enriched with pigeon droppings. A related species, *Cryptococcus gattii*, is in a more geographically restricted region of the US Pacific Northwest. Infection with both species is acquired by inhalation of the yeast cells followed by an initial mild or asymptomatic process in the lungs. The fungi have a predisposition to disseminate to the central nervous system in susceptible patients. Indeed, *Cryptococcus* is the most common fungal pathogen responsible for **meningitis**. Although both species can cause disease in immunocompetent patients, *C. neoformans* is most commonly observed as an opportunistic pathogen in patients with underlying defects in cellular immunity, such as HIV-infected patients and solid organ transplants. The incidence of cryptococcosis has decreased in recent years with the use of prophylactic antifungal agents (e.g., fluconazole) in high-risk patients. Diagnosis of disease is generally made by observation of encapsulated yeast in spinal fluid or detection of the **capsular polysaccharide** by a specific antigen test (positive for both cryptococcal species). Occasionally, yeasts are detected in the blood of infected patients, but blood culture alone is an unreliable diagnostic test because relatively few organisms may be circulating in the blood and culture will require 3 to 7 days before growth is detected.

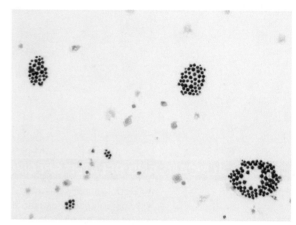

Cryptococcus neoformans in cerebrospinal fluid. Note the clusters of individual cells separated by clear spaces occupied by the unstained surrounding envelope.

CRYPTOCOCCUS NEOFORMANS

Epidemiology	• Worldwide distribution, commonly in soil contaminated with avian excreta; *Cryptococcus gattii* more restricted to tropical and subtropical regions (associated with eucalyptus and fir trees) • Infections typically acquired by inhalation • Prevalence of infections less common with the use of prophylactic antifungals such as fluconazole in immunocompromised patients
Clinical Disease	• Infections initially develop in **lungs** although dissemination in the blood, particularly to the central nervous system, is common • **Meningitis** is usually the presenting disease
Diagnosis	• Definitive diagnosis by culture of the organism in blood, sputum, or cerebrospinal fluid (CSF) (most reliable source) • Microscopic examination of CSF may demonstrate characteristic budding cells (**India ink** is used as a contrasting dye to detect the presence of a clear capsule surrounding the yeast cell) • Use of antigen tests to detect the polysaccharide capsular material; this is more reliable than stains for CSF (white blood cells may be misidentified as *Cryptococcus* by an inexperienced microscopist)
Treatment, Control, Prevention	• Meningitis uniformly fatal if untreated • Amphotericin B and fluconazole used initially, followed by maintenance use of fluconazole or itraconazole; antigen test can be used to monitor response to therapy • Prophylactic use of antifungals recommended for high-risk patients

MISCELLANEOUS YEAST-LIKE FUNGI

The following is a summary of other medically important single-cell fungi that can produce disseminated disease:

Fungus	Diseases and Comments
Malassezia	Catheter-related sepsis, particularly in infants receiving lipid infusions (some species require **lipids** for growth); treatment by removal of line and discontinuation of the lipid infusions
Trichosporon	Catheter-related sepsis in neutropenic patients; **high mortality** because susceptibility to most antifungals including amphotericin B is variable
Rhodotorula	Catheter-related sepsis in immunocompromised patients; amphotericin B and fluconazole with good activity
Microsporidia	Many genera; disease dependent on infecting species; most common diseases following ingestion include chronic diarrhea, hepatitis, or peritonitis in AIDS patients; treatment with albendazole
Pneumocystis	**Common opportunistic pathogen in AIDS patients**; respiratory tract is the main portal of entry and pneumonia the most common presentation, although dissemination occurs less commonly; treatment and prophylaxis of high-risk patients are with trimethoprim-sulfamethoxazole

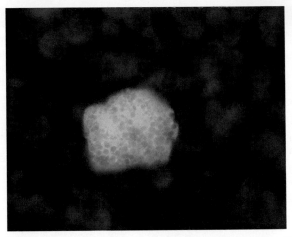

Pneumocystis jiroveci in bronchoalveolar lavage stained with immunofluorescent antibodies.

ASPERGILLUS FUMIGATUS

Aspergillus is the most common mold that causes opportunistic infections. Many species have been described, but the number of species associated with human disease is relatively limited, with *A. fumigatus* by far the most common. Aspergilli are environment fungi whose spores are inhaled, producing a wide range of diseases including allergic hypersensitivity reactions, primary pulmonary disease, or highly aggressive disseminated disease. A preliminary diagnosis of infection is made by observation of the fungus in tissue (typical appearance is branching, septate [divided into compartments], nonpigmented [hyaline] hyphae) and confirmed by growth of the mold in 2 to 5 days in culture. Identification of the individual species is by the morphologic appearance of the mold growing in culture (color of the colonies, arrangement of spores on the fruiting structures attached to the hyphae). The spores are not observed in patient tissues.

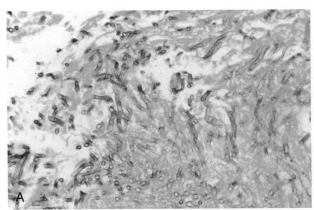
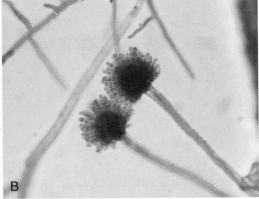

Aspergillus fumigatus. (A) Mold form in lung tissue; (B) mold form with fruiting conidia structure in culture.

ASPERGILLUS FUMIGATUS

Epidemiology	• Worldwide distribution with spores ubiquitous in air, soil, and decaying vegetation • Within the hospital environment, *Aspergillus* may be found in air, showerheads, water storage tanks, potted plants, and in areas of construction and remodeling • Most infections are acquired by inhalation • Most infections are caused by *A. fumigatus* (most common), *Aspergillus flavus*, *Aspergillus niger*, and *Aspergillus terreus*
Clinical Disease	• Disease is a function of the host immune response and, less so, the *Aspergillus* species or strain • Exposure to fungal spores may result in a hypersensitive reaction (**allergic aspergillosis**) or **invasive disease** • Invasive disease marked by **angioinvasion** (invasion of blood vessels) and tissue destruction • Hematogenous dissemination to the brain (most common), heart, kidneys, gastrointestinal tract, liver, spleen
Diagnosis	• Diagnosis is by observation of the mold in tissue and isolation in culture; isolation in asymptomatic patients may represent insignificant colonization so additional cultures and demonstration of tissue involvement is required • Blood cultures are rarely positive • Antigen tests can be used to complement culture • Nucleic acid amplification tests are controversial because environmental contamination of reagents is common
Treatment, Control, Prevention	• Treatment of chronic pulmonary aspergillosis may involve steroids as well as long-term antifungal therapy, usually with an azole agent • Therapy for invasive aspergillosis usually involves administration of voriconazole or amphotericin B; efforts to decrease immunosuppression are generally necessary • Prophylaxis of high-risk neutropenic patients usually with itraconazole, posaconazole, or voriconazole • Exposure is difficult to control because the mold is present in the environment; however, high-risk patients should avoid areas of remodeling, construction, and excavation

MISCELLANEOUS OPPORTUNISTIC MOLDS

The following is a summary of other medically important multicellular molds that can produce disseminated disease:

Fungus	Diseases and Comments
Mucorales (e.g., *Rhizopus, Mucor, and Rhizomucor*)	Genera of nonseptate, nonpigmented molds that cause invasive disease in immunocompromised patients, particularly **diabetes** patients, patients with **metabolic acidosis**, and those with hematologic malignances
Fusarium, Scedosporium, Paecilomyces	Septated, nonpigmented molds that cause disseminated infections in immunocompromised patients; one of the few molds that are isolated in blood cultures
Alternaria, Bipolaris, Curvularia	Septated, pigmented molds that cause either localized subcutaneous disease following trauma or disseminate to multiple organs in immunocompromised patients

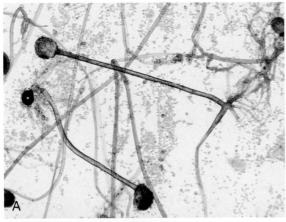

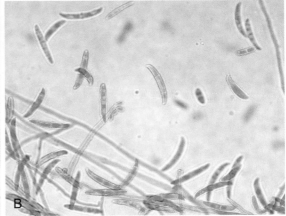

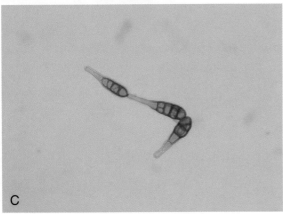

Other opportunistic fungi in culture stained with lactophenol cotton blue dye. (A) *Rhizopus*; (B) *Fusarium*; (C) naturally pigmented (dematiaceous) *Alternaria*.

CLINICAL CASES (REFER TO SECTION VI)

Lower Respiratory Tract Infection
- Invasive aspergillosis in renal transplant patient
- *Pneumocystis* pneumonia in newly diagnosed HIV/AIDS patient

Skin and Soft Tissue Infections
- *Malassezia* infection in patients receiving hyperalimentation
- Cryptococcosis in heart transplant patient
- Mucormycosis in COVID-19 patient

Sepsis and Cardiovascular Infections
- Candidemia in immunocompetent woman
- Catheter-related *Candida auris* sepsis
- Fusariosis in neutropenic leukemia patient

SUPPLEMENTAL READING

1. Kullberg BJ, Arendrup MC. Invasive candidiasis. *N Engl J Med.* 2015;373(15):1445–1456.
2. Du H, et al. *Candida auris*: epidemiology, biology, antifungal resistance, and virulence. *PLoS Pathog.* 2020;16(10), e1008921.
3. Marcon MJ, Powell DA. Human infections due to *Malassezia* spp. *Clin Microbiol Rev.* 1992;5(2):101–119.
4. Maziarz EK, Perfect JR. Cryptococcosis. *Infect Dis Clin North Am.* 2016;30(1):179–206.
5. Latge JP. *Aspergillus fumigatus* and Aspergillosis. *Clin Microbiol Rev.* 1999;12(2):310–350.
6. Nucci M, Anaissie E. *Fusarium* infections in immunocompromised patients. *Clin Microbiol Rev.* 2007;20(4):695–704.
7. Fishman JA. *Pneumocystis jiroveci*. *Semin Respir Crit Care Med.* 2020;41(1):141–157.

23

Introduction to Parasites

OVERVIEW

Parasites are the most complex of all microbes. All parasites are classified as eukaryotic, some are unicellular and others are multicellular, some are as small as 4–5 μm in diameter and others are up to 10 m in length, and some are amorphous with minimal features whereas others have characteristic structures, such as a head, body, and legs. Historically, parasitic infections were viewed as exotic diseases acquired only in remote regions of the world, but the reality is that some of the more common parasitic infections can be acquired in most communities in developed countries, and global transportation can bring diseases restricted to remote regions of the world to anyone's doorsteps. The epidemiology of these diseases is equally challenging, with some parasites spreading from person-to-person while others require a complex series of hosts for development into infectious forms. The difficulties confronting students are not only an understanding of the spectrum of parasites and the disease they cause, but also an appreciation of the epidemiology of these infections, which is vital for developing a differential diagnosis and an approach to the control and prevention of parasitic infections. With literally hundreds of parasites associated with human disease, the student needs some help in organizing the most relevant information. In this chapter and subsequent ones, I will concentrate on only the most common parasites associated with human disease, recognizing that avirulent parasites, particularly those classified in the kingdom Protozoa, can colonize humans and create confusion when detected in clinical specimens. In this chapter, I first provide a classification structure for the parasites and then a view of the parasites from the perspective of the diseases they cause. I also provide an overview of the antiparasitic agents that can be used to treat these infections. In the subsequent chapters, I provide a more detailed view of the biology, epidemiology, clinical disease, diagnosis, and treatment of these organisms.

CLASSIFICATION

The parasites of humans are classified into three kingdoms: Protozoa, Stramenopila, and Animalia. **Protozoa** are simple, unicellular parasites that are microscopic in size. Stramenopila include a number of unicellular plant-like organisms (e.g., algae) and one organism, *Blastocystis*, that is commonly observed in fecal specimens but is of uncertain clinical significance (actually, of controversial significance). The kingdom of Stramenopila will not be discussed further. The last kingdom, Animalia, includes all eukaryotic microorganisms that are not Protozoa, Stramenopila, or Fungi. For our purposes here, this kingdom includes the "**worms**" and the "**bugs**."

Kingdom	General Class	Organism	Disease
Protozoa	Ameba	*Entamoeba histolytica*	Amebiasis (amebic dysentery)
		Acanthamoeba spp.	Keratitis, encephalitis
		Naegleria fowleri	Meningoencephalitis
	Flagellate	*Giardia duodenalis*	Giardiasis (diarrheal disease)
		Trichomonas vaginalis	Trichomoniasis (vaginitis)
		Leishmania spp.	Leishmaniasis (cutaneous or visceral disease)
		Trypanosoma brucei	African sleeping sickness
		Trypanosoma cruzi	Chagas disease
	Sporozoan	*Cryptosporidium* spp.	Diarrheal disease
		Cyclospora cayetanensis	Diarrheal disease
		Cystoisospora belli	Diarrheal disease
		Toxoplasma gondii	Toxoplasmosis (disseminated disease)
		Plasmodium spp.	Malaria
		Babesia spp.	Babesiosis (malaria-like disease)
Animalia	Nematodes (roundworms)	*Enterobius vermicularis*	Enterobiasis (perianal itching)
		Trichuris trichiura	Trichuriasis (diarrheal disease)
		Ascaris lumbricoides	Ascariasis (intestinal disease)
		Strongyloides stercoralis	Strongyloidiasis (intestinal disease)
		Necator americanus	Hookworm (intestinal disease)
		Ancylostoma duodenale	Hookworm (intestinal disease)
		Brugia malayi	Filariasis or elephantiasis
		Wuchereria bancrofti	Filariasis or elephantiasis
		Loa loa	Disseminated disease
		Onchocerca volvulus	Onchocerciasis (disseminated disease with blindness)
		Trichinella spiralis	Trichinosis (disseminated disease)
		Toxocara canis	Visceral larva migrans
		Ancylostoma braziliense	Cutaneous larva migrans
	Trematodes (flatworms)	*Fasciolopsis buski*	Intestinal disease
		Fasciola hepatica	Hepatic disease
		Opisthorchis sinensis (also known as *Clonorchis sinensis*)	Hepatic disease
		Paragonimus westermani	Pulmonary disease
		Schistosoma spp.	Schistosomiasis (disseminated disease)
	Cestodes (tapeworms)	*Taenia saginata*	Intestinal disease
		Taenia solium	Intestinal disease; cysticercosis (disseminated)
		Diphyllobothrium latum	Intestinal disease
		Hymenolepis spp.	Intestinal disease
		Dipylidium caninum	Intestinal disease
		Echinococcus granulosus	Echinococcosis (disseminated disease)
	Arthropods	Mosquito	Vector for many diseases
		Tick	Vector for many diseases
		Flea	Vector for many diseases
		Lice	Vector for many diseases
		Mite	Vector for many diseases
		Fly	Vector for many diseases

ROLE IN DISEASE

In this section, I present a summary of the parasites that are associated with human disease from the perspective of the clinical presentation. This is the view of the physician when presented with an ill patient; however, it is critical that he or she know the most likely parasites responsible for the clinical symptoms. The goal of this section and subsequent chapters is to give the student the tools to develop this differential diagnosis.

	PARASITE			
Disease	**Protozoa**	**Nematode**	**Trematode**	**Cestode**
Systemic				
Dissemination and multiorgan involvement	*Plasmodium falciparum, Toxoplasma, Leishmania*	*Toxocara, Strongyloides, Trichinella*		
Iron deficiency		*Necator, Ancylostoma*		
Vitamin B$_{12}$ deficiency				*Diphyllobothrium*
Blood				
Malaria	*Plasmodium*			
Babesiosis	*Babesia*			
Filariasis		*Brugia, Loa, Wuchereria*		
Lymphatics				
Lymphedema		*Brugia, Loa, Wuchereria*		
Lymphadenopathy	*Toxoplasma, Trypanosoma*			
Bone Marrow				
Leishmaniasis	*Leishmania*			
Central Nervous System				
Meningoencephalitis	*Naegleria, Trypanosoma, Toxoplasma*			
Granulomatous encephalitis	*Acanthamoeba*			
Mass lesion, brain abscess	*Toxoplasma, Acanthamoeba*		*Schistosoma japonicum*	*Taenia solium*
Eosinophilic meningitis	*Plasmodium falciparum*	*Toxocara*		
Cerebral paragonimiasis			*Paragonimus*	
Eye				
Keratitis	*Acanthamoeba*	*Onchocerca*		
Chorioretinitis, conjunctivitis	*Toxoplasma*	*Loa, Onchocerca*		
Ocular cysticercosis				*Taenia solium*
Toxocariasis		*Toxocara*		
Intestinal Tract				
Anal pruritus	*Enterobius*			
Colitis	*Entamoeba histolytica*			
Toxic megacolon	*Trypanosoma cruzi*			

Continued

	PARASITE			
Disease	**Protozoa**	**Nematode**	**Trematode**	**Cestode**
Rectal prolapse		Trichuris		
Abdominal pain, diarrhea, dysentery	Entamoeba histolytica, Giardia, Cryptosporidium, Cyclospora, Cystoisospora	Strongyloides, Trichuris, Necator, Ancylostoma	Schistosoma mansoni	Taenia, Diphyllobothrium, Hymenolepsis, Dipylidium
Obstruction, perforation		Ascaris, Fasciolopsis		
Genitourinary Tract				
Vaginitis, urethritis	Trichomonas	Enterobius		
Cystitis, hematuria	Plasmodium		Schistosoma haematobium	
Renal failure	Plasmodium, Leishmania			
Liver, Spleen				
Abscess	Entamoeba histolytica		Fasciola	
Hepatitis	Toxoplasma			
Biliary obstruction		Ascaris	Opisthorchis, Fasciola	
Cirrhosis	Leishmania	Toxocara	Schistosoma	
Mass lesion				Taenia solium, Echinococcus
Heart				
Myocarditis	Toxoplasma, Trypanosoma cruzi			
Lung				
Abscess	Entamoeba histolytica		Paragonimus	
Nodule, mass				Echinococcus
Pneumonitis	Toxoplasma	Ascaris, Ancylostoma, Strongyloides, Toxocara	Paragonimus	
Muscle				
Generalized myositis		Trichinella, Toxocara		
Myocarditis	Trypanosoma cruzi	Trichinella, Toxocara		
Skin and Subcutaneous Tissue				
Ulcerative lesion	Leishmania			
Nodule, swelling	Trypanosoma cruzi, Acanthamoeba	Onchocerca, Loa, Toxocara		
Rash, vesicles	Toxoplasma	Ancylostoma	Schistosoma	

ANTIPARASITIC AGENTS

Treatment of parasitic infections poses a potential problem. Because both parasites and humans are eukaryotic, many antiparasitic agents also act on human metabolic pathways; that is, these agents can pose a risk of toxicity. Differential toxicity is achieved by preferential uptake, metabolic alteration of the drug by the parasite, or differences in susceptibility between host and parasite. Agents used for the treatment of **protozoan infections** generally target nucleic acid synthesis, protein synthesis, or specific metabolic pathways that are unique for the rapidly proliferating parasites. In contrast, agents used for treatment of the **helminth infections** target unique metabolic pathways in the nonproliferating adult worms. Because the student may not be familiar with the antiparasitic agents, I will first present a listing of the different classes of agents and then summarize the specific agents used to treat each parasite. The following is a summary of the major antiparasitic agents and clinical indications.

Drug Class	Examples	Clinical Indications
Antiprotozoal Agents		
Heavy metals	Melarsoprol, sodium stibogluconate, meglumine antimoniate	Trypanosomiasis, leishmaniasis
Artemisinin derivatives	Artesunate, artemether, arterolane	Malaria
Aminoquinoline analogs	Chloroquine, piperaquine, mefloquine, quinine, primaquine, halofantrine, lumefantrine	Malaria prophylaxis and therapy
Folic acid antagonists	Sulfonamides, pyrimethamine, trimethoprim	Toxoplasmosis, malaria, cyclosporiasis
Inhibitors of protein synthesis	Clindamycin, spiramycin, paromomycin, tetracycline, doxycycline	Malaria, babesiosis, amebiasis, cryptosporidiosis, leishmaniasis
Diamidines	Pentamidine	Leishmaniasis, trypanosomiasis
Nitroimidazoles	Metronidazole, benznidazole, tinidazole	Amebiasis, giardiasis, trichomoniasis, trypanosomiasis
Nitrofurans	Nifurtimox	Trypanosomiasis
Phosphocholine analog	Miltefosine	Leishmaniasis
Sulfated naphthylamine	Suramin	Trypanosomiasis
Thiazolides	Nitazoxanide	Cryptosporidiosis, giardiasis
Antihelminthic Agents		
Benzimidazoles	Mebendazole, thiabendazole, albendazole	Broad-spectrum antihelminthic for nematodes and cestodes
Tetrahydropyrimidine	Pyrantel pamoate	Ascariasis, pinworm, hookworm
Piperazine	Piperazine, diethylcarbamazine	Ascaris and pinworm infections
Avermectins	Ivermectin	Filarial infections, strongyloidiasis, ascariasis, scabies
Prazinoisoquinoline	Praziquantel	Broad-spectrum antihelminthic for cestodes and trematodes
Phenol	Niclosamide	Infesting tapeworm
Quinolone	Bithionol, oxamniquine	Paragonimiasis, schistosomiasis
Organophosphate	Metrifonate	Schistosomiasis
Sulfated naphthylamine	Suramin	Onchocerciasis

The following table is a list of primary and secondary treatments for the most common parasites. Please note that for many of the groups of parasites, the same antiparasitic agents are used for treatment.

Parasite	Primary Antiparasitic Agents	Secondary Antiparasitic Agents
Intestinal Protozoa		
Entamoeba histolytica	Metronidazole + paromomycin	Iodoquinol; tinidazole + paromomycin
Cryptosporidium spp.	Nitazoxanide	Paromomycin + azithromycin
Cystoisospora belli	Trimethoprim-sulfamethoxazole	Ciprofloxacin; pyrimethamine
Cyclospora cayetanensis	Trimethoprim-sulfamethoxazole	Ciprofloxacin
Giardia duodenalis	Metronidazole; nitazoxanide	Furazolidone; paromomycin; quinacrine

Continued

Parasite	Primary Antiparasitic Agents	Secondary Antiparasitic Agents
Urogenital Protozoa		
Trichomonas vaginalis	Metronidazole	
Blood and Tissue Protozoa		
Acanthamoeba spp.	Miltefosine	
Naegleria fowleri	Miltefosine; amphotericin B	
Plasmodium spp.	Chloroquine; refer to current Centers for Disease Control and Prevention recommendations	
Babesia microti	Clindamycin + quinine; atovaquone + azithromycin	
Toxoplasma gondii	Pyrimethamine + sulfadiazine	
Leishmania spp.	Sodium stibogluconate; meglumine antimonite; miltefosine	Pentamidine; amphotericin B
Trypanosoma brucei	Suramin; pentamidine; melarsoprol (for central nervous system disease)	
Trypanosoma cruzi	Benznidazole; nifurtimox	
Intestinal Nematodes		
Ascaris lumbricoides	Albendazole	Mebendazole; pyrantel pamoate
Enterobius vermicularis	Mebendazole	Albendazole; pyrantel pamoate
Ancylostoma duodenale	Albendazole; mebendazole; pyrantel pamoate	
Necator americanus	Albendazole; mebendazole; pyrantel pamoate	
Strongyloides stercoralis	Ivermectin	Albendazole; mebendazole
Trichuris trichiura	Albendazole; mebendazole	
Blood Nematodes		
Brugia malayi	Diethylcarbamazine	Albendazole
Wuchereria bancrofti	Diethylcarbamazine	Albendazole
Loa loa	Diethylcarbamazine	
Onchocerca volvulus	Ivermectin	
Tissue Nematodes		
Trichinella spiralis	Mebendazole (adult worms only)	
Intestinal Trematodes		
Fasciolopsis buski	Praziquantel	Niclosamide
Tissue Trematodes		
Fasciola hepatica	Triclabendazole	Bithionol
Opisthorchis sinensis	Praziquantel	Albendazole
Paragonimus westermani	Praziquantel	Triclabendazole
Blood Trematodes		
Schistosoma mansoni	Praziquantel	Oxamniquine
Schistosoma japonica	Praziquantel	
Schistosoma haematobium	Praziquantel	

Parasite	Primary Antiparasitic Agents	Secondary Antiparasitic Agents
Intestinal Cestodes		
Taenia spp.	Praziquantel	Niclosamide
Diphyllobothrium latum	Praziquantel	Niclosamide
Hymonolepis spp	Praziquantel	Niclosamide
Dipylidium caninum	Praziquantel	Niclosamide
Tissue Cestodes		
Echinococcus spp.	Albendazole	Mebendazole; praziquantel

Protozoa

Protozoa are simple, unicellular parasites that are microscopic in size. Classification of protozoa is complex but the easiest way to organize these parasites is by where they produce disease. It is also useful to understand the reservoirs and vectors of these parasites.

Group	Parasite	Reservoir	Vector
Intestinal amoeba	*Entamoeba histolytica*	Humans	—
Coccidia	*Cyclospora cayetanensis*	Humans	—
	Cryptosporidium spp.	Humans	—
	Cystoisospora belli	Humans	—
Flagellates	*Giardia duodenalis*	Humans, beavers, muskrats	—
	Trichomonas vaginalis	Humans	—
Free-living amoeba	*Naegleria* spp.	Environment	
	Acanthamoeba spp.	Environment	
Blood and Tissue Protozoa	*Plasmodium* spp.	Humans	Mosquito
	Babesia microti	Rodents	Tick
	Toxoplasma gondii	Cat	—
	Leishmania spp.	Rodents, dogs	Sandfly
	Trypanosoma brucei	Domestic animals, humans, cattle, sheep, wild game	Tsetse fly
	Trypanosoma cruzi	Wild animals	Reduviid bug

The protozoa listed in this chapter are certainly not a comprehensive list of all protozoa or even all protozoa associated with human disease; however, the most important species are included in this chapter.

INTESTINAL AMOEBA

The intestinal protozoa can be subdivided into the amebae, coccidia, and flagellates. *E. histolytica* represents the intestinal amebae and must be differentiated from a number of nonpathogenic amebae that can also be found in the intestines (this is done by their morphologic appearance and is not discussed further in this chapter). Although not common in the United States, infections can be acquired when traveling to countries with poor hygienic standards.

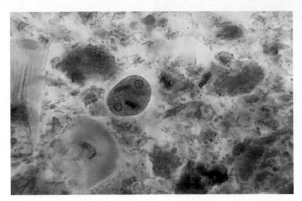

Trichrome stain of *Entamoeba histolytica* cyst with two nuclei and an elongated chromatoidal bar in the cytoplasm.

ENTAMOEBA HISTOLYTICA	
Epidemiology	• Worldwide distribution • Most prevalent in tropical and subtropical regions with poor hygiene • Many asymptomatic carriers serve as reservoirs for disease • Two forms of parasites: infectious cysts and noninfectious, replicating trophozoites • Trophozoites replicate in the lumen of the colon • Transmission through contaminated water and food or through oral-anal sexual practices
Clinical Disease	• **Asymptomatic carriage** • **Intestinal amebiasis**: localized infection of the colon presenting with abdominal pain, cramping, and diarrhea • **Extraintestinal amebiasis**: dissemination to **liver** with abscess formation is most common
Diagnosis	• Intestinal amebiasis most commonly diagnosed by microscopic detection of trophozoites and cysts in stool specimens • Nucleic acid amplification tests (NAATs) available for detection of *E. histolytica* in stool specimens • Parasites may not be observed in stool specimens for patients with extraintestinal infections; serology is the most reliable diagnostic method for these patients
Treatment, Prevention, Control	• Acute, noninvasive intestinal disease treated with metronidazole plus paromomycin • Invasive infections treated with metronidazole or tinidazole plus paromomycin or diloxanide furoate • Prevention and control through implementation of appropriate sanitation standards and use of chlorination and filtration of water where necessary

COCCIDIA

Three **coccidia** are discussed in this chapter: *Cyclospora*, *Cryptosporidium*, and *Cystoisospora*. *Cyclospora* infections in the United States are typically associated with food-related outbreaks such as with raw fruits or vegetables shipped from countries with poor hygienic conditions. *Cryptosporidium* and *Cystoisospora* were initially implicated in intestinal disease in HIV-infected individuals but are now recognized as pathogens of both immunocompetent and immunocompromised individuals. *Cryptosporidium* is associated with large outbreaks when drinking water or recreational waters are contaminated. Many species of *Cryptosporidium* infect a variety of animals, but *Cryptosporidium hominis* and *Cryptosporidium parvum* are most commonly associated with human infections.

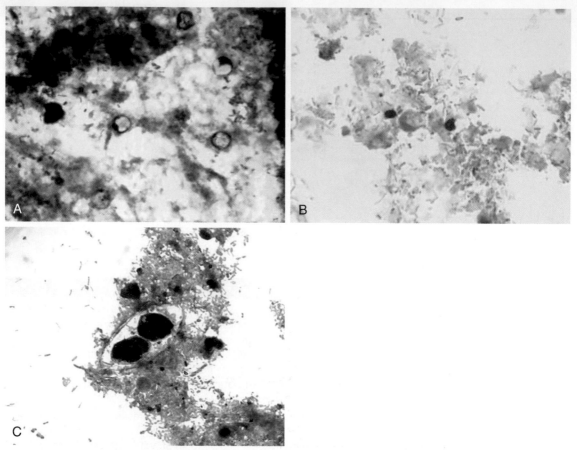

Acid-fast stains of (A) *Cyclospora*, (B) *Cryptosporidium*, and (C) *Cystoisospora*.

CYCLOSPORA CAYETANENSIS	
Epidemiology	<ul><li>Worldwide distribution</li><li>Most prevalent in tropical and subtropical regions with poor hygiene</li><li>Infection from ingestion of contaminated food (e.g., raw fruits and vegetables) or water; person-to-person transmission not observed</li><li>Outbreaks most common during the spring and summer months</li><li>Small (8–10 μm), spherical, noninfectious oocysts are passed in stool; in the external environment they develop two internal sporocysts, each of which contain two sporozoites</li><li>When the oocyst is ingested, the sporozoites are liberated and enter the epithelial cells of the **small intestine** where they establish disease</li></ul>
Clinical Disease	<ul><li>**Asymptomatic carriage**</li><li>**Mild to severe diarrheal disease** with nausea, anorexia, abdominal cramping, and watery diarrhea; self-limiting disease in immunocompetent patients although symptoms may persist for weeks</li><li>**Chronic infection** can occur, particularly in HIV-infected patients</li></ul>
Diagnosis	<ul><li>Infection most commonly diagnosed by microscopic detection of oocysts in stool specimens</li></ul>
Treatment, Prevention, Control	<ul><li>Drug of choice is trimethoprim-sulfamethoxazole; alternative ciprofloxacin or nitazoxanide</li><li>Maintain personal hygiene and high sanitary conditions</li><li>Treatment of water with chlorine or iodine is generally not effective because the oocysts are relatively resistant</li></ul>

CRYPTOSPORIDIUM SPP.

Epidemiology	• Worldwide distribution • Infection most commonly associated with contaminated water or fecal-oral, oral-anal transmission • Small (4–6 μm), spherical, infectious oocysts containing sporozoites are excreted in feces • Ingested sporozoites attach to brush border of epithelial cells lining the **small intestine** where they establish disease • Well-documented outbreaks associated with contaminated water such as in reservoirs or recreational water parks and pools
Clinical Disease	• **Asymptomatic carriage** • Symptomatic disease similar to disease with *Cyclospora* • **Enterocolitis** characterized by watery diarrhea with remission after 10 days in immunocompetent patients • More **severe enterocolitis** in immunocompromised patients (e.g., HIV-infected patients) that can evolve into chronic disease
Diagnosis	• Detection of oocysts in stool specimens by microscopy, immunoassay, or NAATs
Treatment, Prevention, Control	• Infections in immunocompetent patients are self-limiting • Nitazoxanide is used to treat immunocompetent patients; alternative paromomycin plus azithromycin; no effective treatment for immunocompromised patients • Prevention of disease is difficult because widespread distribution in animals and inadvertent contamination of water supplies and recreational waters • Maintain personal hygiene and high sanitary conditions; avoid oral-anal sexual practices

CYSTOISOSPORA BELLI

Epidemiology	• Worldwide distribution • Most prevalent in tropical and subtropical regions with poor hygiene • Infection from ingestion of contaminated food or water, or oral-anal sexual contact • Large, oblong, noninfectious oocysts are passed in stool; in the external environment they develop two internal sporocysts, each of which contain four sporozoites • When the oocyst is ingested, the sporozoites are liberated and enter the epithelial cells of the **small intestine** where they establish disease
Clinical Disease	• **Asymptomatic carriage** • **Mild to severe diarrheal disease**, similar to giardiasis • **Chronic infection** can occur, particularly in HIV-infected patients
Diagnosis	• Infection most commonly diagnosed by microscopic detection of oocysts in stool specimens
Treatment, Prevention, Control	• Drug of choice is trimethoprim-sulfamethoxazole; alternative ciprofloxacin or pyrimethamine • Maintain personal hygiene and high sanitary conditions; avoid oral-anal sexual practices

FLAGELLATES

Two flagellates (so named because their flagella, or hairlike structures, are a key morphologic feature for their identification) are discussed in this chapter: the intestinal protozoa *G. duodenalis* and the urogenital protozoa *T. vaginalis*.

In contrast with most of the other parasites discussed in this chapter, *G. duodenalis* (also called *Giardia lamblia* and *Giardia intestinalis*) is widely disseminated in the United States. Wild animals are an important reservoir for this parasite, and their feces can contaminate many streams and lakes as well as drinking water such as from wells.

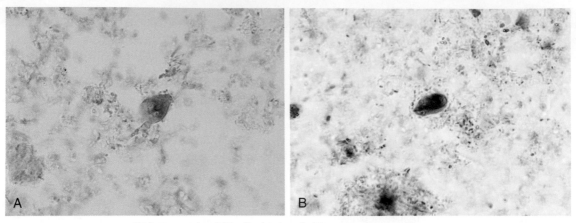

Trichrome stain of *Giardia duodenalis* (A) trophozoite and (B) cyst.

GIARDIA DUODENALIS

Epidemiology	• Worldwide distribution • Animals such as beavers and muskrats serve as the natural reservoir • Asymptomatic human carriers also serve as a reservoir • Two forms of parasite: infectious cysts and noninfectious, replicating trophozoites • Human infections most commonly from ingestion of cyst-contaminated water or food products • Person-to-person spread through fecal-oral contamination • Outbreaks reported in day-care facilities, nurseries, and long-term care institutions
Clinical Disease	• **Asymptomatic carriage** • Infection (**giardiasis**) of **small intestine** with symptoms ranging from diarrhea to malabsorption syndrome • Incubation period on average 10 days; onset sudden with foul-smelling watery diarrhea, abdominal cramps, flatulence • Symptoms persist for 1–2 weeks although chronic disease may develop
Diagnosis	• Intestinal giardiasis most commonly diagnosed by microscopic detection of trophozoites and cysts in stool specimens • NAATs now available for detection of *G. duodenalis* in stool specimens • Immunoassays and fluorescent antibody tests are available but less sensitive than NAATs
Treatment, Prevention, Control	• Drug of choice is metronidazole or nitazoxanide; alternatives furazolidone; paromomycin; quinacrine • Avoid contaminated water and food • Chlorine treatment alone is insufficient because the cysts are relatively resistant; water should be boiled or filtered

The importance of *T. vaginalis* has been underappreciated because most women and men infected with this parasite are asymptomatic. However, carriage of this organism increases the risk of infection and transmission of other sexually transmitted diseases and places pregnant women at increased risk of premature delivery.

TRICHOMONAS VAGINALIS

Epidemiology	• Worldwide distribution • Trophozoite is the only form; colonizes urethra and vagina in women and urethra in men • Person-to-person transmission through sexual intercourse
Clinical Disease	• Most infected individuals are **asymptomatic** • **Vaginitis** and **urethritis**: inflammation of the epithelial lining with associated itching, burning, painful urination, vaginal discharge in women, and urethral discharge • Without treatment, infections can persist for months or years
Diagnosis	• Detection of parasite by microscopic examination, culture, or NAAT of discharge • NAAT is the most sensitive test and preferred for detection of asymptomatic and symptomatic infected individuals
Treatment, Prevention, Control	• Metronidazole is the drug of choice • To avoid reinfection, both sexual partners must be treated • Safe sexual practices must be maintained

FREE-LIVING AMOEBA

Two free-living amebae are discussed in this chapter: *Naegleria* and *Acanthamoeba*. Both are important human pathogens capable of causing overwhelming and rapidly fatal disease but fortunately are relatively uncommon.

NAEGLERIA SPP.

Epidemiology	• Worldwide distribution • Common in soil and freshwater lakes and rivers • Infections are most common after exposure to trophozoites in contaminated waters in the warm summer months • Parasite enters the body through the nose and migrates to the brain; infections are not caused by ingestion of contaminated waters
Clinical Disease	• **Primary amebic meningoencephalitis**: rapidly progressive and fatal destruction of brain tissue
Diagnosis	• Because of the rapid progression of disease, diagnosis by history of exposure and clinical symptoms is confirmed postmortem • Detection of parasite by microscopic examination of cerebrospinal fluid or brain tissue • NAATs available only in reference laboratories
Treatment, Prevention, Control	• Treatment is generally ineffective because of the rapid progression of disease, although the experimental drug miltefosine is available through the Centers for Disease Control and Prevention (CDC); alternative amphotericin B • Prevention is difficult because of the widespread distribution of the parasite

ACANTHAMOEBA SPP.

Epidemiology	• Worldwide distribution • Common in soil and freshwater lakes and rivers; in tap water and bottle water; can contaminate dialysis fluids and contact lens cleaners • Infections of the eye most commonly associated with improperly cleaned contact lenses used by patients with mild preexisting trauma to the cornea (e.g., scratched or irritated cornea)
Clinical Disease	• **Keratitis**: symptoms can range from irritation, redness, and mild eye pain to rapid destruction of the cornea • **Granulomatous amebic encephalitis**: disease primarily in immunocompromised patients with a longer incubation period and slower progression than that observed with *Naegleria* infections

Continued

ACANTHAMOEBA SPP.—cont'd	
Diagnosis	• Culture of eye scrapings is a sensitive and rapid method to diagnose amebic keratitis (specimens are inoculated onto an agar plate covered with a film of gram-negative bacteria; the trail of migrating amebae is easily visualized after overnight incubation) • Detection of the parasite by microscopic examination of the brain tissue is the test of choice for amebic encephalitis
Treatment, Prevention, Control	• Treatment is generally ineffective although the experimental drug miltefosine is available through the CDC • Eye infections are avoided by using sterile cleaning solutions for contact lenses and avoiding the use of lenses if the eye is irritated

BLOOD PROTOZOA

Two protozoa are important blood-borne parasites: *Plasmodium* and *Babesia*. In contrast with the protozoa discussed previously, all the blood and tissue protozoa require important vectors for transmission of disease: the *Anopheles* mosquito for malaria (*Plasmodium*) and the tick for babesiosis (*Babesia*).

Five species of *Plasmodium* are responsible for malaria in humans: *Plasmodium falciparum*, *Plasmodium vivax*, *Plasmodium ovale*, *Plasmodium malariae*, and *Plasmodium knowlesi*, with the first two species the most common. In 2019, the World Health Organization estimated that there were almost 230 million cases of malaria and more than 400,000 deaths, primarily children in Africa. Approximately 2000 cases of malaria occur in the United States each year, mainly in travelers and immigrants from endemic areas, although transmission in the United States is well documented.

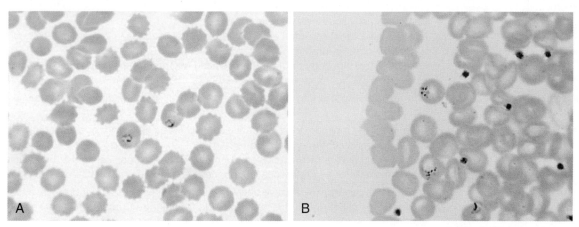

Giemsa stain of peripheral blood with infection with (A) *Plasmodium falciparum* and (B) *Babesia microti*.

PLASMODIUM SPP.	
Epidemiology	• Tropical and subtropical regions of Africa, India, Southeast Asia, Russia, China • Individual species can be geographically restricted • *Plasmodium* species share a similar lifecycle • Human infection initiated by the bite of the *Anopheles* **mosquito** which transmits infectious sporozoites into the blood; sporozoites are carried to the liver cells where replication occurs; when the hepatocytes rupture, infectious merozoites are released into the blood and the merozoites attach, penetrate, and replicate in erythrocytes • Mosquitos are infected when they ingest sexually mature forms of the parasite—gametocytes

PLASMODIUM SPP.—cont'd

Clinical Disease	• The clinical presentation of **malaria** is a function of the individual species of *Plasmodium* (e.g., *Plasmodium falciparum* produces the most severe symptoms) and preexisting exposure (milder disease can occur in patients with partial immunity)
	• Onset of disease can be acute following a period of replication in the liver cells; symptoms include chills, fever, and myalgias and can progress to nausea, vomiting, and diarrhea; symptoms can be periodic (a day of acute symptoms followed by a few days of mild symptoms) corresponding to synchronized infection and rupture of erythrocytes
	• *Plasmodium vivax* and *Plasmodium ovale* can establish a **dormant liver phase** that can be activated months or years after the primary infection, producing symptoms of an acute infection
Diagnosis	• Detection of the parasite in infected erythrocytes by microscopy (Giemsa stain)
	• Detection of characteristic forms in infected cells is used to differentiate the individual species
	• NAAT is the most sensitive method for detection and identification of parasites but these tests are not currently widely available
	• Immunoassays are available; these tests are rapid but not as sensitive as microscopy
Treatment, Prevention, Control	• Treatment is complicated because resistance to the most commonly used drug, chloroquine, is widespread; the CDC (or similar organization) guidelines should be followed for treatment of infections with known or suspected resistant strains
	• Risk of infection can be reduced through the use of protective clothing, mosquito repellants on exposed skin, and prophylactic antibiotics when traveling in endemic regions
	• Vaccines for prevention of infections are under investigation

Many species of *Babesia* cause human disease worldwide, but the focus in this chapter is the most common species in the United States responsible for disease, with more than 2000 cases reported annually.

BABESIA MICROTI

Epidemiology	• Northeastern and upper Midwestern states in the United States
	• Wild rodents (e.g., white footed mouse) are the primary reservoir
	• *Ixodes* (deer) **ticks** are the vector of disease and either become infected by feeding on an infected rodent or transovarially; humans are accidental hosts
	• Most infections result from the nymph stage of the tick so a history of a tick bite may not be elicited (nymphs are very tiny [size of poppy seed])
	• Most infections are during the spring and summer months
	• During the blood meal, infectious sporozoites are released into the human blood stream and enter into erythrocytes where the parasites replicate
Clinical Disease	• **Babesiosis** is characterized by the onset of malaise, fever, headache, chills, sweating, and fatigue; more severe disease occurs in immunocompromised patients
Diagnosis	• Detection of the parasite in infected erythrocytes by microscopy (Giemsa stain)
	• NAATs are available primarily in reference laboratories
Treatment, Prevention, Control	• Atovaquone plus azithromycin is used for mild disease; clindamycin plus quinine, and exchange transfusion is used for severe disease
	• Infections are prevented by use of protective clothing and insect repellents; prompt removal of ticks (although they may not be noticed) because they must feed for several hours to transmit disease

TISSUE PROTOZOA

Three genera of tissue protozoa are discussed here: *Toxoplasma* which is found worldwide including in the United States, and *Leishmania* and *Trypanosoma* which have a more restricted geographic distribution.

Unfortunately, we do not have to travel very far to be exposed to *Toxoplasma*—it is as close as the pet cat.

The parasitic lifecycle is maintained in cats, who shed *T. gondii* oocysts that mature into infectious forms in a few days. The infectious forms are consumed by rodents, which in turn are consumed by cats. Humans are the unfortunate accidental hosts.

TOXOPLASMA GONDII	
Epidemiology	• Worldwide distribution • Domestic **cats** serve as the reservoir • Parasite replicates in the intestinal epithelial cells; noninfectious oocysts are passed in cat feces; the oocysts mature over 2–3 days forming two sporocysts, each containing four sporozoites • Human infections develop following exposure to infectious oocysts following handling cat feces or ingestion of **oocysts** in improperly cooked meat from infected animals (e.g., pork, lamb); transplacental transmission can also occur
Clinical Disease	• **Asymptomatic infection** • Symptoms of **toxoplasmosis** are dependent on the immune status of the host (disease most severe for the fetus *in utero* and in immunocompromised patients) and the tissues involved (e.g., lung, heart, lymphoid organs, and central nervous system) • Disease characterized by tissue destruction with abscess formation and formation of cysts • Encephalopathy, meningoencephalitis, and cerebral mass lesion can develop in immunocompromised patients
Diagnosis	• Most infections diagnosed by serology or microscopic detection of cysts in infected tissue • NAATs available in reference laboratories
Treatment, Prevention, Control	• Mild infections can be managed symptomatically; severe or disseminated infections treated with pyrimethamine plus sulfadiazine; treatment may be lifelong • Pregnant women and immunocompromised patients should avoid exposure to cat feces or consumption of under-cooked meat

The taxonomy of *Leishmania* is in a state of flux and the names of the individual species are not critical for understanding the diseases they produce.

LEISHMANIA SPP.	
Epidemiology	• Individual species restricted to specific geographies • Parasites found in Southern Europe and tropical and subtropical regions including Africa, Asia, Middle East, Latin America • Reservoir hosts include rodents and dogs; transmission from host-to-humans or human-to-human is through the bite of a sandfly (smaller than a mosquito) • **Promastigote** stage of the parasite is in the saliva of an infected sandfly; after injection, the promastigote transforms into the **amastigote** stage and invades the human reticuloendothelial cells where they multiply; rupture of the cells and further replication produces localized or disseminated disease • Sandflies become infected when they ingest a blood meal with amastigotes; these transform to infectious promastigotes in the fly midgut and migrate to the salivary gland during a blood meal • Clinical manifestations are a function of the species of parasite and immune status of patient
Clinical Disease	• **Cutaneous leishmaniasis**: a localized ulcer at the site of the bite • **Mucocutaneous leishmaniasis**: progression of disease with destruction of adjacent mucous membranes • **Disseminated or visceral leishmaniasis**: self-limited mild disease; fulminant disease with multiorgan destruction (e.g., liver, spleen, kidneys); or chronic process
Diagnosis	• Clinical diagnosis in endemic region confirmed by demonstration of amastigotes in tissue by microscopy, immunoassay, or NAATs
Treatment, Prevention, Control	• Treatment of choice for all forms of leishmaniasis is sodium stibogluconate, meglumine antimonite, or miltefosine; alternatives pentamidine or amphotericin B • Prevention by control of vector and treatment of infected humans

Two species of *Trypanosoma*, *Trypanosoma brucei* and *Trypanosoma cruzi*, produce very different diseases in different regions of the world, so they are presented separately. Additionally, *T. brucei* is subdivided into subspecies that are geographically restricted to regions of Africa and produce variants on the disease most commonly called **African Sleeping Sickness** due to the parasites' effects on the central nervous system.

TRYPANOSOMA BRUCEI	
Epidemiology	• *T. brucei gambiense* in tropical West and Central Africa (Democratic Republic of Congo, Angola, Sudan, Central African Republic, Chad, northern Uganda) • *T. brucei rhodesiense* in East Africa (Tanzania, Uganda, Malawi, Zambia) • Animal reservoir for *T. b. gambiense* is most likely domestic animals and humans; reservoirs for *T. b. rhodesiense* are cattle, sheep, and wild game • Transmission by **tsetse flies** (*Glossina*) • An infected tsetse fly injects **trypomastigotes** into skin tissue during a blood meal; these mature and are transported by blood to other body fluids (cerebrospinal fluid, lymph) where replication continues • Tsetse flies become infected when they ingest bloodstream trypomastigotes that will multiply in the fly midgut; this form transforms into the **epimastigote** and migrates to the salivary glands where replication continues

Continued

TRYPANOSOMA BRUCEI—cont'd

Clinical Disease	• **African sleeping sickness**: *T. b. gambiense* disease develops after an incubation period of days to a few weeks; an ulcer may develop at the site of the bite; fever, myalgia, arthralgia, and lymph node enlargement; chronic disease progresses to central nervous system, involvement with lethargy, tremors, meningoencephalitis, mental retardation, and eventual death • *T. b. rhodesiense* disease has a more acute progression with death occurring in the first year in untreated patients
Diagnosis	• Detection of trypomastigotes in blood and spinal fluid is the diagnostic test of choice • Immunoassays and NAATs are insensitive
Treatment, Prevention, Control	• Suramin or pentamidine is used to treat acute infections; if central nervous system involvement is suspected, melarsoprol is the drug of choice • Control by reducing the human reservoir and insect control, although this is difficult in resource-limited countries

TRYPANOSOMA CRUZI

Epidemiology	• Mexico, Central America, and South America • Reservoir is a variety of wild animals and the vector for transmission is the **reduviid bug** (kissing bug) • Vector nests in homes, particularly with mud walls and thatched roofs • Human infections can also be transmitted congenitally, in contaminated blood products and following organ transplantation • Transmission occurs during a blood meal when **trypomastigotes** in the bug feces contaminate the bite wound; the parasites invade cells at the bite wound, transform into the **amastigote** stage, and replicate; the amastigote stage transforms in the trypomastigote stage and exits the cell to either reinfect other cells or be ingested by a feeding bug • In the reduviid bug, the trypomastigotes are transformed into epimastigotes and replicate in the midgut, which in turn are transformed into trypomastigotes in the hindgut
Clinical Disease	• **Asymptomatic disease** • **Acute Chagas disease**: characterized by erythema and induration at the site of the bug bite; followed by fever, chills, malaise, myalgia, and fatigue • **Chronic Chagas disease**: progression to chronic stage characterized by hepatosplenomegaly, myocarditis, and enlargement of the esophagus and colon; central nervous system involvement with meningoencephalitis may also occur
Diagnosis	• Detection of trypomastigotes in blood in the early stages of disease or amastigotes in infected tissues • Serology and NAATs are insensitive
Treatment, Prevention, Control	• All infected patients should be treated; the drugs of choice are benznidazole and nifurtimox, although these are less effective for chronic disease • Bug control through use of insecticides and quality home construction will reduce exposure

CLINICAL CASES (REFER TO SECTION VI)

Gastrointestinal Tract Infections
- Amoebic liver abscess in HIV patient
- Cryptosporidiosis outbreak in university students
- Cyclospora infection in immunocompetent traveler
- Drug-resistant giardiasis in an AIDS patient

Central Nervous System Infections
- Toxoplasmosis in woman with Hodgkin Disease

Sepsis and Cardiovascular Infections
- Malaria
- Trypanosomiasis in an 18-month-old boy

SUPPLEMENTAL READING

1. Haque R, et al. Amoebiasis. *N Engl J Med.* 2003;348(16):1565–1573.
2. Minetti C, et al. Giardiasis. *Brit Med J.* 2016;355:i5369.
3. Bouzid M, et al. *Cryptosporidium* pathogenicity and virulence. *Clin Microbiol Rev.* 2013;26(1):115–134.
4. Almeria S, Cinar H, Dubey J. *Cyclospora cayetanensis* and cyclosporiasis: an update. *Microorganisms.* 2019;7(9):317–350.
5. Garcia LS. Malaria. *Clin Lab Med.* 2010;30(1):93–129.
6. Young KM, et al. Zoonotic *Babesia*: a scoping review of the global evidence. *PLoS One.* 2019;14(12), e0226781.
7. Saadatnia G, Golkar M. A review of human toxoplasmosis. *Scand J Infect Dis.* 2012;44(11):805–814.
8. Echeverria LE, Morilla CA. American trypanosomiasis. *Infect Dis Clin North Am.* 2019;33(1):119–134.
9. Buscher P, et al. Human African trypanosomiasis. *Lancet.* 2017;390(10110):2397–2409.
10. Burza S, Croft SL, Boelaert M. Leishmaniasis. *Lancet.* 2018;392(10151):951–970.

25

Nematodes

The helminths or "worms" are subdivided into three groups: nematodes ("roundworms"), trematodes ("flatworms"), and cestodes ("tapeworms"). Roundworms are presented in this chapter, and the flatworms and tapeworms in the following two chapters. It is easiest to remember roundworms based on where they are found in human infections.

Intestinal Nematodes	*Enterobius vermicularis* ("pinworm")
	Trichuris trichiura ("whipworm")
	Ascaris lumbricoides ("roundworm")
	Strongyloides stercoralis ("threadworm")
	Necator americanus and *Ancylostoma duodenale* ("hookworm")
Blood Nematodes	*Brugia malayi* ("Malayan filariasis" or "elephantiasis")
	Wuchereria bancrofti ("Bancroft filariasis" or "elephantiasis")
	Loa loa ("African eye worm")
	Onchocerca volvulus (onchocerciasis or "river blindness")
Tissue Nematodes	*Trichinella spiralis* ("trichinosis")
	Toxocara canis ("visceral larva migrans")
	Ancylostoma braziliense ("cutaneous larva migrans")

INTESTINAL NEMATODES

These nematodes share several important features. They have a simple lifecycle with **humans as their only hosts**, and infections are the result of ingestion of infectious eggs containing larvae (*Enterobius, Trichuris, Ascaris*) or exposure to larvae (*Strongyloides, Necator, Ancylostoma*) present in the soil that invade through exposed skin (i.e.,

bare feet). Because their lifecycles involve shedding of eggs or (with *Strongyloides*) larvae in feces, these are diseases in communities with poor sanitary conditions. The exception to this is infection with *Enterobius* where the adult worms deposit eggs on the anal folds at night and the eggs are infectious within a few hours. Enterobius infections are readily spread person-to-person, so they are common in most communities. Except for *Enterobius*, asymptomatic infections with intestinal nematodes are common in residents of communities where the worms are endemic, while acute symptomatic disease is more common in previously unexposed visitors. Diagnosis is made by detecting characteristic eggs or larvae in fecal specimens, again except for *Enterobius* where the eggs are deposited on the skin surrounding the anus and are not found in feces. Treatment for all these infections is the same, as are preventive measures. The following are some important general facts about the intestinal nematodes:

Intestinal Nematode	Route of Infection	Migration Through Lungs (Pneumonitis)	Diagnosis	Primary Treatment
Enterobius vermicularis	Ingestion of eggs	No	Eggs in anal folds	Albendazole, mebendazole
Trichuris trichiura	Ingestion of eggs	No	Eggs in stool	Albendazole, mebendazole
Ascaris lumbricoides	Ingestion of eggs	Yes	Eggs in stool	Albendazole, mebendazole
Necator americanus	Larvae penetrate skin	Yes	Eggs in stool	Albendazole, mebendazole
Ancylostoma duodenale	Larvae penetrate skin	Yes	Eggs in stool	Albendazole, mebendazole
Strongyloides stercoralis	Larvae penetrate skin	Yes	Larvae in stool	Ivermectin

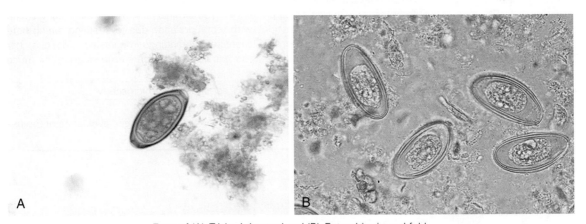

Eggs of (A) *Trichuris* in stool and (B) *Enterobius* in anal fold.

ENTEROBIUS VERMICULARIS	
Epidemiology	• Worldwide distribution • Humans are the only host for "pinworm" infections; no animal reservoir or insect vector • Infection through ingestion of eggs • Adults mature in 3–4 weeks, and female worms migrate to the anus to discharge their eggs; the embryonated eggs develop to the infective stage in 4–6 h • Infections most common in children, members of a household with children, and residents of institutionalized care facilities • Highly infectious for humans; pets and other animals are not susceptible to this parasite
Clinical Disease	• **Enterobiasis** characterized by irritation of the anal fold by the migrating adult worms when they deposit their eggs leading to severe itching and loss of sleep

ENTEROBIUS VERMICULARIS—cont'd

Diagnosis	• Detection and identification of worm eggs at the anus; eggs are collected on a sticky paddle and examined by microscopy; occasionally small adult worms will also be observed • Eggs are not typically observed in stool specimens
Treatment, Prevention, Control	• The drug of choice is mebendazole, alternatives are albendazole or pyrantel pamoate; treatment consists of a single dose followed by another dose 2 weeks later • The entire household should be treated to reduce the risk of reinfections

TRICHURIS TRICHIURA

Epidemiology	• Worldwide, particularly in tropical regions where sanitation is poor • Humans are the only hosts for "whipworm" infections; no animal reservoir or insect vector • Human infection by ingestion of embryonated egg, primarily from food products grown in soil contaminated with human feces • Eggs hatch in the small intestine, releasing the larval form that migrates to the **colon** where it develops into an adult worm; egg production begins after about 2 months; eggs are passed in the stool and require 2–4 weeks in soil to develop into infective forms
Clinical Disease	• **Asymptomatic infection** is the most common condition in endemic areas • Symptomatic **trichuriasis** may present with abdominal pain, bloody diarrhea, weakness, and weight loss; severe infections with rectal prolapse due to straining during defecation, and anemia and eosinophilia (characteristic findings in parasitic infections characterized by tissue invasion—in this case, the adult worms are embedded in the mucosal layer of the large intestine)
Diagnosis	• Detection of characteristic eggs in stool specimens by microscopy
Treatment, Prevention, Control	• The drug of choice is albendazole or mebendazole • Good personal hygiene, maintenance of sanitary conditions, and avoidance of the use of human feces as fertilizer

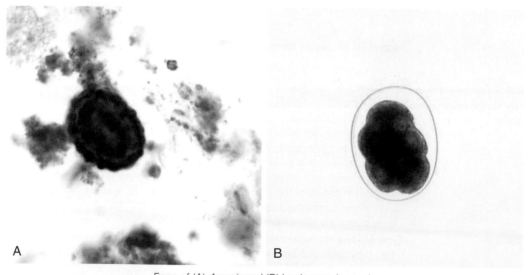

Eggs of (A) *Ascaris* and (B) hookworm in stool.

ASCARIS LUMBRICOIDES

Epidemiology	• Worldwide distribution, particularly in tropical regions where sanitation is poor • Humans are the only hosts for "roundworm" infections; no animal reservoir or insect vector • Human infection by ingestion of embryonated egg, primarily from food products grown in soils contaminated with human feces • Eggs hatch in the **small intestine**, releasing the larval form that invades the intestinal mucosa and is carried by the circulatory system to the lungs, where larvae mature for approximately 2 weeks; they then penetrate the alveolar walls, ascend to the throat, and are swallowed; the larvae mature into adult worms in the small intestine and initiate egg production approximately 3 months after the eggs were initially ingested
Clinical Disease	• **Asymptomatic infection** is the most common condition in endemic areas • Migration of the larvae through the lungs can produce an irritation (**pneumonitis**) with cough and eosinophilia • Symptomatic **ascariasis** can be mild abdominal discomfort (light infections) or intestinal obstruction (heavy infections with these very large adult worms)
Diagnosis	• Detection of characteristic eggs in stool specimens by microscopy • Passage of an adult worm can be alarming because of the size (20–35 cm; 8–14 in) but is diagnostic because it is the largest of the intestinal helminths
Treatment, Prevention, Control	• The drug of choice is albendazole; alternatives are mebendazole or pyrantel pamoate • Good personal hygiene, maintenance of sanitary conditions, and avoidance of the use of human feces as fertilizer

NECATOR AMERICANUS AND ANCYLOSTOMA DUODENALE

Epidemiology	• Worldwide although the individual parasites differ geographically • *N. americanus* distribution in the United States more limited with improved hygienic conditions • Present in warm, moist climates where the soil is contaminated with human feces • Humans are the only hosts for "hookworm" infections; no animal reservoir or insect vectors • Human infections occur when infectious larvae (**filariform larvae**) present in the soil penetrate exposed skin, migrate in the blood to the lungs, penetrate into the pulmonary alveoli, ascend to the pharynx and are swallowed; in the **small intestine** the larvae mature to adult worms, attach to the intestinal wall, and initiate egg production; eggs are passed in the stool and when in contact with the soil, release their immature larvae (**rhabditiform larvae**) which mature into the infectious filariform larvae in approximately 2 weeks
Clinical Disease	• **Asymptomatic infection** is the most common condition in endemic areas • Migration of the larvae through the lungs can produce an irritation (**pneumonitis**) with cough and eosinophilia • **Hookworm infections** can produce symptoms of nausea, vomiting, and diarrhea, as well as anemia from the feeding adult worms
Diagnosis	• Detection of characteristic eggs in stool specimens by microscopy • The eggs of both hookworms cannot be differentiated
Treatment, Prevention, Control	• The drugs of choice are albendazole, mebendazole, or pyrantel pamoate • Good personal hygiene, maintenance of sanitary conditions, and avoidance of contamination of soil with human feces

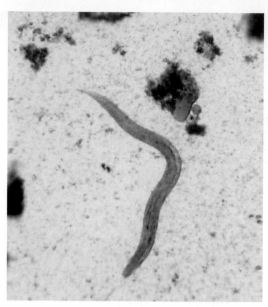

Strongyloides larva in stool.

STRONGYLOIDES STERCORALIS

Epidemiology	• Worldwide distribution, particularly in tropical regions where sanitation is poor • Estimated between 30 and 100 million persons are infected worldwide • Humans are the only hosts for "threadworm" infections; no animal reservoir or insect vectors • Lifecycle is very similar to hookworms; infectious filariform larvae present in the soil penetrate through exposed skin and migrate to the small intestine either directly or through the lungs; the worms mature into adults, attach to the wall of the **small intestine**, and produce eggs • In contrast with hookworms, the rhabditiform larvae in the eggs are released into the lumen of the intestine and that is the form detected in stool specimens • Rhabditiform larvae mature to filariform larvae in the soil; alternatively, rhabditiform larvae can mature to filariform larvae in patients with heavy worm burdens and reinfect the patient (**autoinfection**) without undergoing a stage of external development • Infections can persist for many years
Clinical Disease	• **Asymptomatic infection** is the most common condition in endemic areas • Migration of the larvae through the lungs can produce an irritation (**pneumonitis**) with cough and eosinophilia • Symptomatic **strongyloidiasis** can produce symptoms of epigastric pain and tenderness, vomiting, diarrhea, and malabsorption • Severe, chronic infections can develop in immunocompromised patients
Diagnosis	• Detection of larvae in stool specimens by microscopy; multiple specimens may need to be examined because shedding may be infrequent • Larvae can also be detected by spreading a stool specimen in the center of an agar plate; after overnight incubation, larvae can be detected by a trail of bacteria on the agar surface as the larvae migrates to the periphery of the plate
Treatment, Prevention, Control	• The drug of choice is ivermectin; alternatives are albendazole or mebendazole • Good personal hygiene, maintenance of sanitary conditions, and avoidance of contamination of soil with human feces

BLOOD NEMATODES

The blood nematodes are grouped together because dissemination of **microfilariae** in the blood is an important feature of human disease. These nematodes have a more complex lifecycle with an **insect vector** important for transmission of all four parasites, but **humans are the only hosts**. Like the intestinal nematodes, there is **no animal reservoir** so control and elimination of disease is focused on rapid diagnosis and treatment of human disease, with insect control playing a secondary role. These diseases are also much more restricted in their geographic distributions, which offers a realistic opportunity to focus public health efforts on elimination of these diseases. However, it must be realized that a significant proportion of the population in endemic regions is infected asymptomatically. Disease is associated with migration of microfilariae in the blood and tissues and, with *Brugia* and *Wuchereria*, the obstruction of lymphatic flow with subsequent enlargement of distal tissues ("elephantiasis"). Diagnosis of disease is by detecting microfilariae in the blood of individuals (*Brugia*, *Wuchereria*, and *Loa*) or in the skin of patients infected with *Onchocerca*. The microfilariae have a characteristic morphology, which allows differentiation of individual species. The following are some important general facts about the blood nematodes:

Blood Nematode	Vector	Location of Adult Worm	Diagnosis	Treatment (Microfilariae)
Brugia malayi	Mosquito	Lymphatics, lymph nodes	Microfilariae in blood	Diethylcarbamazine
Wuchereria bancrofti	Mosquito	Lymphatics, lymph nodes	Microfilariae in blood	Diethylcarbamazine
Loa loa	Deerfly	Subcutaneous tissues	Microfilariae in blood	Diethylcarbamazine
Onchocerca volvulus	Blackfly	Subcutaneous tissues	Microfilariae in skin	Ivermectin

BRUGIA MALAYI AND *WUCHERERIA BANCROFTI*	
Epidemiology	• Broad geographic distribution in tropical and subtropical areas of Africa, Mediterranean coast, India, Southeast Asia, Japan, parts of the Caribbean, and South America • An estimated 120 million people are infected worldwide • Infectious larvae transmitted to humans by **mosquito** bite; larvae migrate to **lymphatics and lymph nodes** where they develop into adult worms; female worm produces microfilariae, which circulate in the blood and can infect a biting mosquito; after 1–2 weeks in the mosquito, the microfilariae develop into infectious filariform larvae
Clinical Disease	• Early symptoms of **filariasis** are fever, lymphangitis and lymphadenitis with chills, and recurrent fevers • Progressive infection with lymph node swelling leading to obstruction by adult worms with subsequent enlargement of distal tissues (**elephantiasis**)
Diagnosis	• Demonstration of microfilariae in the peripheral blood by microscopy
Treatment, Prevention, Control	• Diethylcarbamazine is the drug of choice for treating microfilariae but is not effective against the adult worms; alternative is albendazole • Mosquito control and use of protective clothing and insect repellents reduce the risk of exposure • Treatment of patients reduces the risk of human-to-mosquito-to-human transmission

LOA LOA

Epidemiology	• West and Central African countries where as many as 80% of the residents in the rain forests in some countries report a history of infection • Human infection (**loiasis** or **African eye worm** infection) from the bite of the **deerfly** in the genus *Chrysops* • Deerflies most active in the day during the rainy season • Infectious larvae are transmitted to humans by the bite of the infected fly; larvae develop into adults in the subcutaneous tissues and produce microfilariae; during the day (corresponding to the feeding patterns of the fly) the microfilariae are in the patient's blood; flies ingest the microfilariae during their blood meal and these will migrate to the thoracic muscles of the fly where they develop into infectious larvae; larvae then migrate to the fly's proboscis from where they can then be transmitted during the next meal
Clinical Disease	• **Asymptomatic infection** is the most common condition in endemic areas • Symptomatic **loiasis** most commonly presents with itching over the entire body, muscle and joint pains, and tiredness • **Calabar swellings**: localized, nontender swellings that occur most commonly on the extremities; associated with itching • **Eye worm**: migration of an adult worm across the surface of the eye, associated with eye pain, itching, and light sensitivity; permanent damage to the eye does not occur
Diagnosis	• Diagnosis by clinical signs (Calabar swellings with associated pruritus; observation of adult worm in the eye) confirmed by the presence of microfilariae in the blood during daytime hours
Treatment, Prevention, Control	• Diethylcarbamazine is the drug of choice for treating microfilariae and adult worms but may result in severe allergic reaction • Protection from fly bites and use of insect repellents • Prompt treatment of infected individuals

ONCHOCERCA VOLVULUS

Epidemiology	• Distribution in sub-Saharan Africa, Yemen, Brazil, and Venezuela • Human infection (**onchocerciasis** or **"river blindness"**) from the bite of the **blackfly** in the genus *Simulium* • Blackflies are active around streams and rivers • Multiple bites are generally necessary for transmission so infections are rare in short-term visitors • Infectious larvae are transmitted to humans by the bite of the infected fly; larvae develop into adults in the subcutaneous connective tissues and produce microfilariae; microfilariae are primarily in the skin and lymphatics of connective tissues, but also occasionally in the blood, urine, and sputum; flies ingest the microfilariae during their blood meal, and these will migrate to the thoracic muscles of the fly where they develop into infectious larvae; larvae then migrate to the fly's proboscis from where they can then be transmitted during the next meal
Clinical Disease	• **Onchocerciasis** characterized by involvement of the skin, subcutaneous tissue, lymph nodes, and eyes; acute and chronic inflammation in response to microfilariae as they migrate through the skin; infection of the cornea leads to conjunctivitis progressing to sclerosing keratitis and eventual **blindness** • **Skin nodules** with loss of elasticity and depigmentation; pruritus, hyperkeratosis, and thickening
Diagnosis	• Demonstration of microfilariae in the skin; skin surface shaved with a razor, placed in saline, and after a few hours examined for microfilariae
Treatment, Prevention, Control	• Surgical removal of encapsulated nodules with adult worms; single dose of ivermectin to reduce the microfilariae but does not kill the adult worms • Humans are the reservoir of infections so control of human infections will control disease; mass chemotherapy of populations in endemic regions with ivermectin reduces the burden of disease and reduces the risk of transmission • Control of the insect vector is difficult

TISSUE NEMATODES

Tissue nematodes differ from the other roundworms in that humans are dead-end, accidental hosts and animal reservoirs are important for these diseases. In these infections, the complete lifecycle occurs within the host so transmission to humans is by accidental exposure to infectious larvae in meat (*Trichinella*) or eggs (*Toxocara*, dog roundworm; *Ancylostoma braziliense*, dog hookworm). In infections with *Toxocara* and *A. braziliense*, the eggs are not passed in feces to complete their lifecycle in the environment; instead, the eggs hatch and the larvae wander in tissues producing their disease. With *Trichinella* infections, the larvae move through tissues and become encysted, primarily in muscles. Because *Trichinella* infections are the most common, these are summarized here.

TRICHINELLA SPIRALIS	
Epidemiology	• Worldwide distribution • Human disease produced when eating raw or undercooked meat from an infected animal with encysted larvae in striated muscle • Transmission most commonly associated with ingestion of undercooked pork although many carnivorous animals are infected • The larvae leave the meat in the small intestine, develop into adults within 2 days, and initiate production of larvae within 3 months; larvae migrate to **striated muscles** and encyst • The lifecycle of *T. spiralis* in pigs and other animals is identical to human disease
Clinical Disease	• Acute, early symptoms of **trichinosis** are fever, lymphangitis, and lymphadenitis with chills, recurrent febrile attacks, and eosinophilia • Symptoms in progressive disease related to the host inflammatory response to migrating microfilariae, obstruction of lymphatics by the worms with subsequent enlargement of tissues (e.g., **filarial elephantiasis**) and muscle pain
Diagnosis	• Clinical symptoms and a history of consumption of improperly cooked pork or bear meat, confirmed by serology or observation of encysted larvae in a muscle biopsy
Treatment, Prevention, Control	• Symptomatic because there are no effective treatments for larvae in tissues; mebendazole is used to treat adult worms • Disease in the United States has been significantly reduced by implementation of controls in the domestic pork industry; however, pigs raised on farms with exposure to rodents are at significant risk of acquiring infections • Pork and bear meat should be cooked thoroughly; microwave, smoking, or drying meat does not kill all larvae

CLINICAL CASES (REFER TO SECTION VI)

Skin and Soft Tissue Infections
• Onchocerciasis

Miscellaneous Infections
• Hepatitis ascariasis
• *Strongyloides* hyperinfection
• *Loa loa* Infection is a U.S. College Student

SUPPLEMENTAL READING

1. Else KJ, et al. Whipworm and roundworm infections. *Nat Rev Dis Primers*. 2020;6(1):44.

2. Dold C, Holland CV. *Ascaris* and ascariasis. *Microbes Infect*. 2011;13(7):632–637.

3. Loukask A, et al. Hookworm infection. *Nat Rev Dis Primers*. 2016;2:16088.

4. Nutman TB. Human infection with *Strongyloides stercoralis* and other related *Strongyloides* species. *Parasitology*. 2017;144(3):263–273.

5. Babu S, Nutman TB. Immunology of lymphatic filariasis. *Parasite Immunol*. 2014;36(8):338–346.

6. Metzger WG, Mordmuller B. *Loa loa*—does it deserve to be neglected? *Lancet Infect Dis*. 2014;14(4):353–357.

Trematodes

The trematodes (also called **flatworms** or **flukes**, based on the shape of the adult worms) are more geographically restricted compared with other parasites. This is because of the complexity of their lifecycle. All these parasites have a **primary host** where adult worms are found and an **intermediate host** where larval forms mature. In each example in this chapter, the intermediate host is a snail. In the cases of the intestinal and tissue trematodes, there is a second intermediate host (this does not exist with the blood trematodes).

Site of Infection	Flatworm	Primary Host	First Intermediate Host	Second Intermediate Host	Treatment
Intestinal Trematode	*Fasciolopsis buski* ("giant intestinal fluke")	Pigs, dogs, rabbits; **humans are accidental hosts**	Snail	Aquatic plants (e.g., water chestnuts)	Praziquantel
Tissue Trematodes	*Fasciola hepatica* ("sheep liver fluke")	Herbivores (sheep, cattle); **humans are accidental hosts**	Snail	Aquatic plants (e.g., watercress)	Triclabendazole
	Clonorchis sinensis ("Chinese liver fluke")	Dogs, cats, fish-eating mammals; **humans are accidental hosts**	Snail	Freshwater fish	Praziquantel
	Paragonimus westermani ("oriental lung fluke")	Wild boars, pigs, monkeys; **humans are accidental hosts**	Snail	Freshwater crustaceans (e.g., crabs, crayfish)	Praziquantel

Site of Infection	Flatworm	Primary Host	First Intermediate Host	Second Intermediate Host	Treatment
Blood Trematodes	Schistosoma mansoni ("intestinal bilharziasis")	Primates, rodents, marsupials; **humans are accidental hosts**	Snail	None	Praziquantel
	Schistosoma japonica ("oriental blood fluke")	Cats, dogs, cattle, horses, pigs; **humans are accidental hosts**	Snail	None	Praziquantel
	Schistosoma haematobium ("urinary bilharziasis")	Monkeys, baboons, chimpanzees; **humans are accidental hosts**	Snail	None	Praziquantel

INTESTINAL TREMATODE

A number of intestinal flukes exist in different regions of Southeast Asia and China, with *F. buski* the largest and most common. Epidemiology, disease, and treatment of these flukes are similar, so *F. buski* is presented as a model for these infections.

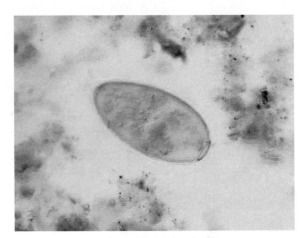

Egg of *Fasciolopsis*.

FASCIOLOPSIS BUSKI

Epidemiology	• Present in China, Vietnam, Thailand, Indonesia, Malaysia, and India • Reservoir hosts are pigs, dogs, and rabbits; humans are accidental hosts • Human exposure to encysted larvae (**metacercariae**) when the husks from aquatic vegetables (e.g., **water chestnuts**) are peeled with the teeth; larvae are swallowed and develop into immature flukes in the duodenum; attach to mucosa of the small intestine and develop into adults; eggs are produced and passed in feces • Adults have a life span of about one year • Free-swimming larvae (**miracidia**) hatch from the eggs, penetrate snails, and undergo maturation; final stage (**cercariae**) released from snails and encyst on aquatic vegetation
Clinical Disease	• Attachment of adult worms to the small intestine produces inflammation, ulceration, and hemorrhage; abdominal discomfort and diarrhea; **malabsorption syndrome** • Marked eosinophilia
Diagnosis	• Detection of characteristic eggs in feces; adult flukes are rarely observed in feces
Treatment, Prevention, Control	• The drug of choice is praziquantel; niclosamide is an alternative • Implementation of proper sanitation and control of human feces reduces the incidence of infections

TISSUE TREMATODES

The tissue trematodes have a very similar lifecycle to *F. buski* except the adult worm does not reside in the intestines. The adult forms of two worms reside in the gall bladder (*F. hepatica* and *C. sinensis*), and their characteristic eggs are found in the feces, while the third worm (*P. westermani*) lives in the lungs and the eggs are expectorated in sputum (if swallowed they would be found in stool specimens).

FASCIOLA HEPATICA	
Epidemiology	• Worldwide distribution in sheep- and cattle-raising areas, including former Soviet Union, Japan, Egypt, and many Latin American countries • Reservoir hosts are herbivores, particularly sheep and cattle; humans are accidental hosts • Human exposure to ingestion of **watercress** with encysted metacercariae; flukes migrate through the duodenal wall to the liver and then to the **gallbladder** where they mature into adults; eggs are produced and passed in the feces • Free-swimming larvae (miracidia) hatch from the eggs, penetrate snails, and undergo maturation; final stage (cercariae) released from snails and encyst on aquatic vegetation
Clinical Disease	• Migration of worms through the liver produces inflammation, tenderness, and hepatomegaly; right upper quadrant pain, fever, and eosinophilia • Severe infection with biliary obstruction, hepatitis, and cirrhosis
Diagnosis	• Detection of characteristic eggs in the feces; eggs indistinguishable from *F. buski* so detection of eggs in gallbladder confirms diagnosis of *F. hepatica* infection
Treatment, Prevention, Control	• Poor response to praziquantel (reason important to differentiate from *F. buski*); treat with triclabendazole; alternative is bithionol • Avoid ingestion of watercress and uncooked aquatic vegetation in endemic areas

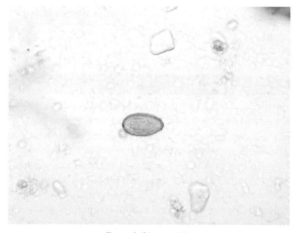

Egg of *Clonorchis*.

CLONORCHIS SINENSIS

Epidemiology	• Present in China, Japan, Korea, and Vietnam • Reservoir hosts are dogs, cats, and fish-eating mammals; humans are accidental hosts • Human exposure to ingestion of **uncooked freshwater fish** with encysted metacercariae; flukes migrate through the duodenal wall to the liver and then to the **gallbladder** where they mature to adults; eggs are produced and passed in feces • In contrast with *F. hepatica*, the eggs are ingested by snails and undergo maturation; final stage (cercariae) released from snails and penetrate under the scales of **freshwater** fish where they develop into metacercariae • Adult worms can persist for up to 30 years if untreated
Clinical Disease	• Usually asymptomatic or mild • Severe infections of the **gallbladder** results in fever, diarrhea, epigastric pain, hepatomegaly, anorexia, and jaundice; eosinophilia; biliary obstruction • Chronic infection can result in **adenocarcinoma** of bile ducts
Diagnosis	• Detection of characteristic small eggs in feces
Treatment, Prevention, Control	• The drug of choice is praziquantel; alternative is albendazole • Avoid eating uncooked freshwater fish; implement proper sanitation policies including disposal of human, dog, and cat feces in sites that avoid contamination of water

PARAGONIMUS WESTERMANI

Epidemiology	• Present in many countries in Asia, Africa, and Latin America • Many immigrants to the United States, particularly from Indonesia, are infected • Reservoir hosts are shore-feeding animals (wild boars, pigs, monkeys) that ingest infected crustaceans (**crabs, crayfish**); humans are accidental hosts with infections following ingestion of **inadequately cooked or pickled crustaceans** with encysted metacercariae • In humans, the metacercariae hatch in the stomach and migrate through the intestinal wall to the abdominal cavity, through the diaphragm, to the pleural cavity; adult worms in lungs produce eggs that appear in sputum or are swallowed and found in feces • Embryonated eggs passed by the reservoir hosts hatch releasing miracidia that penetrate snails; after maturation in the snail, cercariae are released, invade crustaceans, and develop in metacercariae that encyst in the tissues
Clinical Disease	• Symptoms correspond to migration of larvae through tissues and are associated with fever, chills, and high eosinophilia • Adult worms stimulate an inflammatory response with fever, cough, and increased sputum production • Progressive infections lead to cavitary **lung disease** and fibrosis of lung tissues • Infections in humans may persist for 20 years
Diagnosis	• Detection of characteristic eggs in sputum or pleural effusion
Treatment, Prevention, Control	• Drug of choice is praziquantel; alternative is triclabendazole • Avoid consumption of uncooked or pickled crabs and crayfish, as well as meat from animals in the endemic regions • Proper sanitation and control of the disposal of human feces are essential

BLOOD TREMATODES

Schistosomes differ from the other flukes in that male and female worms exist, and they are **intravascular parasites**—the adult worms are not found in the intestines, tissues, or cavities. As with the other flukes, snails are an important intermediate host, but the free-swimming cercariae that are released from the snails directly penetrate human skin rather than establishing residence on a secondary host. Disease is related to where the adults establish residence in the circulatory system and release their eggs.

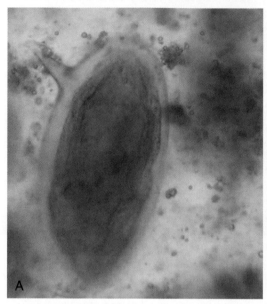
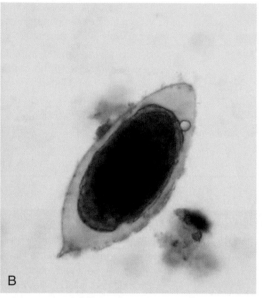

(A) *Schistosoma mansoni* (note lateral spine) and (B) *Schistosoma haematobium* (note terminal spine).

SCHISTOSOMA MANSONI	
Epidemiology	• *S. mansoni* is the most widespread schistosome; endemic in southern and sub-Saharan Africa, the Nile River valley in Sudan and Egypt, South America including Brazil, Suriname, and Venezuela, and the Caribbean West Indies • Waters of lakes and rivers where host snail is present and sanitation is poor • Reservoir host include primates, marsupials, and rodents; snails are intermediate hosts • Residents (and tourists), particularly children, at risk when swimming or bathing in waters contaminated with free-swimming cercariae • After skin penetration, the parasites enter the circulatory system and migrate to portal blood in the liver and mature to adults; paired adult male and female worms migrate to the **inferior mesenteric vein** near the lower colon, laying eggs that circulate to the liver and are shed in stools
Clinical Disease	• Penetration through the skin results in itching, allergic reaction, and dermatitis • Migration through the lungs and liver results in cough and hepatitis, respectively • Egg laying by adult worms produces fever, malaise, abdominal pain, and liver tenderness; inflammation and thickening of the bowel wall is related to inflammatory response to deposited eggs with abdominal pain, diarrhea, and bloody stools • Chronic infections with hepatosplenomegaly
Diagnosis	• Detection of characteristic eggs in feces
Treatment, Prevention, Control	• The drug of choice is praziquantel; alternative is oxamniquine; treatment terminates egg production but does not alleviate the host response to deposited eggs • Implementation of proper sanitation and control of human feces reduces the incidence of infections

SCHISTOSOMA JAPONICA

Epidemiology	• Present in Indonesia and part of China and Southeast Asia • Waters of lakes and rivers where host snail is present and sanitation is poor • Reservoir hosts include cats, dogs, cattle, horses, and pigs • Residents (and tourists), particularly children, at risk when swimming or bathing in waters contaminated with free-swimming cercariae • After skin penetration, the parasites enter the circulatory system and migrate to portal blood in the liver and mature to adults; paired adult male and female worms migrate to the **superior mesenteric vein** near the small intestine and the **inferior mesenteric vein**, laying eggs that circulate to liver and are shed in stools
Clinical Disease	• Similar to *S. mansoni* infections; however, smaller eggs and higher egg production can lead to more severe disease and dissemination to other organs including the brain
Diagnosis	• Detection of characteristic eggs in feces
Treatment, Prevention, Control	• Drug of choice is praziquantel • Implementation of proper sanitation and control of human feces reduces the incidence of infections

SCHISTOSOMA HAEMATOBIUM

Epidemiology	• Present throughout Africa; also in Cyprus, southern Portugal, and India • Waters of lakes and rivers where host snail is present and sanitation is poor • Reservoir hosts include monkeys, baboons, and chimpanzees • Residents (and tourists), particularly children, at risk when swimming or bathing in waters contaminated with free-swimming cercariae • After skin penetration, the parasites enter the circulatory system and migrate to vesical, prostatic, and uterine plexuses of the venous circulation and mature into adults; large eggs are produced and deposited in the bladder wall as well as uterine and prostatic tissues
Clinical Disease	• Early stages of disease as with other schistosomes with dermatitis, allergic reactions, fever, and malaise • Disease progresses to urinary symptoms including hematuria, dysuria, and urinary frequency • Chronic infections associated with **bladder carcinoma**
Diagnosis	• Detection of characteristic eggs in urine; eggs not found in the feces
Treatment, Prevention, Control	• Drug of choice is praziquantel

CLINICAL CASES (REFER TO SECTION VI)

Lower Respiratory Tract Infections
- Paragonimiasis

Genitourinary Tract Infections
- *Schistosoma haematobium* infection in Italian family

Central Nervous System Infections
- Schistosomiasis

Miscellaneous Infections
- Fascioliasis
- Cholangitis caused by *Clonorchis sinensis*
- Liver cirrhosis and splenomegaly in Sudanese woman

SUPPLEMENTAL READING

1. Mas-Coma S, Valero MA, Bargues MD. Fascioliasis. *Adv Exp Med Biol.* 2019;1154:71–103.
2. Na BK, Pak JH, Hong SJ. *Clonorchis sinensis* and clonorchiasis. *Acta Trop.* 2020;203, 105309.
3. Yoshida A, Doanh PN, Manuyama H. *Paragonimus* and paragonimiasis in Asia: an update. *Acta Trop.* 2019;199, 105074.
4. McManus DP, et al. Schistosomiasis. *Nat Rev Dis Primers.* 2018;4(1):13.
5. Gryseels B. Schistosomiasis. *Infect Dis Clin North Am.* 2012;26(2):383–397.

Cestodes

Cestodes are flat, ribbon-like worms (the reason they are called "**tapeworms**") that have a head (**scolex**) with suckers and hooks for attachment to the intestinal wall and a long segmented body (**proglottids**). The worms are hermaphroditic, so as they develop, the segments closest to the head are immature and the most distal proglottids are gravid (filled with eggs). These gravid proglottids break off from the worm and are shed in the feces. The morphologic features of the proglottids and eggs are the diagnostic clues that are used to distinguish these worms. The size of these worms is impressive, with *T. saginata* and *D. latum* up to 30 feet long and *H. nana* and *Dipylidium caninum* only a few inches long. The lifecycles of tapeworms generally involve at least two hosts, with the adult worms developing in the primary host and the larval forms developing in the intermediate host. Human disease is primarily restricted to intestinal symptoms, except for infection where humans are accidental intermediate hosts.

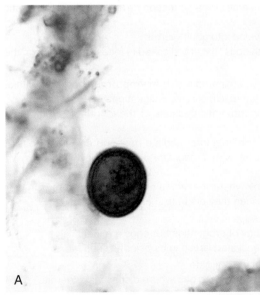
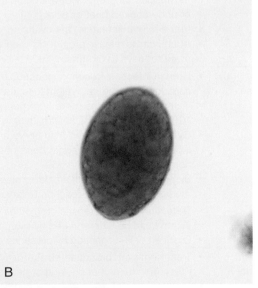

Eggs of (A) *Taenia* and (B) *Diphyllobothrium*.

175

Site of Infection	Tapeworm	Primary Host	Intermediate Host	Treatment
Intestinal Cestodes	*Taenia saginata* ("beef tapeworm")	Humans	Cattle	Praziquantel, niclosamide
	Taenia solium ("pork tapeworm")	Humans	Pigs	Praziquantel, niclosamide
	Diphyllobothrium latum ("fish tapeworm")	Humans	Copepods (1st stage), fish (2nd stage)	Praziquantel, niclosamide
	Hymenolepis nana ("dwarf tapeworm")	Mice; **humans are accidental hosts**	Beetles	Praziquantel, niclosamide
	Hymenolepis diminuta ("rat tapeworm")	Rats; **humans are accidental hosts**	Beetles	Praziquantel, niclosamide
	Dipylidium caninum ("dog tapeworm")	Dogs, cats; **humans are accidental hosts**	Fleas	Praziquantel, niclosamide
Tissue Cestodes	*Taenia solium* ("cysticercosis")	Humans	**Humans are accidental hosts**	Praziquantel, niclosamide
	Echinococcus granulosus ("unilocular cystic hydatid disease")	Dogs	Sheep, cattle, goats, pigs; **humans are accidental hosts**	Albendazole
	Echinococcus multilocularis ("alveolar hydatid disease")	Wolves, foxes, dogs (uncommon)	Rodents; **humans are accidental hosts**	Albendazole

INTESTINAL CESTODES

TAENIA SAGINATA AND *TAENIA SOLIUM*

Epidemiology	<ul><li>*T. saginata* in Eastern Europe, Eastern Africa, Latin America</li><li>*T. solium* in Eastern Europe, India, Asia, sub-Saharan Africa, Latin America, and the United States</li><li>Animals (cattle, *T. saginata*; pigs, *T. solium*) infected when eggs or proglottids (tapeworm segments with mature eggs) are ingested; eggs hatch in intestine releasing oncospheres (larvae) that migrate to muscles where they develop into cysticerci; human infection develops following ingestion of raw or undercooked **beef or pork**</li><li>In the human intestine, the cysticerci develop into adult worms</li><li>Adult worms release proglottids filled with eggs that are released in feces; can survive in the environment for days to months</li></ul>
Clinical Disease	<ul><li>Human infection following ingestion of contaminated meat; **Asymptomatic** or **mild** with abdominal pain, loss of appetite, weight loss, upset stomach, chronic indigestion</li><li>*T. saginata* infections more commonly symptomatic because of the length of the tapeworm (up to 10 m compared with *T. solium*, 3 m)</li><li>**Cysticercosis**—humans may serve as accidental intermediate host and develop disease following ingestion of *T. solium* eggs; does not occur with *T. saginata* eggs; lifecycle similar as with animal hosts</li><li>Symptoms of cysticercosis determined by where the larvae encyst; most severe is in brain or eye; marked inflammatory reaction to larvae when they die in tissues</li></ul>
Diagnosis	<ul><li>Detection of characteristic proglottids or eggs in feces</li><li>Worms can be differentiated by morphology of proglottids but eggs are identical</li><li>Cysticercosis diagnosed by presence of encysted larvae in biopsied tissues</li></ul>
Treatment, Prevention, Control	<ul><li>Treatment with praziquantel; alternative is niclosamide</li><li>Prevention by proper cooking of beef and pork in regions where disease is endemic</li><li>Maintenance of good sanitary conditions</li></ul>

DIPHYLLOBOTHRIUM LATUM

Epidemiology	• Worldwide distribution, particularly in western Europe, eastern Europe, Asia, and the United States • Broader geographic distribution related to regional or international transport of fish • Infection associated with eating raw or undercooked **fish**; freezing for 7 days or proper cooking will kill the parasite • Humans ingest undercooked fish with larvae in the tissues; larvae develop into mature adults in the small intestine and develop to up to 10 m in length; immature eggs are released from the proglottids and passed in feces • Eggs contaminating fresh waters require 2–4 weeks to develop into free-swimming larvae (coracidium) that are ingested by small crustaceans (copepods); these are ingested by large fish and the larvae migrate to the flesh where they develop into infectious plerocercoid larvae
Clinical Disease	• Most infections are **asymptomatic** • **Symptoms** include epigastric pain, abdominal cramping, nausea, vomiting, and weight loss • **Vitamin B12 deficiency** with anemia and neurologic symptoms
Diagnosis	• Detection of characteristic proglottids or eggs in feces
Treatment, Prevention, Control	• Treatment with praziquantel; alternative is niclosamide • Prevention by proper cooking of fish in regions where disease is endemic

The lifecycles and diseases caused by *H. nana* (mouse or dwarf tapeworm) and *Hymenolepis diminuta* (rat tapeworm) are similar, with humans serving as accidental primary hosts following ingestion of infected beetles in flours and cereals. A summary of *H. nana* is presented here.

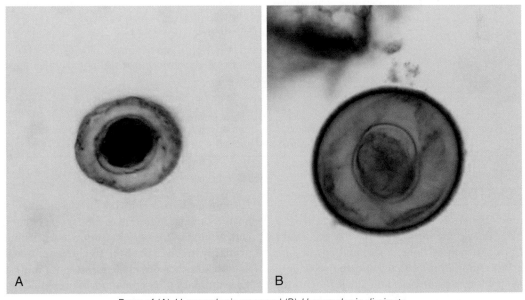

Eggs of (A) *Hymenolepis nana* and (B) *Hymenolepis diminuta*.

HYMENOLEPIS NANA

Epidemiology	• Worldwide distribution • **Most common tapeworm infection** in North America; common parasite of mice • Human and mouse infections following ingestion of infective eggs in contaminated food; hatch in small intestine releasing larva that develop into the cysticercoid stage; attach to small intestine and mature into adult; eggs are infectious at the time of passing in feces; can be ingested directly or by **beetles** who can serve as an intermediate host for humans or rodents • Adult worms are small (<5 cm) and short lived, although **autoinfection** (direct ingestion of passed infectious eggs) can lead to hyperinfection
Clinical Disease	• Infections with small numbers of tapeworms are **asymptomatic** • Symptoms with large number of worms include diarrhea, abdominal pain, headache, and anorexia
Diagnosis	• Detection of characteristic eggs in feces
Treatment, Prevention, Control	• Treatment with praziquantel; alternative is niclosamide • Prevention by maintenance of sanitary conditions and personal hygiene

DIPYLIDIUM CANINUM

Epidemiology	• Worldwide distribution • Parasite of dogs and cats with the flea as the intermediate host; human infections most common in children • Ingestion of a flea with infectious cysticercoid larvae initiates disease in a dog or cat; larvae develops into an adult that sheds proglottids containing packets of eggs; eggs are released and ingested by dog or cat larval fleas; the oncosphere in the egg is released in the flea intestine; penetrates through intestinal wall to body cavity, where it develops into a cysticercoid larva • Human infections occur when crushed **fleas** on the animal's mouth are transmitted accidentally when the animal licks a child or is kissed • Adult worms are about 15 cm in length
Clinical Disease	• Infections with small numbers of tapeworms are **asymptomatic** • Heavier infections produce abdominal discomfort, pruritus, and diarrhea; anal pruritus due to active mobility of proglottids
Diagnosis	• Detection of gravid proglottid in feces; egg packets containing embryonated eggs are rarely observed in feces
Treatment, Prevention, Control	• Treatment with praziquantel; alternatives are niclosamide and paromomycin • Deworm pets and eliminate fleas

TISSUE CESTODES

Echinococcus granulosus and *E. multilocularis* have a similar lifecycle varying primarily by the secondary hosts. Carnivores such as dogs, foxes, and coyotes are the primary host for *Echinococcus*, and the secondary hosts are sheep for *E. granulosus* and small rodents for *E. multilocularis*. Humans are accidental secondary hosts following ingestion of food or water contaminated with *Echinococcus* eggs in canine feces. Human disease primarily involves the liver and lungs, although dissemination to other organs (e.g., spleen, brain) can occur. The summary of *E. granulosus* is presented here.

ECHINOCOCCUS GRANULOSUS

Epidemiology	• Present in sheep- and cattle-raising countries including Australia, New Zealand, southern Africa, and parts of Europe, South America, and North America • Infection acquired by dogs when they ingest the organs of animals with encysted parasite; develop into adults (less than 1 in.) in the intestine and eggs shed in feces; sheep, cattle, goats, and pigs ingest eggs which hatch in the small intestine • Human infection following accidental ingestion of **eggs in food or water contaminated with dog feces**; the oncosphere is released and penetrates the human intestinal wall, enters the circulation and is carried to tissues, primarily the liver and lung (less commonly to central nervous system and bones)
Clinical Disease	• Human infection (**echinococcosis**) characterized by a slow-growing (5–20 years before symptomatic), tumor-like, unilocular cyst filled with tapeworm heads (hydatid sand) and fluid • Fluid potentially toxic if the cyst ruptures
Diagnosis	• Clinical, radiologic, and epidemiologic data confirmed at surgery • Serologic tests supportive but relatively insensitive
Treatment, Prevention, Control	• Surgical resection of the cyst is the treatment of choice plus albendazole • If in an inoperable location, treatment with albendazole; alternatives are mebendazole or praziquantel • Control of infections in dogs by preventing them from eating animal viscera and proper personal hygiene

CLINICAL CASES (REFER TO SECTION VI)

Lower Respiratory Tract Infections
• Echinococcosis in Pregnant Woman

Central Nervous System Infections
• Neurocysticercosis in Italian Traveler

Gastrointestinal Tract Infections
• Diphyllobothriasis
• *Hymenolepis nana* infection in a pregnant woman

SUPPLEMENTAL READING

1. Gonzales I, et al. Pathogenesis of *Taenia solium* taeniasis and cysticercosis. *Parasite Immunol.* 2016;38(3):136–146.
2. Scholz T, et al. Update on the human broad tapeworm *Diphyllobothrium*, including clinical relevance. *Clin Microbiol Rev.* 2009;22(1):146–160.
3. Schantz PM. Tapeworms (cestodiasis). *Gastroenterol Clin North Am.* 1996;25(3):637–653.
4. Higuita NIA, Brunetti E, McCloskey C. Cystic echinococcosis. *J Clin Microbiol.* 2016;54(3):518–523.
5. Deplazes P, et al. Global distribution of alveolar and cystic echinococcosis. *Adv Parasitol.* 2017;95:315–493.

28

Arthropods

Arthropods serve an important role as vectors of many bacterial, viral, and parasitic diseases.

The list below is a general summary of the most common human diseases associated with arthropod vectors.

Arthropod	Organism	Disease
Tick	*Anaplasma phagocytophilum*	Human anaplasmosis
	Borrelia burgdorferi	Lyme disease
	Borrelia, other species	Endemic relapsing fever
	Coxiella burnetii	Q fever
	Ehrlichia chaffeensis	Human monocytic ehrlichiosis
	Ehrlichia ewingii	Human granulocytic ehrlichiosis
	Francisella tularensis	Tularemia
	Orbivirus	Colorado tick fever
	Rickettsia rickettsii	Rocky Mountain spotted fever
Flea	*Dipylidium caninum*	Dog tapeworm
	Rickettsia prowazekii	Sporadic typhus
	Rickettsia typhi	Murine typhus
	Yersinia pestis	Plague
Lice	*Bartonella quintana*	Trench fever
	Borrelia recurrentis	Epidemic relapsing fever
	Rickettsia prowazekii	Epidemic typhus
Mite	*Orientia tsutsugamushi*	Scrub typhus
	Rickettsia akari	Rickettsialpox
Fly	*Bartonella bacilliformis*	Bartonellosis
	Hymenolepis nana	Dwarf tapeworm
	Leishmania species	Leishmaniasis
	Onchocerca volvulus	Onchocerciasis "river blindness"
	Trypanosoma brucei	African trypanosomiasis
	Trypanosoma cruzi	Chagas disease
Mosquito	*Alphavirus*	Eastern equine encephalitis
		Venezuelan equine encephalitis
		Western equine encephalitis
	Brugia species	Malayan filariasis
	Bunyavirus	La Crosse encephalitis
	Dirofilaria immitis	Dirofilariasis
	Flavivirus	Dengue fever
		St. Louis encephalitis
		Yellow fever
	Plasmodium species	Malaria
	Wuchereria bancrofti	Bancroftian filariasis

Clinical Cases—Introduction to Infectious Diseases

SECTION OVERVIEW

First and foremost, I want to say this is not a comprehensive review of clinical infectious diseases. For that, I refer the student to excellent textbooks that thoroughly discuss these diseases in pediatric and adult patients.[1,2] My intention in this section is to provide clinical examples of infections so that the student may be better able to apply the foundational knowledge they gained in the first 5 sections of this textbook to clinical diagnosis. The following eight chapters will present a brief overview of specific clinical syndromes and then illustrate them with clinical cases. My recommendation is that after you have read the clinical case history, return to the chapter that discussed the pathogen and review the summary table. This will help link the microbiology of the organism with the infectious disease it causes.

REFERENCES

1. Long SS, Prober CG, Fischer M. *Principles and Practice of Pediatric Infectious Diseases.* 5th ed. Philadelphia, PA: Elsevier; 2018.
2. Bennett JE, Dolin R, Blaser MJ. *Mandell, Douglas, and Bennett's Principles and Practice of Infectious Diseases.* 9th ed. Philadelphia, PA: Elsevier; 2020.

29

Upper Respiratory Tract Infections

Upper respiratory tract infections can be subdivided by clinical presentation:

Common cold	Sore throat, sneezing, rhinorrhea, nasal congestion, cough
Pharyngitis	Inflammation of pharynx
Epiglottitis	Inflammation of supraglottis structures
Laryngitis	Inflammation of larynx resulting in hoarse voice
Otitis	Inflammation of auditory canal
Sinusitis	Inflammation of paranasal sinuses

Common colds are primarily viral infections with rhinovirus the most common pathogen. Other common viruses include coronavirus, parainfluenza virus, respiratory syncytial virus (RSV), adenovirus, and human metapneumovirus. Infections in children are more common than in adults and immunity is generally short-lived so recurrent infections are common. **Pharyngitis** is defined as inflammation of the pharynx combined with fever and sore throat. Again, this disease is most often observed in children and young adults, and the majority of infections are caused by viruses, particularly adenovirus. Group A *Streptococcus* (*S. pyogenes*) is the most recognized bacterial pathogen, although infections with other bacteria may also present with symptoms of pharyngitis. These can include Groups C and G *Streptococcus*, *Neisseria gonorrhoeae* (oral gonorrhoea), *Corynebacterium diphtheriae* (diphtheria), *Bordetella pertussis* (whooping cough), *Fusobacterium necrophorum* (Lemierre syndrome),

Arcanobacterium haemolyticum (illness resembling *S. pyogenes* scarlet fever), *Mycoplasma pneumoniae*, and *Chlamydia psittaci* (psittacosis). The epidemiology of epiglottitis has changed with the introduction of the type B *Haemophilus influenzae* vaccine. Prior to the vaccine, most infections of the epiglottis were in children and caused by *H. influenzae*. Infections in vaccinated children are now rare, and most adult infections are caused by *Streptococcus pneumoniae*, *S. pyogenes*, and *Neisseria meningitidis*. **Laryngitis** is primarily an infection caused by respiratory viruses, with bacteria and fungi less commonly implicated. *Pseudomonas aeruginosa* is a frequent pathogen responsible for infections of the outer ear (**external otitis**) that can range from mild inflammation ("swimmer's ear") to a rapidly destructive process ("malignant" otitis). Middle ear infections (**otitis media**) are commonly initiated with a respiratory virus infection leading to an inflammatory process of the eustachian tube. Trapped bacteria can then multiply and produce increased pressure and pain in the ear canal. *S. pneumoniae*, nontypeable *H. influenzae*, and *M. catarrhalis* are the most common bacterial pathogens. Lastly, the pathogenesis of **sinusitis** is similar to otitis media, with infections initiated by a respiratory virus infection and then progressing to a bacterial infection. Again, *S. pneumoniae*, nontypeable *H. influenzae*, and *M. catarrhalis* are prominent pathogens in sinusitis, as well as anaerobic bacteria originating from the nasal passages. *Staphylococcus aureus* can produce an acute presentation of sinusitis, and fungal pathogens can play a prominent role in some specific patient populations (e.g., *Mucor*, *Rhizopus*, and *Rhizomucor* in diabetic patients; *Aspergillus fumigatus* in allergic sinusitis).

The following are a series of case reports that illustrate upper respiratory tract infections.

STREPTOCOCCUS PYOGENES PHARYNGITIS AND SCARLET FEVER

A 20-year-old man presented to his primary care physician with a 3-day history of swollen tonsils, sore throat, fevers, chills, and rash. The nonpruritic rash had started on his abdomen, spread to his chest and back, and then appeared on his arms, legs, and face. He had no known allergies or exposures to new medications and had no history of similar rash. Examination revealed exudative tonsillitis, strawberry tongue, and cervical adenopathy with tenderness. Skin examination revealed diffuse blanching erythema with punctate papules that caused the skin on his chest, abdomen, back, arms, and legs to have a sandpaper-like quality. His neck and right flank had linear petechial patches. A rapid test for streptococcal pharyngitis was positive. The finding of acute streptococcal pharyngitis along with the diffuse rash led to a diagnosis of scarlet fever. The rash of scarlet fever is a delayed-type hypersensitivity to an exotoxin and therefore occurs in persons who have had a previous exposure to *Streptococcus pyogenes*. The rash classically manifests with linear petechial confluences (Pastia's lines), which were seen in this patient. The patient was treated with antibiotic agents and had complete resolution of his symptoms within 3 days. One other bacterial pathogen, *Arcanobacterium haemolyticum*, can have an identical presentation. Treatment for this infection is also with penicillin. (Brinker. *New Engl J Med*. 2017;376:1972.)

STREPTOCOCCUS DYSGALACTIAE PHARYNGITIS

A 35-year-old woman presented to her physician with acute exudative tonsillopharyngitis with sore throat, enlarged tonsils and anterior cervical lymph nodes, and elevated temperature and antistreptolysin O titers. Group G beta-hemolytic *Streptococcus dysgalactiae* subsp. *equisimilis* was isolated from her throat, susceptible to multiple antibiotics including amoxicillin. She was treated with amoxicillin for 10 days with prompt resolution of symptoms, but 2 weeks after antibiotics were discontinued, the antistreptolysin O titers were persistently elevated and cultures remained positive. The patient was retreated for 10 days and again 15 days after antibiotics were discontinued the antistreptolysin O titers were elevated and cultures positive. Finally, after a 10-day course of clarithromycin, the antibody titers and cultures reverted to negative. The most common cause of bacterial pharyngitis is *Streptococcus pyogenes* but *S. dysgalactiae* is associated with a clinically similar presentation and has been responsible for epidemic tonsillopharyngitis in adults and children and sporadic episodes in adults. This pathogen is frequently overlooked by laboratories that commonly screen throat specimens for only group A *Streptococcus pyogenes*. (Savini et al. *J Clin Microbiol*. 2008;46:814–816.)

RESPIRATORY DIPHTHERIA

Lurie and associates reported the last patient with respiratory diphtheria seen in the United States. An unvaccinated 63-year-old man developed a sore throat while on a week-long trip in rural Haiti. Two days after he returned home to Pennsylvania, he visited a local hospital with complaints of a sore throat and difficulties in swallowing. He was treated with oral antibiotics but returned 2 days later with chills, sweating, difficulty swallowing and breathing, nausea, and vomiting. He had diminished breath sounds in the left lung, and radiographs confirmed pulmonary infiltrates as well as enlargement of the epiglottis. Laryngoscopy revealed yellow exudates on the tonsils, posterior pharynx, and soft palate. He was admitted to the intensive care unit and treated with azithromycin, ceftriaxone, nafcillin, and steroids, but over the next 4 days became hypotensive with a low-grade fever. Cultures were negative for *Corynebacterium diphtheriae*. By the 8th day of illness, a chest radiograph showed infiltrates in the right and left lung bases, and a white exudate consistent with *C. diphtheriae* pseudomembrane was observed over the supraglottic structures. At this time, cultures remained negative for *C. diphtheriae*, but polymerase chain reaction testing for the exotoxin gene was positive. Despite aggressive therapy, the patient continued to deteriorate, and on the 17th day of hospitalization, the patient developed cardiac complications and died. This patient illustrates: (1) the risk factor of unimmunized patients traveling to an endemic area; (2) the classic presentation of severe respiratory diphtheria; (3) delays associated with the diagnosis of an uncommon disease; and (4) the difficulties that most laboratories would now have isolating the organism in culture. Although *C. diphtheriae* will grow readily in culture, differentiation from other corynebacteria normally present in the upper respiratory tract is difficult. (Luria et al. *MMWR*. 2004;52:1285–1286.)

FATAL *CORYNEBACTERIUM DIPHTHERIAE* INFECTION

A 14-year-old girl living in Nepal presented to the Emergency Department with a 3-day history of neck swelling, fever, throat pain, and difficulty swallowing. Examination of the oropharynx revealed a grayish-white membrane. According to her mother, the patient had received three doses of the diphtheria-pertussis-tetanus vaccine during her first year of life with no additional doses. Diphtheria was suspected, and treatment with penicillin G and anti-diphtheria serum was initiated. A throat culture grew *Corynebacterium diphtheriae*. On the third day of hospitalization, chest discomfort, palpitations, and elevated troponin 1 levels developed, along with electro-cardiographic abnormalities. These signs and symptoms aroused concern about diphtheria-associated myocarditis. The girl continued to have ventricular arrhythmias despite receiving treatment in the pediatric ICU and she died 2 days later. This case illustrates a well-known but infrequent complication of diphtheria. The child had not been fully vaccinated. The current recommendations are one dose at each of the following ages: 2 months, 4 months, 6 months, 15 to 18 months, and 4 to 6 years. (Sah. *N Engl J Med.* 2019; https://doi.org/10.1056/NEJMicm1814405.)

BORDETELLA PERTUSSIS OUTBREAK IN HEALTHCARE WORKERS

Pascual and associates reported an outbreak of pertussis among hospital workers. The index case, a nurse anesthetist, presented acutely with cough, paroxysms followed by vomiting, and apneic episodes that led to loss of consciousness. Surgical service personnel, exposed patients, and family members were surveyed, and cultures, polymerase chain reaction tests, and serology were obtained from patients with respiratory symptoms. Twelve (23%) healthcare workers and 0 of 146 patients had clinical pertussis. The lack of disease in patients was attributed to mask use, cough etiquette, and limited face-to-face contact. This outbreak emphasizes the susceptibility of adults to infection and the highly infectious nature of *B. pertussis*. Although the clinical presentation of this patient is characteristic of pertussis (whooping cough) observed in children, adult patients typically present with a chronic cough because their larger open airways result in less frequent apneic episodes. Thus, diagnosis of pertussis in adults may be delayed. The organism requires specialized media for growth so the most common diagnostic test is use of specific PCR tests that are now available commercially. (Pascual et al. *Infect Control Hosp Epidemiol.* 2006;27:546–552.)

BORDETELLA PERTUSSIS WHOOPING COUGH

A 16-month-old girl was hospitalized after suffering with a 2-week chronic cough. She was unresponsive to common antibiotics and anti-inflammatory treatment. On admission, she presented with a low-grade fever, normal blood pressure, and elevated heart rate. The mother reported a similar episode in her 6-year-old son, and neither child had received the pediatric vaccines including the pertussis vaccine. A gradual improvement was noted after the child was started on clarithromycin. The method for diagnosis of *Bordetella pertussis* infection ("whooping cough") is not specifically mentioned in this case report but it is most common accomplished by nucleic acid amplification tests with respiratory secretions. The organism is difficult to grow, with blood and respiratory secretions typically culture negative. This child presented with relatively mild symptoms as did her brother. A more typical presentation in children with narrow airways is violent coughs followed by inspiratory whoops. The child was successfully treated with a macrolide although it should be noted that macrolide-resistance has been observed. Vaccination can effectively eliminate this disease. (Brindicci et al. *Infect Med.* 2018;1:85–88.)

HSV-1 GINGIVOSTOMATITIS

Mohan et al. described a 32-year-old man with primary gingivostomatitis caused by herpes simplex virus-1 (HSV-1). He presented to an outpatient clinic with complaints of a burning sensation in his mouth that worsened when eating hot or spicy foods. He reported the appearance of ulcers in his mouth over the previous 2 days. Upon intra-oral examination, the gingiva was inflamed with multiple ulcers and vesicles on the tongue and buccal mucosa. The clinical diagnosis of HSV gingivostomatitis was made, treatment with acyclovir was initiated, and the patient responded well with complete healing within 2 weeks. HSV infections characteristic present with painful vesicular lesions and, although patients respond to antiviral treatment, the virus will remain latent in the sensory nerve ganglion and can reactivate in the future. The most common laboratory tests for confirming the clinical diagnosis are culture of respiratory secretions in viral cell cultures or nucleic acid amplification tests. (Mohan et al. *BMJ Case Rep.* 2013; https://doi.org/10.1136/bcr-2013-200074.)

HAEMOPHILUS INFLUENZAE TYPE B EPIGLOTTITIS

A 4-year-old boy presented to the Emergency Department with characteristics of systemic illness combined with respiratory distress. His mouth was open, his neck hyperextended, and his voice hoarse. The diagnosis of epiglottitis was established based on physical examination, lateral neck X-ray, and the finding of an enlarged swollen, erythematous epiglottis on flexible fiberoptic laryngoscopy. Blood culture was positive for gram-negative coccobacilli identified as *Haemophilus influenzae* type B (Hib). The child was treated with a 10-day course of ceftriaxone with full recovery. Widespread vaccination for this pathogen has essentially eliminated disease in pediatric patients but this child had not received the Hib vaccine and was susceptible to this infection.

HPV-ASSOCIATED OROPHARYNGEAL CARCINOMAS

Huang and Seow described two patients with HPV-associated cervical cancer and synchronous diagnoses of HPV-related head and neck cancer in their husbands. Both patients were reported to have active oral sex for more than 20 years. The first patient was a 64-year-old woman who had an abnormal Papanicolaou smear and was found to have squamous cell carcinoma of the cervix on cervical punch biopsy. Her husband was diagnosed with laryngeal squamous cell carcinoma one year previously and was treated with total laryngectomy and adjuvant radiation. HPV type 16 was detected in both their tumor specimens using PCR. The second patient was a 50-year-old woman with cervical carcinoma treated surgically and with chemo-radiotherapy. HPV-31 was detected in her tumor specimen. Three years later, her husband presented with nasopharyngeal carcinoma. DNA from a different human papillomavirus, HPV type 18, was detected in his tumor specimen. It is unclear if his wife was infected with multiple HPVs or if his infection was from another source. These two case reports illustrate the role HPV plays in both cervical and oropharynx carcinoma. (Huang, Seow. *Gynecol Obstet Invest.* 2010;70:73–75.)

PSEUDOMONAS AERUGINOSA EAR INFECTION

A 74-year-old man with type 2 diabetes presented with hearing loss, right ear discharge, ipsilateral nasal obstruction, and worsening symptoms for the last 5 months. Physical examination revealed a slight facial palsy on the right side. Laboratory studies showed uncontrolled diabetes and elevation of inflammatory indices. Otoscopic examination showed right ear external otitis and the ear swab was positive for *Pseudomonas aeruginosa* sensitive to ciprofloxacin. Rhino-pharyngo-laryngoscopy examination revealed right nasopharyngeal swelling, and CT and contrast-enhanced MRI of the petrous bone showed an asymmetric nasopharynx air lumen due to prominent soft tissue swelling. Extensive erosion of the petrous bone and the pterygoid process was also visible, along with areas of thickening of the mastoid. Imaging was consistent with external malignant otitis extending to the cranial base. The patient was treated with i.v. ciprofloxacin and piperacillin-tazobactam for 6 weeks. The patient's symptoms regressed and CT performed 3 months later showed resolution of the inflammatory process of the external ear and the temporal bone. Follow-up at 1 year was negative for recurrence. Although *P. aeruginosa* can cause external otitis (frequently called "swimmer's ear"), this patient's underlying uncontrolled diabetes predisposed him to an aggressive otitis infection. The prompt diagnosis and appropriate long-term therapy had a successful resolution. (Di Lullo et al. *Am J Case Rep* 2020;21:e925060.)

30

Lower Respiratory Tract Infections

Lower respiratory tract infections include infections of the bronchi, lungs, and pleural space surrounding the lungs. Infections of the bronchi are primarily caused by viruses including rhinovirus, influenza viruses, respiratory syncytial virus, metapneumovirus, coronaviruses, and adenovirus. A small proportion of bronchial infections are caused by Mycoplasma pneumoniae and Bordetella pertussis. Numerous viruses, bacteria, fungi, and some parasites cause infections of the lungs. It is not worthwhile creating a differential diagnostic list of these pathogens without consideration of the patient's risk factors, such as underlying lung disease, immune status, and epidemiologic exposure. For example, patients with chronic obstructive pulmonary disease (COPD) are at greater risk for colonization with microbes from the upper airways and inflammatory exacerbations of their chronic disease with *Haemophilus influenzae*, *Streptococcus pneumoniae*, and *Moraxella catarrhalis*. Patients with cystic fibrosis are prone to chronic lung infections with *Staphylococcus aureus*, *Pseudomonas aeruginosa*, *Burkholderia cepacia*, *Stenotrophomonas maltophilia*, *Mycobacterium avium*, rhinovirus, and influenza viruses. Immunocompromised patients with HIV/

AIDS suffer from pulmonary infections with *Pneumocystis jirovecii*, *Nocardia* species, *Rhodococcus equi*, *M. avium*, and *Mycobacterium tuberculosis*. Individuals with chronic alcoholism can develop pulmonary disease with aspirated oral anaerobic bacteria and *Klebsiella pneumoniae*. Immunocompromised or malnourished individuals living in countries with endemic *M. tuberculosis* are at increased risk for severe disease. Likewise, all individuals are at risk for exposure and infection during epidemic or pandemic outbreaks with influenza virus or SARS coronaviruses. While community-acquired pneumonias are commonly caused by *S. pneumoniae*, *S. aureus*, *H. influenzae*, *M. catarrhalis*, and influenza viruses, hospital-acquired infections are more commonly caused by gram-negative rods such as *Klebsiella pneumoniae*, *Pseudomonas aeruginosa*, and *Acinetobacter baumannii*, many of which are resistant to multiple antibiotics.

It should be clear from this discussion that many organisms are capable of causing lower tract respiratory disease, but this list can be refined by carefully considering the risk factors for the individual patients. The following are a series of case studies that illustrate this principle.

HAEMOPHILUS INFLUENZAE PNEUMONIA

Holmes and Kozinn described a 61-year-old woman with pneumonia caused by *H. influenzae* serotype d. The patient had a long history of smoking, chronic obstructive lung disease, diabetes mellitus, and congestive heart failure. She presented with left upper lobe pneumonia, producing purulent sputum with many small gram-negative coccobacilli. Both sputum and blood cultures were positive for *H. influenzae* serotype d.

The organism was susceptible to ampicillin, to which the patient responded. This case illustrates the susceptibility of patients with chronic underlying pulmonary disease to infections with nonserotype b strains of *H. influenzae*. The Gram stain morphology of this organism is characteristic and should be sufficient for a rapid preliminary diagnosis. (Holmes, Kozinn. *J Clin Microbiol.* 1983;18:730–732.)

MORAXELLA CATARRHALIS BRONCHOPNEUMONIA

A 63-year-old alcoholic man was admitted to the hospital with fever and productive cough of a few days' duration. His temperature was 39°C, and he appeared malnourished. Examination of the chest showed an increased anteroposterior diameter with diffuse hyperresonance and rhonchi; diminished breath sounds over the right lower lung. A right lower lobe infiltrate was noted on chest radiography. Gram stain of the transtracheal aspirate showed abundant gram-negative coccobacilli and polymorphonuclear cells. Culture of the specimen yielded abundant *Moraxella catarrhalis* and a moderate number of *Haemophilus influenzae*. The patient was treated with ampicillin for 10 days. Defervescence and a pronounced decrease in sputum production were noted after 48 h of therapy and imaging at 12 days after admission to the hospital showed only mild right pleural thickening. *M. catarrhalis* is recognized as an important respiratory pathogen that mimics *Neisseria meningitidis* when observed in Gram stain (originally classified as a *Neisseria*). Although this patient was treated with ampicillin in 1978, most strains isolated today are beta-lactamase producers and resistant to ampicillin. (Louie et al., *West J Med.* 1983;138:47–49.)

ACINETOBACTER BAUMANNII PNEUMONIA

A 41-year-old man was admitted to the hospital with a 2-day history of productive cough, shortness of breath and fever. He presented with septic shock, hypoxemic respiratory failure, and bilateral pulmonary infiltrates. Laboratory results were notable for neutropenia, thrombocytopenia, and acute kidney failure. He had a history of long-term cigarette smoking and alcohol abuse. Antibiotic therapy with vancomycin, piperacillin-tazobactam, levofloxacin, and oseltamivir was started, and hypoxemia progressed rapidly necessitating intubation with high ventilatory support. Blood cultures collected at the time of admission grew gram-negative rods that were identified as *Acinetobacter baumannii* susceptible to all antimicrobials tested. Antimicrobials were changed to meropenem and levofloxacin. After 14 days of treatment, he still required ventilatory support so he was transferred to a subacute rehabilitation facility with eventual recovery. This presentation of pneumonia is unusual because most infections with *A. baumannii* are hospital-acquired, and the pathogen is now frequently resistant to all antibiotics including the carbapenems and colistin. (Serota et al. *Open Forum Infect Dis.* 2018;doi:10.1093/ofid/ofy044.)

KLEBSIELLA PNEUMONIAE PNEUMONIA

A 39-year-old previously healthy man living in Japan was admitted to the Emergency Department with fever and sudden-onset chest pain. He had no medical or travel history within the previous 6 months. Upon initial examination, the patient had a blood pressure of 153/111 mm Hg, high-grade fever (38.0°C), tachycardia, and tachypnea. Laboratory tests revealed elevated white blood cell count with 84% neutrophils, and elevations of C-reactive protein, hepatic enzymes, and blood glucose. A chest X-ray revealed a focal consolidation in the left lower lung field. The patient was hospitalized with the diagnosis of community-acquired pneumonia and promptly treated with ampicillin/sulbactam. However, his condition rapidly deteriorated and he had a cardiac arrest. Cardiopulmonary resuscitation was promptly initiated, and the patient was intubated for mechanical ventilation. His circulation was re-established, and he was transferred to the intensive care unit. Follow-up X-rays revealed rapidly progressive infiltration and CT scan demonstrated hyperdense infiltrates in the lower left lobe and multiple patchy infiltrates in both lung fields, suggestive of invasive pulmonary infection with septic emboli. Abdominal CT scan showed severe fatty infiltration of the liver suggestive of chronic alcoholic change. Despite intensive treatment, the patient continued to decline and died of multiorgan failure and disseminated intravascular coagulopathy. Blood and sputum cultures collected at admission grew *Klebsiella pneumoniae* susceptible to all conventional antimicrobials. *K. pneumoniae* is a common cause of community-acquired pneumonia, particularly in adults with underlying pulmonary disease or chronic alcoholism. This pathogen has also become more prominent in recent years as a cause of hospital-acquired infections and can be difficult to treat because multidrug-resistant strains are common. (Yamamoto et al. *Medicine.* 2020;99:21[e20360].)

PSEUDOMONAS AERUGINOSA PNEUMONIA

A 63-year-old-woman presented to her primary care physician with a 6-day history of fever, cough, and dyspnea. Her cough was productive of green sputum that was occasionally streaked with blood. She had mild chest discomfort but no chest pain or pleurisy. Review of systems was otherwise unremarkable. Her medical history was significant for chronic obstructive lung disease (COPD), hypothyroidism (well-controlled), hypertension, and a long history of smoking and alcohol abuse. Two years ago, she had a chest CT scan that showed evidence of emphysematous changes. On examination, the patient was not in any distress and she did not want further testing. She was prescribed a 5-day course of levofloxacin. Two weeks later, she returned to her physician with worsening cough,

increased hemoptysis, and respiratory distress. Chest X-ray revealed right upper lobe opacification with a large air-fluid level suggestive of cavitating pneumonia. Sputum was collected and Gram stain reveals abundant gram-negative rods and few neutrophils. *Pseudomonas aeruginosa* grew within 24h, resistant to levofloxacin. Therapy was initiated with ceftazidime and, despite susceptibility to the antibiotic, she continued to deteriorate and two weeks after admission she died from progressive respiratory and multiorgan failure. This case illustrates the progression of a community-acquired pneumonia with *P. aeruginosa* in a woman with compromised pulmonary function with a fatal outcome of necrotizing pneumonia. (Maharaj et al. *Case Reports Infect Dis.* 2017: doi:10.1155/2017/1717492)

HISTOPLASMOSIS

Geurkink and Cler described a 60-year-old woman with a history of alcoholic cirrhosis and long-standing tobacco use who presented to their facility in Dallas with complaints of an acute onset of dyspnea and dry cough, with a sharp pain sensation on inspiration. In the Emergency Department, she was found to have oxygen saturation of 79% on room air and was placed on supplemental oxygen. A chest X-ray revealed a large left-sided pneumothorax with nearly complete collapse of the left lung. A chest tube was placed, and she was admitted to the general medical floor. Chest X-ray 24h later showed only a mild decrease in the size of the pneumothorax, and CT scan revealed the presence of a left upper lobe cavitary lesion. Cardiothoracic surgery was consulted, and a surgical biopsy was sent for bacterial, mycobacterial, and fungal stains and culture. The fungal culture was positive for *Histoplasma capsulatum*. An infectious disease consult felt the pneumothorax was likely due to chronic cavitary pulmonary histoplasmosis. Itraconazole was started, and the patient underwent a thoracotomy.

During the procedure, she was noted to have adhesions of both the upper and lower lobes of the left lung which were resected. She was discharged to a long-term acute care facility and after prolonged treatment with itraconazole, chest X-ray showed resolution of her left-sided pneumothorax. This presentation of histoplasmosis is unusual because pneumothorax is not a common complication with this disease. However, this patient illustrates that the initial infection with histoplasmosis is by the respiratory route. Most infections in the United States occur to exposure to the fungus in the Mississippi and Ohio river valleys, although reports of histoplasmosis have been reported globally. Most exposure leads to an asymptomatic infection or only mild pulmonary symptoms; however, this patient's history of alcoholic cirrhosis and tobacco use puts her at increased risk for severe disease. Severe infections in both immunocompetent and immunocompromised patients can disseminate to any organ. (Gerukink, Cler. *J Comm Hosp Intern Med Perspectives.* 2020;10:483–487.)

STREPTOCOCCUS PNEUMONIAE PNEUMONIA

Costa and associates described a 68-year-old woman who was in good health until 3 days before hospitalization. She developed fever, chills, increased weakness, and a productive cough with pleuritic chest pain. On admission, she was febrile, had an elevated pulse and respiration rate, and was in moderate respiratory distress. Initial laboratory values showed leucopenia, anemia, and acute renal failure. Chest radiograph demonstrated infiltrates in the right and left lower lobes with pleural effusions. Therapy

with a fluoroquinolone was initiated, and blood and respiratory cultures were positive for *S. pneumoniae*. Additional tests (serum and urine protein electrophoresis) revealed the patient had multiple myeloma. The patient's infection resolved with a 14-day course of antibiotics. This patient illustrates the typical picture of pneumococcal lobar pneumonia and the increased susceptibility to infection in patients with defects in their ability to clear encapsulated organisms. (Costa et al. Am J Hematol. 2004;77:277–281.)

BURKHOLDERIA CEPACIA PULMONARY INFECTION

Mclean-Tooke and associates described a 21-year-old man with granulomatous lymphadenitis. The man presented with a history of weight loss, fevers, hepatosplenomegaly, and cervical lymphadenopathy. During the preceding 3 years, he had presented on two occasions with enlarged lymph nodes that were biopsied, and histologic examination revealed granulomatous lymphadenitis. A clinical diagnosis of sarcoidosis was made, and the man was discharged on 20 mg prednisolone. Over the next 24 months, the patient remained clinically well; however, he developed pancytopenia, and granulomas were observed on a bone marrow biopsy. During the current hospitalization, the patient developed a cough. Chest radiograph revealed consolidation in the base of the lungs. A lung biopsy and bronchoalveolar lavage was submitted for culture, and *Burkholderia cepacia* was isolated from both specimens. A subsequent immunologic evaluation of the patient confirmed that he had a genetic disease, chronic granulomatous disease (CGD). This case illustrates the specific susceptibility of CGD patients to infections with *Burkholderia*. Patients with *Burkholderia* infections should be evaluated for specific genetic diseases including CGD and cystic fibrosis. (Mclean-Tooke et al. *BMC Clin Pathol.* 2007;7:1.)

CMV PNEUMONIA POST-BONE MARROW TRANSPLANT

Nagafuji and associates reported a 52-year-old woman who developed fatal CMV interstitial pneumonia following autologous bone marrow transplantation for a myeloblastic leukemia. The woman was documented to be CMV-serology positive before transplantation. Following transplantation, her leukocytosis resolved at day 11. On day 25, bone marrow aspiration showed marked hemophagocytosis; treatment with prednisolone was initiated. On day 35, she was noted to be febrile and her CMV antigenemia assay was strongly positive. Ganciclovir and anti-CMV hyperimmune globulin were administered. On day 48, ganciclovir was withdrawn because of myelotoxicity. On day 56, hemorrhagic cystitis developed and CMV was cultured from the urine. Foscarnet was administered and the CMV antigenemia resolved. Foscarnet was discontinued on day 84, but the CMV-associated hemophagocytic syndrome was again documented on day 116. This was again managed with foscarnet, but on day 158 progressive CMV pneumonia developed and the patient died on day 171. The case illustrates the difficulty of managing CMV infections in immunocompromised bone marrow transplant patients. (Nagafuji et al. *Bone Marrow Transpl.* 1998;21:301–303.)

INVASIVE ASPERGILLOSIS IN RENAL TRANSPLANT PATIENT

Guha and associates described a case of invasive aspergillosis in a renal transplant recipient. The patient was a 34-year-old woman who presented with 2-day history of weakness, dizziness, left calf pain, and black tarry stools. She denied chest pain, cough, or shortness of breath. Her past medical history was significant for diabetes leading to renal failure, for which she received a cadaveric renal transplant in 2002. Three weeks before presentation, acute graft rejection developed. She was placed on an immunosuppressive regimen of alemtuzumab, tacrolimus, sirolimus, and prednisone. On admission, she was tachycardic, hypertensive, and febrile. Physical examination revealed a tender venous cord palpable in the popliteal fossa. An initial chest radiograph showed no abnormalities. Laboratory studies showed anemia and azotemia. The white cell blood count was 4800/μL with 80% neutrophils. The patient was given four units of packed red blood cells, and empirical treatment with gatifloxacin. On hospital day 6, vesicular rash developed on the buttocks and left calf, cultures of which were positive for herpes simplex virus, and she was placed on acyclovir. The patient's clinical condition stabilized except for her renal function, and intermittent hemodialysis was started on hospital day 8. On hospital day 12, the patient exhibited decreased responsiveness, became obtunded, and was intubated for respiratory distress. A chest radiograph showed diffuse bilateral lung nodules. Culture of bronchoalveolar lavage fluid was positive for *Aspergillus* species, and viral inclusion bodies suggestive of cytomegalovirus were seen. Her immunosuppression was decreased, and liposomal amphotericin B was started. The patient experienced an acute myocardial infarction and became comatose. Multiple acute infarcts in the frontal lobe and cerebellum were seen on a magnetic resonance imaging scan of the brain. The patient's condition continued to deteriorate, and multiple skin nodules developed on her arm and trunk. Biopsy specimens of the skin nodules grew *Aspergillus flavus* on culture. The patient subsequently died on hospital day 23. At autopsy, *A. flavus* was detected in multiple organs, including heart, lung, adrenal gland, thyroid, kidney, and liver. This case serves as an extreme example of disseminated aspergillosis in an immunocompromised host. (Guha. *Infect Med.* 2007;24(suppl 8):8–11.)

DRUG-RESISTANT *MYCOBACTERIUM TUBERCULOSIS*

The risk of active tuberculosis is significantly increased in HIV-infected individuals. Unfortunately, this problem is complicated by the development of drug-resistant *M. tuberculosis* strains in this population. This was illustrated in the report by Gandhi and associates, who studied the prevalence of tuberculosis in South Africa from January 2005 to March 2006. They identified 475 patients with culture-confirmed tuberculosis, of whom 39% had multidrug-resistant strains (MDR TB) and 6% with extensively drug-resistant strains (XDR TB). All patients with XDR TB were co-infected with HIV, and 98% of these patients died. The high prevalence of MDR TB and the evolution of XDR TB pose a serious challenge for tuberculosis treatment programs and emphasize the need for rapid diagnostic tests. (Gandhi et al. *Lancet.* 2006;368:1575–1580.)

MYCOBACTERIUM AVIUM INFECTION IN AN AIDS PATIENT

Woods and Goldsmith described a patient with advanced AIDS who died of disseminated *M. avium* infection. The patient was a 27-year-old man, who initially presented in October 1985 with a 2-week history of progressive dyspnea and a nonproductive cough. *Pneumocystis* was detected in a bronchoalveolar lavage, and serology confirmed the patient had an HIV infection. The patient was successfully treated with trimethoprim-sulfamethoxazole and discharged. The patient remained stable until May 1987, when he presented with persistent fever and dyspnea. Over the next week, he developed severe substernal chest pain, and a pericardial friction rub. Echocardiogram revealed a small effusion. The patient left the hospital against medical advice but returned 1 week later with a persistent cough, fever, and pain in the chest and left arm. A diagnostic pericardiocentesis was performed, and 220 mL of fluid was aspirated. Tuberculous pericarditis was suspected, and appropriate antimycobacterial therapy was initiated. However, over the next 3 weeks the patient developed progressive cardiac failure and died. *M. avium* was recovered from the pericardial fluid, as well as autopsy cultures of the pericardium, spleen, liver, adrenal glands, kidneys, small intestine, lymph nodes, and pituitary gland. Although *M. avium* pericarditis was unusual, the extensive dissemination of the mycobacteria in patients with advanced AIDS was common before azithromycin prophylaxis became widely used. (Woods, Goldsmith. *Chest.* 1989;95:1355–1357.)

RHODOCOCCUS EQUI PULMONARY INFECTION

A 34-year-old Albanian man was admitted to a regional hospital presenting with dry cough, fever, progressive dyspnea, night sweats, and a thick-walled cavitary lesion of the left lung, associated with bilateral pulmonary infiltrates on radiologic examination. He had been well until 15 days before presentation, except that he had lost more than 20 lbs in the last 6 months. On admission, he was ill-looking, had a low-grade fever, tachycardia and a respiratory rate of 30 breaths per minute. Physical examination revealed diffuse crackles in both lungs, and lesions on the oral mucous membrane and lower extremities consistent with Kaposi's sarcoma. Microscopic examination of sputum revealed acid-fast bacteria and normal respiratory tract flora was isolated on bacterial culture of the sputum. Specimens were subsequently cultured for acid-fast organisms, and empiric therapy was initiated for the preliminary diagnosis of *Mycobacterium tuberculosis* infection. He continued to deteriorate so additional blood cultures and sputum cultures were collected. After 2 days of incubation, gram-variable, pleomorphic, coccobacillary were isolated in the blood cultures and small, whitish colonies were observed in the sputum cultures. After 3–4 days, the colonies developed a salmon-pink color and the organisms in both the blood and sputum cultures were identified as *Rhodococcus equi*. Antimycobacterial treatment was discontinued, and treatment with ertapenem and ciprofloxacin was initiated. Three days later, he became afebrile, with gradual improvement over the next 15 days. Unfortunately, the patient died one month later due to CMV pneumonia. This case is an example of *Rhodococcus* pulmonary infection with abscess formation in a patient with previously undiagnosed HIV infection. *Rhodococcus* is a slow-growing, partially acid-fast coccobacillus that will assume a reddish color with prolonged incubation. The acid-fast property initially led to the misdiagnosis of a mycobacterial infection. (Spiliopoulou et al. *J Med Case Reports.* 2014;8:423.)

FIRST REPORT OF AIDS IN LOS ANGELES

On June 5, 1981, the Centers for Disease Control and Prevention published the first report of five homosexual men in Los Angeles with *Pneumocystis* (*carinii*) *jiroveci* pneumonia with concurrent cytomegalovirus (CMV) infection and candida mucosal infection. Patient 1 was a previously healthy 33-year-old man who developed *P. jiroveci* pneumonia and oral mucosal candidiasis after a 2-month history of fever associated with elevated liver enzymes, leukopenia, and CMV viruria. The patient's condition continued to deteriorate despite treatment with trimethoprim-sulfamethoxazole (TMP-SXT), pentamidine, and acyclovir, and he died on May 3. Patient 2 was a 30-year-old man who developed *P. jiroveci* pneumonia in April 1981 after a 5-month history of daily fevers and of elevated liver function tests and CMV viruria. He also had leukopenia and mucosal candidiasis. His pneumonia responded to TMP-SXT but his fevers persisted. He was lost to follow-up. Patient 3 was well until January 1981 when he developed esophageal and oral candidiasis that responded to amphotericin B treatment. He was hospitalized in February for *P. jiroveci* pneumonia that responded to TMP-SXT. His esophageal candidiasis recurred and was again treated with amphotericin B. An esophageal biopsy was positive for CMV. Patient 4 was a 29-year-old man who developed *P. jiroveci* pneumonia in February 1981. His pneumonia did not respond to TMP-SXT, and he died in March. Both *P. jiroveci* and CMV were found in the lung tissue. Patient 5 was a previously healthy 36-year-old man, clinically diagnosed with CMV infection in September 1980. He was seen in April 1981 because of a 4-month history of fever, dyspnea, and cough. On admission, he was found to have *P. jiroveci* pneumonia, oral candidiasis, and CMV retinitis. His pneumonia was treated with TMP-SXT and topical nystatin was used to treat the *Candida* infection. All five patients had profound immunosuppression and multiple opportunistic infections. This report documented not an isolated focal epidemic but rather the first patients of the AIDS pandemic.

PNEUMOCYSTIS PNEUMONIA IN NEWLY DIAGNOSED HIV/AIDS PATIENT

Kayik et al. described a 50-year-old man who presented with a 1-week history of pleuritic chest pain and fever. He was also hypoxic with oxygen saturation of 86% on room air. His clinical history revealed that he had fatigue, dyspnea, night sweats, generalized bone pain and a loss of about 10 kg over the past six months. Chest X-ray showed diffuse bilateral infiltrates. Bronchoscopy was performed and transbronchial biopsy and bronchoalveolar lavage was submitted for diagnostic testing. Gomori's methenamine silver stain demonstrated the presence of *Pneumocystis jirovecii* in the clinical specimens. Additional testing also revealed the patient had cytomegalovirus (CMV) co-infection. The patient was positive for HIV antibodies with a CD4+ cell count of 48/µL. Infections with *Pneumocystis* and CMV frequently are the initial infections in HIV patients with low CD4+ cell counts. The fungal infection typically responds well to trimethoprim-sulfamethoxazole (TMP-SXT) and pentamidine treatment, and TMP-SXT is commonly used for prophylaxis in HIV/AIDS patients. Detection using silver stains has now been replaced with immunofluorescent microscopy or more sensitive PCR tests. (Kayik et al. *Turk J Pathol.* 2020;36(3):246–250.)

STAPHYLOCOCCUS AUREUS PNEUMONIA

Bacterial pneumonia is a well-described complication of influenza virus infection. Murray et al. described the clinical features of severe pneumonia in five patients. Two patients died at home with the dual infection confirmed by postmortem cultures. The remaining three patients had an influenza-like illness 3–5 days before hospitalization confirmed by the detection of influenza virus A (H1N1) in respiratory secretions. The patients presented with symptoms of fever, productive cough, dyspnea, and pleuritic chest pain, with chest radiographs consistent with lobar pneumonia. All three patients had methicillin-resistant *Staphylococcus aureus* (MRSA) recovered in sputum and blood collected within the first 24 h of hospitalization. All patients were treated with oseltamivir for the influenza virus infection and antibacterials including ceftriaxone (ineffective against MRSA) and azithromycin. All three patients recovered after prolonged hospital stays. These patients represent the complications of influenza virus infection when pathogenic organisms normally resident in the oropharynx (e.g., *S. aureus*, *Streptococcus pneumoniae*) can invade into the lower airways following the viral destruction of the protective ciliated epithelial cells in the throat and establish pneumonia. (Murray et al. *PLoS One.* 2010;5:e8705.)

PREVIOUSLY HEALTHY PATIENT WITH SARS INFECTION

Luo and colleagues[1] described a previously healthy patient who was transferred to their hospital after a 9-day history of persistent fevers, myalgias, and headache. At the time of admission, the patient presented with a fever of 39.4°C, chills, a dry cough, shortness of breath, and diarrhea. Chest X-ray showed inflammation in the right upper lung fields. White blood cells and chemistries were normal. The patient failed to respond to antibiotic treatment, and on day 3, he developed a deep cough and dyspnea along with diffuse pulmonary inflammation. The diagnosis of SARS was made in view of his severe hypoxemia with PaO_2 of 60 mmHg and PaO_2/FiO_2 of 150 mmHg, and a clinical picture consistent with other hospitalized patients with SARS-CoV-1. The patient was transferred to the intensive care unit and placed on ventilatory support but continued to deteriorate into multiorgan dysfunction syndrome involving the kidney, liver, and heart. The medical staff initiated molecular adsorbent recirculating system therapy (extracorporeal liver support utilizing albumin dialysis for 8h) and after four consecutive days of therapy, clinical improvement was noted. After 13 days, ventilatory support was withdrawn and the patient continued to improve. The patient was discharged after 44 days of hospitalization. This case illustrates the severe infection caused by SARS-CoV-1. It is remarkable that within the same virus family, most strains are responsible for mild upper respiratory infections while others such as SARS-CoV-2 and MERS-CoV can cause devastating pneumonia with multiorgan involvement. (Luo et al. *Artif Organs*. 2003;27:847–849.)

H5N1 AVIAN INFLUENZA INFECTION

The first case of H5N1 avian influenza in a human was described by Ku and Chan. After a 3-year-old boy from China developed a fever of 40°C and abdominal pain, he was given antibiotics and aspirin. On the third day, he was hospitalized with a sore throat, and his chest radiograph demonstrated bronchial inflammation. Blood studies showed a left shift with 9% band forms. On the sixth day, the boy was still febrile and fully conscious, but on the seventh day his fever increased, he was hyperventilating, and his blood oxygen levels decreased. A chest radiograph indicated severe pneumonia. The patient was intubated. On the eighth day, the boy was diagnosed with fulminant sepsis and acute respiratory distress syndrome. Therapy for acute respiratory distress syndrome and other attempts to improve oxygen uptake were unsuccessful. He was treated empirically for sepsis, herpes simplex virus infection (acyclovir), methicillin-resistant *S. aureus* (vancomycin), and fungal infection (amphotericin B), but his condition deteriorated further, with disseminated intravascular coagulation and liver and renal failure. He died on the 11th day. Laboratory results indicated evaluated influenza A antibody on the eighth day, and influenza A was isolated from a tracheal isolate taken on the ninth day. The isolate was sent to the Centers for Disease Control and Prevention and elsewhere, where it was typed as H5N1 avian influenza and named *A/Hong Kong/156/97* (*H5N1*). The child may have contracted the virus while playing with pet ducklings and chickens at his kindergarten. Although the H5N1 virus still has difficulty infecting humans, this case demonstrates the speed and severity of the respiratory and systemic manifestations of avian influenza H5N1 disease. (Ku, Chan. *J Paediatr Child Health*. 1999;35:207–209.)

ADENOVIRUS 14 PNEUMONIA

The Centers for Disease Control and Prevention reported that analysis of isolates from trainees during an outbreak of febrile respiratory infection at Lackland Air Force Base showed 63% resulted from adenovirus, and 90% of these were adenovirus 14. Of the 423 cases, 27 were hospitalized with pneumonia, 5 required admission to the intensive care unit, and 1 patient died. In an analogous case reported by Cable News Network, an 18-year-old high-school athlete complained of flulike symptoms with vomiting, chills, and fever of 40°C that progressed to life-threatening pneumonia within days. The adenovirus causing these infections is a mutant of the adenovirus 14 that was identified in 1955. The adenovirus 14 mutant has spread around the United States, putting adults at risk for severe disease. Adenovirus 14 infection usually causes a benign respiratory infection in adults, with newborns and the elderly at higher risk for severe outcomes. Although most virus mutations produce a weaker virus, occasionally a more virulent antibody-escape or antiviral drug-resistant virus may occur. (*MMWR Morb Mortal Wkly Rep*. 2007;56:1181–1184.)

REINFECTION IN A PATIENT WITH SARS-COV-2

Selvaraj et al. described a man with a second episode of SARS-CoV-2 disease. The man was in his 70s and had multiple risk factors for disease including his age, hypertension, obesity, and asthma. He tested positive for SARS-CoV-2 in early April 2020 and presented to the hospital 12 days later with worsening shortness of breath. Chest X-ray showed mild, patchy mid- and lower-lung airspace disease bilaterally. He was able to maintain oxygen saturation levels >90% on room air and was discharged with medications for symptomatic relief. Follow-up 3 weeks later showed resolution of this disease. Seven months later, he returned to the hospital with shortness of breath, fever, body aches, nausea, and malaise. He reported that two family members reported positive for SARS-CoV-2 10 days before he presented to the hospital. On physical examination, he was hypoxic on ambient air (87% oxygen saturation), and lung examination revealed rales at the bases. He was hospitalized and started on supplemental oxygen. A respiratory viral panel was performed and returned positive for SARS-CoV-2. X-ray findings revealed multifocal airspace disease, greatest in the left lung. He was treated with dexamethasone and Remdesivir as well as empiric ceftriaxone. After 3 days of improvement, he was discharged on supplemental air. Recurrent infections with SARS-CoV-2 are noted to be more common in patients who were initially infected with the original strain of virus and then exposed to a variant mutant strain. Currently, this is most common with the Delta variant but was also reported with the Beta variant that was responsible for a second wave of infections in Brazil. Both of these variants have been shown to be partially refractory to antibodies developed either during the initial infection or after vaccination. (Selvaraj et al. *Rhode Island Med J.* 2020;103:24–26.)

MERS-COV INFECTION IN VISITOR TO SAUDI ARABIA

Cha et al. reported the clinical history of a 68-year-old man who developed respiratory symptoms one week after visiting Bahrain and Saudi Arabia. He initially developed fever, myalgia, shortness of breath, coughing, and general weakness. After a progression of his symptoms, he visited a primary care hospital and CT scan of his chest revealed ground glass opacity in the right upper lobe. MERS-CoV PCR test was positive. He was transferred to a tertiary care hospital after 4 days of ineffective response to treatment and progression of his respiratory symptoms. Upon admission, he complained of myalgia, dry cough, dyspnea, and nausea and vomiting. He was initially treated with interferon and ribavirin but this was discontinued on hospital day 7 because of sustained fever and thrombocytopenia. He was placed on mechanical ventilation which was accompanied by a progression of multiple pneumonic infiltrates. Blood and urine cultures remained negative during hospitalization, but sputum cultures were positive for multidrug-resistant *Acinetobacter baumannii*, *Pseudomonas aeruginosa* and *Enterobacter aerogenes*, as well as methicillin-resistant *Staphylococcus aureus*. These were treated with a variety of antibiotics. MERS-CoV PCR tests of sputum, urine, and stool specimens on hospital day 37 were negative. His hospitalization was complicated by acute renal tubular necrosis. The patient's prognosis was not reported but this case illustrates the complexity of managing MERS-CoV disease, with secondary bacterial infections and multiorgan dysfunction. (Cha et al. *J Korean Med Soc.* 2016;31:635–640.)

NEISSERIA MENINGITIDIS PNEUMONIA

A 17-year-old boy, in previous good health, presented to the Emergency Department with a 7-day history of productive cough, right pleural pain, fever, and dyspnea. He was admitted to the ICU due to septic shock and respiratory distress. He was managed with vasoactive drugs and prone positioning ventilation for 48 h. Chest radiography showed a right superior lobe condensation. The electrocardiogram and echocardiogram suggested septic myocarditis. Blood cultures were collected and became positive within 24 h with gram-negative diplococci, which was subsequently identified as *Neisseria meningitidis* serogroup W135. A lumbar puncture ruled out meningitis and a 10-day treatment with ceftriaxone was completed with full recovery. *N. meningitidis* meningitis and meningococcemia are life-threatening illness with high morbidity and mortality. In contrast, pneumonia caused by this organism is typically milder with generally good response to antimicrobial therapy. (Yubini et al. *Rev Med Chile.* 2018;146:doi:10.4067/s0034-9887201800200249.)

FRANCISELLA TULARENSIS PNEUMONIA

In June 1978, three cases of tularemia pneumonia occurred in men residing in the Washington DC area. All three men became ill three to four days after a brief session training their hunting dogs in an undeveloped wooded area adjacent to a housing complex. One of the dogs, which later died, had captured a wild rabbit during the training session. All three men had handled the rabbit while familiarizing their dogs with the rabbit's scent. The men had no other common exposure that was a likely source of infection. Most of my career was spent in Saint Louis, Missouri where infections with *Francisella tularensis* are relatively common in the area. Although ulceroglandular disease is the most common presentation, infections presenting primarily as pneumonia are not uncommon. Pulmonary infections are most commonly acquired by exposure to aerosolized blood from an infected rabbit while ulceroglandular disease is typically associated with the bite of an infected tick. It was often said that the slow rabbits are the sick rabbits which is why the dog may have captured the wild rabbit. When I moved from Missouri to the Washington DC area, another case of tularemia pneumonia was presented during a clinical conference. This case was identical to another patient that was seen in Saint Louis where exposure to the infected rabbit occurred when the patient was mowing an open field and accidentally ran over a family of rabbits. Although some believe it is difficult to grow the organism, I have found this is not the case. These are extremely small, gram-negative coccobacilli and in my experience when such an organism is observed in the Gram stain of a blood culture, the technologist should strongly suspect either *Francisella* or *Brucella*.

PSITTACOSIS IN A PREVIOUSLY HEALTHY MAN

Scully and associates described a 24-year-old man who was admitted into a local hospital in acute respiratory distress. Several days before his hospitalization, he developed nasal congestion, myalgia, dry cough, mild dyspnea, and a headache. Immediately before admission, the cough became productive and he developed pleuritic pain, fever, chills, and diarrhea. Radiographs demonstrated consolidation of the right upper lobe of the lungs and patchy infiltrates in the left lower lobe. Despite the fact his antibiotic treatment included erythromycin, doxycycline, ceftriaxone, and vancomycin, his pulmonary status did not begin to improve for 7 days, and he was not discharged from the hospital until a month after his admission. A careful history revealed the man had been exposed to parrots in a hotel lobby while vacationing. The diagnosis of *Chlamydia psittaci* pneumonia was made by growing the organism in cell culture and serologic tests. Culture is rarely performed in most clinical laboratories so serology is the test of choice or more recently detection of the bacterial DNA by PCR tests. (Scully et al. *N Engl J Med*. 1998;338:1527–1535.)

COCCIDIOIDOMYCOSIS

Stafford and colleagues describe a 31-year-old African American US Army soldier who presented with fever, chills, night sweats, and a nonproductive cough of 4 weeks' duration. In addition, he had recently detected a painless right breast mass. His past medical history was unremarkable. He was stationed at Fort Irwin, California, where he was working as a telephone repairman. His physical examination was unremarkable except for a firm, nontender, 3-cm subcutaneous mass overlying the right breast. Multiple small (<1 cm) nontender lymph nodes were palpable in the axillae and groin. Laboratory studies revealed a white blood count of 11.9/μL, with 30% eosinophils. Serum chemistries were notable for an elevated alkaline phosphate level. Results of blood cultures, tests for serum *Cryptococcus* antigen, urinary *Histoplasma* antigen, and HIV antibody were negative, as was a tuberculin skin test. A chest radiograph showed bilateral interstitial micronodules in a military pattern, as well as a right-sided paratracheal fullness. A CT scan of the chest confirmed the presence of diffuse 1- to 2-mm micronodules in all lobes. The CT scan also showed a lobular parenchymal mass lesion in the right middle lobe and a right chest wall mass. A fine-needle aspiration of the right breast mass revealed spherules filled with endospores, consistent with coccidioidomycosis. Culture of the material grew *C. immitis*. A serology panel for *C. immitis* was positive and revealed immunoglobulin G complement fixation titers at a dilution of greater than 1:256. Cerebrospinal fluid analysis was normal, but a bone scan revealed multiple regions of increased osteoblastic activity involving the left scapula, right anterior fifth rib, and midthoracic vertebral regions. Treatment was initiated with amphotericin B, but

Continued

COCCIDIOIDOMYCOSIS—cont'd

increasing neck pain prompted further imaging, which demonstrated a lytic lesion of the C1 vertebral body and a paravertebral mass. Despite antifungal therapy, progressive enlargement of the mass necessitated surgical debridement. The patient was continued on amphotericin B lipid formulation, with plans for long-term, perhaps lifelong, antifungal therapy.

This is an example of the serious problems posed by coccidioidomycosis. Clues leading to diagnosis of disseminated coccidioidomycosis in this patient included an infectious prodrome, peripheral eosinophilia, hilar lymphadenopathy, characterization of pattern of organ involvement (lungs, bones, soft tissues), residence in an endemic area, and African American ethnicity (higher risk group of dissemination). (Stafford et al. *Infect Med.* 2007;24(suppl 8):23–25.)

PARAGONIMIASIS

Singh and colleagues described a case of pleuropulmonary paragonimiasis mimicking pulmonary tuberculosis. The patient was a 21-year-old man who was admitted to the hospital for progressive dyspnea, with a 1-month history of headache, fever, cough with scant hemoptysis, fatigue, pleuritic pain, anorexia, and weight loss. He had a history of antituberculous therapy for 6 months without clinical improvement. Two months before admission, after ingesting three raw crabs, he had a 3-day episode of watery diarrhea. On hospital admission, the patient was cachectic and afebrile. There was bilateral dullness to percussion and absent breath sounds in the lower two-thirds of the chest. He was found to be anemic and had clubbing without lymphadenopathy, cyanosis, or jaundice. A chest radiograph showed bilateral pleural effusions that were also confirmed by computed tomography. Ultrasound-guided thoracentesis of the right lung yielded about 200 mL of yellowish fluid. The fluid was exudative and contained 2700 white blood cells/mL, 91% of which were eosinophils. Gram stain of the fluid was negative, as was culture for bacteria and fungi. Sputum smears revealed operculated yellowish eggs consistent with *Paragonimus westermani* infection. The patient was treated with a 3-day course of praziquantel and responded well. Of note, the right-sided plural effusion did not recur after the thoracentesis and praziquantel treatment. This case emphasizes the importance of making an etiologic diagnosis of a pleuropulmonary process to differentiate paragonimiasis from tuberculosis in regions where both are endemic infectious diseases. (Singh et al. *Indian J Med Microbiol.* 2005;23:131–134.)

ECHINOCOCCOSIS IN A PREGNANT WOMAN

Yeh and colleagues described a 36-year-old pregnant woman at 21 weeks of gestation who presented with a 4-week history of a dry nonproductive cough. The patient denied any constitutional symptoms and had no new pets, environmental exposures, or sick contacts. It was her first pregnancy, and there were no complications. She had no medical conditions and did not smoke or drink alcohol. She was a financial consultant and enjoyed running and hiking. She had traveled to Australia, Central Asia, and sub-Saharan Africa in the past. The patient appeared well, with appropriate weight gain for the second trimester of her pregnancy. Her physical examination, including auscultation of her lungs, was normal. Her cough did not improve with use of an inhaled bronchodilator. Imaging studies were not performed because of her pregnancy. She had a normal uncomplicated vaginal delivery 4 months later. She continued to have a dry cough and presented to her physician months after delivery for a reevaluation of her cough. At that time, her physical graph revealed a soft-tissue mass, 7 cm in diameter, adjacent to the right heart border. High-resolution computed tomography (CT) scans of the chest confirmed the presence of a homogeneous and fluid-filled structure without septa, thought to be in the mediastinum. Subsequent echocardiography also confirmed a simple cystic structure with thin walls surrounding echo-free fluid that was indenting the right atrium. Based on the radiographic and echocardiography findings, the clinicians caring for the patient thought that the mass was most likely a benign pericardial cyst. Because she was not experiencing dyspnea, the patient declined surgical removal. However, because of worsening cough over the next few months, she consulted a thoracic surgeon for elective resection. Intraoperative findings revealed an intraparenchymal

ECHINOCOCCOSIS IN A PREGNANT WOMAN—cont'd

pulmonary cyst in the right lung that was not attached to the pericardium or bronchus. The cyst was removed intact without gross spillage of the contents. Staining of the cyst wall with hematoxylin and eosin after cross sectioning showed an acellular laminated layer. Microscopic examination of the cyst contents showed protoscolices with hooklets and suckers in a background of histiocytes and eosinophilic debris, consistent with *E. granulosus*. CT of the abdomen after removal of the thoracic cyst revealed no hepatobiliary disease. Postoperative screening for serum antibody against *Echinococcus* was positive. Praziquantel was administered for 10 days after surgery and albendazole for 1 month after surgery, with no complications. After this course of therapy, the patient had resolution of her cough and returned to her normal level of activity. There was no evidence of recurrent disease on CT follow-up 6 months after surgery. (Ye et al. *N Engl J Med.* 2007;357:489–494.)

CHLAMYDIA TRACHOMATIS PNEUMONIA IN NEWBORN INFANTS

Niida and associates described two female infants with *C. trachomatis* pneumonia. The first infant was born by vaginal delivery after 39 weeks' gestation and the second by caesarean section at 40 weeks' gestation because of fetal distress. The infants were in good condition until fever and tachypnea developed at 3 and 13 days, respectively. Chest radiographs showed infiltrates over the whole lungs. Cultures of blood, urine, throat, feces, and cerebrospinal fluid were negative, but antigen tests for *C. trachomatis* were positive from conjunctival and nasopharyngeal swabs. These cases illustrate the presentation of pneumonia in infants infected with *C. trachomatis* at or near birth, although the characteristic staccato cough was not described in these patients, complicating a rapid, clinical diagnosis. (Niida et al. *Eur J Pediatr.* 1998;157:950–951.)

OUTBREAK OF PARAINFLUENZA VIRUS (PIV) IN NEONATAL INTENSIVE CARE UNIT

Maeda et al. reported an outbreak of PIV infections in a neonatal ICU. The index patient was a newborn girl who was delivered at 28 weeks. Shortly after birth, she was intubated and ventilated for respiratory distress syndrome. She remained on the ventilatory for 37 days and required nasal continuous positive airway pressure until day 75. On hospital day 114, she developed apnea, fever, and cough, and pulmonary infiltrates were seen on chest radiography. PIV3 was detected on virus culture. Her respiratory symptoms persisted for 17 days and she required supplemental oxygen for 13 days. She was discharged on hospital day 136, with recurrent wheezing that persisted and common cold symptoms until 1-year of age. Two other babies in the ICU also developed respiratory infections with PIV3 during the index patient's infection. PIV is a common cause of respiratory infections in infants and young children and PIV3 is commonly associated with more severe symptoms as observed in this child. (Maeda et al. *Ped Intern.* 2017;59:1219–1222.)

RESPIRATORY SYNCYTIAL VIRUS (RSV) INFECTION IN ELDERLY IMMUNOCOMPETENT PATIENT

Yoon and Lee reported a previously healthy 81-year-old man presented to their hospital with fever, cough, and dyspnea. He was hypoxemic and had a ground glass opacity in both lung fields and right-side pleural effusion evident on chest radiography. His pulmonary symptoms progressed and he required mechanical ventilation. All cultures and serology were negative, but multiplex NAAT was positive for RSV and negative for all other respiratory pathogens. Thoracentesis was required on hospital day 2, and turbid yellowish fluid was extracted. On hospital day 3, his condition worsened and he had to be intubated and mechanically ventilated. The initial PaO_2/FiO_2 was 65, compatible with severe ARDS (acute respiratory distress syndrome). He was started on methylprednisolone and the antiviral ribavirin. The hypoxemia and lung lesions gradually improved, and he was extubated on hospital day 17. He was maintained on ribavirin until he was discharged on day 27. Although RSV infections are most common in children, severe infections as observed in this elderly man do occur. (Yon, Lee. *J Med Case Reports* 2017;11:353–358.)

31

Gastrointestinal Tract Infections

As with respiratory infections, there is a long list of viruses, bacteria, fungi, and parasites responsible for gastrointestinal disease. For the student, it is best to classify these infections based on clinical symptoms and then subdivide the infections by patient age, underlying risk factors, and epidemiologic exposure. For this discussion, I will subdivide the infections into gastritis, secretory or noninflammatory intestinal infection, inflammatory intestinal infections, and intoxications.

Gastritis is primarily caused by *Helicobacter pylori*, as discussed in Chapter 10. Likewise, there is a limited number of microbes associated with intoxications; that is, disease caused by ingestion of toxins. Characteristic of intoxications, the onset is relatively rapid after ingestion of contaminated food and the duration of symptoms is generally less than 24 h. *Staphylococcus aureus* and *Bacillus cereus* are the most common intoxications, while other organisms such as *Clostridium perfringens* and *Bacteroides fragilis* are less commonly implicated.

Noninflammatory intestinal infections are characterized by watery diarrhea with or without vomiting, and low-grade fever. Many of these infections are restricted to pediatric patients because repeated exposure to the pathogens provides immunity to adults. This is not true for some pathogens where multiple strains may circulate in a community, immunity may be short-lived, or an adult travels from a nonendemic region to an endemic one. Viruses responsible for noninflammatory gastroenteritis include norovirus, sapovirus, rotavirus, astrovirus, and adenovirus. Except for norovirus, these are primarily pediatric diseases and the use of vaccines has significantly reduced disease caused by rotavirus. Bacteria responsible for noninflammatory disease are more numerous and include enterotoxigenic *Escherichia coli* (ETEC), enteropathogenic *E. coli* (EPEC), enteroaggregative *E. coli* (EAEC), shiga toxin-producing *E. coli* (STEC), *Shigella*, *Salmonella*, *Campylobacter*, *Vibrio cholerae*, and other *Vibrio* species. It should be noted here that some of these pathogens (e.g., STEC, *Shigella*, *Salmonella*, and *Campylobacter*) can progress to inflammatory disease characterized by diarrhea with or without blood, abdominal cramps, fever, and the absence of vomiting. Fungal enteric pathogens are relatively uncommon; however, microsporidia are a collection of more than 200 genera that are currently placed in the kingdom of Fungi. Many of the microsporidial genera are associated with self-limited watery diarrhea in immunocompetent patients and persistent, profuse, watery diarrhea in immunocompromised patients. Protozoa associated with noninflammatory disease include *Cryptosporidium*, *Giardia*, *Cystoisospora*, and *Cyclospora*.

Bacteria that can present with symptoms consistent with inflammatory disease are mentioned above. Additionally, *Clostridioides difficile* is a common enteric pathogen that can present with fever, bloody or nonbloody diarrhea, and abdominal cramps. Likewise, the protozoa *Entamoeba histolytica* is responsible for inflammatory disease. Finally, many intestinal helminths (nematodes, trematodes, cestodes) may present with enteric symptoms where diagnosis is guided by a careful travel history and examination of stool specimens for the parasitic eggs.

The following clinical cases should illustrate many of the clinical and epidemiological signs that can guide a specific diagnosis.

STAPHYLOCOCCAL FOOD POISONING

A report published in the CDC Morbidity and Mortality Weekly Report illustrates many important features of staphylococcal food poisoning. A total of 18 persons attending a retirement party became ill approximately 3–4 h after eating. The most common symptoms were nausea (94%), vomiting (89%), and diarrhea (72%). Relatively few individuals had fever or headache (11%). The symptoms lasted a median of 24 h. The illness was associated with eating ham at the party. A sample of the cooked ham tested positive for staphylococcal enterotoxin type A. A food preparer had cooked the ham at home, transported it to her workplace, sliced it while it was still hot, and then refrigerated the ham in a large plastic container covered with foil. The ham was served cold the next day. Cooking the ham would kill any contaminating *S. aureus*, so it is likely the ham was contaminated after it was cooked. The delays involved in refrigerating the ham and the fact it was stored in a single container allowed the organism to proliferate and produce enterotoxin. Type A toxin is the most common toxin associated with human disease. The rapid onset and short duration of nausea, vomiting, and diarrhea are typical of this disease because symptoms result from the preformed toxin and not the presence of this organisms in the food. Care must be used to avoid contamination of salted meats such as ham because reheating the food at a later time will not inactivate the heat-stable toxin. (*MMWR.* 1997;46:1189–1191.)

BACILLUS CEREUS FOOD POISONING

A 30-year-old woman developed abdominal cramping and 2 episodes of vomiting approximately 1 h after eating reheated fried rice that was taken home from a restaurant the night before. There was no fever or diarrhea, and she felt fine within 24 h. *Bacillus cereus* food poisoning is one of the most common causes of foodborne illnesses worldwide but is rarely diagnosed because the symptoms are short-lived and self-limited, and diagnosis would require isolating the organism or its toxins from the implicated food. Rice is a common source of infections. Both spores and vegetative cells may be found in foods. Although the vegetative cells are rapidly killed with cooking, the spores will survive and can germinate if the food is left for a prolonged period unrefrigerated. During this time, enterotoxins are produced and will not be killed with reheating. Because the disease is an intoxication, the onset of symptoms is rapid and persist for less than 24 h.

CLOSTRIDIUM PERFRINGENS FOOD POISONING

The Centers for Disease Control and Prevention (CDC) reported two outbreaks of *C. perfringens* gastroenteritis associated with corned beef served at St. Patrick's Day celebrations. On March 18, 1993, the Cleveland City Health Department received telephone calls from 15 persons who became ill after eating corned beef purchased from one delicatessen. After publicizing the outbreak, 156 persons contacted the Health Department with a similar history. In addition to a history of diarrhea, 88% complained of abdominal cramps and 13% with vomiting, which developed an average of 12 h after eating the implicated meat. An investigation revealed the delicatessen had purchased 1400 pounds of raw, salt-cured meat, and beginning on March 12, portions of the corned beef were boiled for 3 h, allowed to cool at room temperature, and then refrigerated. On March 16 and 17, the meat was removed from the refrigerator, heated to 48.8°C, and served. Cultures of the meat yielded greater than 10^5 colonies of *C. perfringens* per gram. The Health Department recommended that if the meat could not be served immediately after cooking, it should be rapidly cooled in ice and refrigerated. Before it is served, it should be warmed to at least 74°C to destroy the heat-sensitive enterotoxin. In contrast to intoxications caused by *Staphylococcus aureus* and *Bacillus cereus*, the delay in disease onset is more prolonged, vomiting is not a prominent symptom, and meats and gravies are commonly implicated. (*MMWR.* 1994;43:137–144.)

CLOSTRIDIUM PERFRINGENS GASTROENTERITIS

Gastroenteritis caused by *Clostridium perfringens* typically occurs when the bacteria contaminate meats and gravies and are able to grow to the high concentrations ($>10^6$ vegetative cells per gram food) required to initiate infections. When the food is ingested, most of the vegetative cells will die during passage through the acidic stomach to the small intestine, hence the requirement for large numbers of organisms to establish disease. After transit to the small intestine, the organisms are stimulated to form spores ("sporulation"). *C. perfringens* enterotoxin is released only in sporulating bacteria, with the enterotoxin binding to and damaging the small intestine villi. Clinically, *C. perfringens* food poisoning usually involves diarrhea and abdominal cramps developing 8–12 h after ingestion of the food and symptoms persist for 12–24 h before self-resolving. The rapid onset and short duration of illness is typical of "bacterial intoxication" as a cause for gastroenteritis, similar to what is observed with *Staphylococcus aureus* and *Bacillus cereus*. (Shrestha et al. *Microbiol Spectr.* 2018;6:doi:10.1128/microbiolspec.GPP#-0003-2017.)

HELICOBACTER PYLORI PEPTIC ULCERS

Helicobacter pylori colonizes the mucus layer of the human stomach, neutralizing the acidic environment by hypersecretion of urease. In developing countries, 50%–90% of the population are infected with the organism, typically in childhood. In contrast, colonization in developed countries does not occur until after 40 years of age and is much less common (<10%). Most gastric diseases (duodenal ulcer, gastric ulcer, gastric cancer) are associated with *H. pylori*. More than half the gastric adenocarcinomas in the world are related to *H. pylori* infection. Diagnosis of *H. pylori* infection is based on the high concentration of urease produced by these organisms and the subsequent accumulation of ammonia from hydrolysis of urea. (Marshall. *Clin Med JRCPL.* 2002;2:147–152.)

OUTBREAK OF ACUTE ROTAVIRUS INFECTION

Mikami and associates described an outbreak of acute gastroenteritis that occurred over a 5-day period in 45 of 107 children (aged 11–12 years) after a 3-day school trip. The source person for the outbreak was ill at the start of the trip. A case of acute gastroenteritis caused by rotavirus is defined as three or more episodes of diarrhea and/or two or more episodes of vomiting per day. Other symptoms included fever, nausea, fatigue, abdominal pain, and headache. The rotavirus responsible for the outbreak was identified from stools of several individuals as serotype G2 group A rotavirus by comparison of the genomic RNA migration pattern by electrophoresis, by reverse transcriptase-PCR, and by enzyme-linked immunosorbent assay of virus obtained from stool samples. Although rotavirus is the most common cause of infantile diarrhea, this virus, especially the G2 strain, also causes gastroenteritis in adults. (Mikami et al. *J Med Virol.* 2004;73:460–464.)

SEVERE ROTAVIRUS INFECTION IN AN INFANT

Bharwani and colleagues described a 10-month-old infant who developed a severe rotavirus infection. The previously healthy girl presented to the hospital emergency department with two brief generalized tonic-clonic convulsions after 2 days of vomiting, diarrhea, and a low-grade fever. Upon arrival, her blood pressure was 102/54 mm Hg, heart rate was 150 beats/minute, respiratory rate was 34 breaths/minute, body temperature was 37.8°C, and oxygen saturation was 94% on room air. She was lethargic and dehydrated. Blood tests revealed hyponatremia, hypoproteinemia, leukocytosis, and thrombocytosis. After initial stabilization (hydration, correction of electrolyte imbalances, seizure control), bacterial cultures of blood, cerebrospinal fluid, and urine were performed (all were negative). Over the next 24 h, the patient developed generalized edema with ascites and pleural effusion. Because of labored breathing, dyspnea, and continued acidosis, the patient was transferred to the intensive care unit where thoracentesis was performed to relieve the accumulated fluids. Stool tested positive for red and white blood cells and for rotavirus; no bacterial pathogens were recovered. Methylprednisolone was administered

SEVERE ROTAVIRUS INFECTION IN AN INFANT—cont'd

on Day 4 due to persistent hypoalbuminemia and on Day 6 because the patient was tachycardic and hypotensive. Blood tests showed neutropenia, thrombocytopenia, anemia, and coagulopathy, with increased prothrombin and partial prothrombin times. Bacterial cultures remained negative throughout the hospitalization, and over the next 2 weeks, the patient gradually improved. The infant was fully recovered at follow-up at 2 months post-discharge. This case demonstrates a severe episode of rotavirus infection that would have been fatal without the aggressive medical support that was available. This is a reminder that rotavirus is responsible for many of the fatalities associated with infant diarrhea in unvaccinated children. (Bharwani et al. *BMJ Case Rep.* 2011–2011.)

NOROVIRUS OUTBREAK

Evans and associates described an outbreak of gastroenteritis in children who attended a concert. Infection was traced back to contamination of a specific seating area, bathrooms, and other areas visited by one individual. The male individual was ill before attending a concert and then vomited four times in the concert hall: in a waste bin in the corridor, into the toilets, onto the floor of the fire escape, and on a carpeted area in the walkway. His family members showed symptoms within 24 h. A children's concert for several schools was held the next day. Children sitting in the same section as the incident case and those who traversed the contaminated carpet had the highest incidence of disease, characterized by watery diarrhea and vomiting for approximately 2 days. Reverse transcriptase-PCR analysis of fecal samples from two ill children detected norovirus genomic RNA. Infected vomit may have up to a million viruses per milliliter, and only 10–100 viruses are required to transmit the disease. Contact with contaminated shoes, hands, clothing, or aerosols may have infected the children. Norovirus is resistant to routine cleansers; disinfection usually requires freshly prepared hypochlorite bleach-containing solutions or steam cleaning. (Evans et al. *Epidemiol Infect.* 2002;129:355–360.)

NOROVIRUS TRANSMISSION ON CRUISE SHIP

Noroviruses are the most common cause of infectious acute gastroenteritis. Isakbaeva et al. described a norovirus outbreak of gastroenteritis on a cruise ship that affected six consecutive cruises. In the initial outbreak, 84 passengers (4% of all passengers) developed acute gastroenteritis. The outbreak continued on the subsequent cruise, after which the ship was taken out of service and aggressively sanitized. Despite the cleaning, gastroenteritis developed in 215 passengers and crew members on the next cruise. The investigation of the outbreak identified the most likely source of the initial outbreak was consumption of norovirus-contaminated food or water and then spread person-to-person because of the high viral shedding and infectivity of noroviruses. On subsequent cruises (4–6) the number of ill persons reporting to the infirmary remained above background levels. Stool cultures collected on cruises 1 and 2 yielded identical strains of norovirus and subsequent cruises yield this strain plus at least three newly introduced norovirus strains. This outbreak illustrates the challenges in controlling norovirus infections in a closed population, such as on a cruise ship. Infection control management in this setting requires a combination of measures including extensive disinfection, good food and water handling practices, isolation of ill persons, and promoting hand washing among passengers and crew members. (Isakbaeva et al. *Emerg Infect Dis.* 2005;11:154–157.)

ADENOVIRUS GASTROENTERITIS IN IMMUNOCOMPROMISED CHILD

Johansson et al. described episodes of severe gastroenteritis in an immunocompromised 5-year-old girl. The girl initially presented to her pediatrician with complaints of leg pains and lethargy over the previous 2 weeks. Her medical work-up revealed her condition was due to pre-B cell, acute lymphatic leukemia. She was subsequently treated with vincristine, adriamycin, oral prednisolone, and intrathecal methotrexate. On Day 3, after the first injection, she developed fever to 40°C. Blood cultures were collected, and cefuroxime was added to her treatment regimen. On Day 5, she developed abdominal pain, liver enlargement, and diarrhea. During the ensuing 6 weeks, her high fevers and diarrhea recurred accompanied by occasional vomiting. At 8 weeks, her gastrointestinal symptoms decreased. All bacterial cultures of blood, urine, and feces were negative but viral cultures of feces, urine, and blood were positive for adenovirus type 5. This child's immunosuppressive therapy made her particularly vulnerable to the adenovirus gastroenteritis. The most common adenovirus types associated with this condition are 40 and 41; however, adenovirus type 5 has been implicated in infections in immunocompromised patients, particularly pneumonia. (Johansson et al. *Pediatr Infect Dis J.* 1990;9:449–450.)

VIBRIO PARAHAEMOLYTICUS GASTROENTERITIS

One of the largest known outbreaks of *V. parahaemolyticus* infection in the United States was reported in 2005. On July 19, the Nevada Office of Epidemiology reported isolation of *V. parahaemolyticus* from a person who developed gastroenteritis 1 day after eating raw oysters served on an Alaskan cruise ship. Epidemiologic investigations determined that 62 individuals (29% attack rate) developed gastroenteritis following consumption of as few as one raw oyster. In addition to watery diarrhea, the ill individuals reported abdominal cramping (82%), chills (44%), myalgias (36%), headache (32%), and vomiting (29%), with symptoms lasting a median of 5 days. None of the persons required hospitalization. All oysters were harvested from a single farm, where the water temperatures in July and August were recorded at 16.6°C and 17.4°C. Water temperatures above 15°C are considered favorable for growth of *V. parahaemolyticus*. Since 1997, the mean water temperatures at the oyster farm have increased by 0.21°C per year, and now remain consistently above 15°C. Thus, this seasonal warming has extended the range of *V. parahaemolyticus* and the associated gastrointestinal disease. This outbreak illustrates the role of contaminated shellfish in *V. parahaemolyticus* disease and the clinical symptoms typically observed. (McLaughlin et al. *N Engl J Med.* 2005;353:1463–1470.)

VIBRIO CHOLERAE GASTROENTERITIS

Harris and colleagues describe a 4-year-old Haitian boy who was admitted to a Haiti hospital because of vomiting and persistent diarrhea. The boy was healthy until about 10 h before admission. He was extremely dehydrated, not producing urine, and passed a clear, watery stool during his initial examination. Oral rehydration solution was administered, but little fluid was retained because of vomiting and numerous episodes of diarrhea. Intravenous lines were established, and 2 L of isotonic crystalloid solution was infused over a 2-h period. Approximately 4 h after admission, episodes of diarrhea were occurring too often to count and no urine output had occurred; however, the patient was able to drink an oral rehydrating solution and his mental status had improved. Azithromycin was administered orally, and fluids continued to be administered orally and intravenously. During the remainder of the day, the frequency of diarrhea decreased and vomiting ceased; however, the patient appeared dehydrated on the morning of the second day. Additional fluids were administered with resolution of the dehydration. The patient remained in the hospital for an additional day before discharge, with instructions to the parents about the need for adequate oral hydration. This is a classic example of cholera caused by *Vibrio cholerae*. This patient illustrates the severity of diarrhea caused by cholera and the difficulty in managing the fluid loss. This patient was fortunate to have received treatment in the hospital because it was highly likely that he would not have survived without the medical care. This is illustrated by how rapidly he became dehydrated during the first night of hospitalization. (Harris et al. *N Engl J Med.* 2011;364:2452–2461.)

ENTEROTOXIGENIC *ESCHERICHIA COLI* GASTROENTERITIS

Enterotoxigenic *E. coli* (ETEC) produces a watery diarrhea with a similar presentation as cholera. Although it is commonly referred to as traveler's diarrhea, infections do occur in high income countries but are underappreciated. In recent years, infections have been more frequently recognized with the introduction of molecular diagnostic panels for detection of the most common bacterial and viral causes of diarrhea. This was illustrated in a study by Buuck et al. where they reviewed the frequency of all diarrheagenic *E. coli* reported to the Minnesota Department of Public Health over a 2-year period (2016–2017). A total of 244 cases were identified. Of the confirmed cases, watery diarrhea (97%) and cramps (81%) were reported most frequently, followed by headache (55%), fever (40%), and bloody stools (13%). Only about one-third of the patients reported international travel during the 1-week period before symptom onset, with Mexico the most frequent destination for travelers. ETEC strains produce both a heat-labile and heat-stable toxin that disrupt the lining of the small intestine resulting in a watery diarrhea, in contrast with other diarrheal *E. coli* strains such at STEC and EIEC that disrupt the lining of the large intestine resulting in a bloody diarrhea (Buuck et al. *Epid Infect.* 148;e206:1–7).

CAMPYLOBACTER JEJUNI ENTERITIS AND GUILLAIN-BARRÉ SYNDROME

Scully and associates described the clinical history of a 74-year-old woman who developed Guillain-Barré syndrome following an episode of *Campylobacter jejuni* enteritis. After 1 week of watery diarrhea, fever, nausea, abdominal pain, weakness, and fatigue, the patient's speech was noted to be severely slurred. She was taken to the hospital where it was noted she was unable to speak, although she was oriented and able to write coherently. She had perioral numbness, bilateral ptosis, and facial weakness, and her pupils were nonreactive. Neurologic examination revealed bilateral muscle weakness in her arms and chest. On the 2nd hospital day, the muscle weakness extended to her upper legs. On the 3rd hospital day, the patient's mental status remained normal, but she could only move her thumb minimally and could not lift her legs. Sensation to light touch was normal, but deep-tendon reflexes were absent. *C. jejuni* was recovered from this patient's stool culture, collected at the time of admission, and the clinical diagnosis of Guillain-Barré syndrome was made. Despite aggressive medical treatment, the patient had significant neurologic deficits 3 months after discharge to a rehabilitation facility. This woman illustrates one of the significant complications of *Campylobacter* enteritis. *Campylobacter* infections are the most commonly identified cause of Guillain-Barré syndrome. (Scully et al. *N Engl J Med.* 1999;341:1996–2003.)

CRYPTOSPORIDIOSIS OUTBREAK IN UNIVERSITY STUDENTS

Quiroz and colleagues described an outbreak of cryptosporidiosis that was linked to a food handler. In the fall of 1998, an outbreak of gastroenteritis among university students was reported to the Department of Health. Preliminary findings suggested that the illness was associated with eating at one of the campus cafeterias; four employees of this cafeteria had a similar illness. The outbreak was thought to be caused by a viral agent until *C. parvum* was detected in the stool specimens of several cafeteria employees. In a case-control study of 88 case patients and 67 control patients, eating in 1 or 2 cafeterias was associated with diarrheal illness. *C. parvum* was detected in stool samples of 16 (70%) of 23 ill students and 2 of 4 ill employees. One ill food handler with laboratory-confirmed cryptosporidiosis prepared raw produce on the days surrounding the outbreak. All 25 *C. parvum* isolates submitted for DNA analysis, including 3 from the ill food handler, were genotype 1. This outbreak illustrates the potential for cryptosporidiosis to cause foodborne illness. Epidemiologic and molecular evidence indicates that an ill food handler was the likely outbreak source. (Quiroz et al. *J Infect Dis.* 2000;181:695–700.)

DRUG-RESISTANT GIARDIASIS INFECTION IN AIDS PATIENT

Abboud and colleagues described a case of metronidazole- and albendazole-resistant giardiasis that was successfully treated with nitazoxanide. The patient was a 32-year-old homosexual man with AIDS, who was admitted to the hospital because of intractable watery diarrhea with low-grade fever and abdominal cramps. Examination of stool revealed the presence of numerous cysts of *G. duodenalis* (*G. lamblia*). The patient was unsuccessfully treated five times with metronidazole and albendazole without improvement of diarrhea or cyst shedding. Although combined antiretroviral therapy was also administered, it was ineffective, and viral genotypic analysis found mutations associated with high resistance to most antiretroviral drugs. The patient was subsequently treated for giardiasis with nitazoxanide, which resulted in resolution of the diarrhea and negative results of tests for stool cyst shedding. Resistance of the infecting strain of *G. duodenalis* to both metronidazole and albendazole was confirmed by *in vivo* and *in vitro* studies. Nitazoxanide may be considered as a useful alternative therapy for resistant giardiasis. (Abboud et al. *Clin Infect Dis*. 2001;32:1792–1794.)

CYCLOSPORA INFECTION IN IMMUNOCOMPETENT TRAVELLER

Kansouzidou et al. described a 44-year-old immunocompetent man who developed diarrheal disease caused by *Cyclospora cayetanensis*. He had traveled extensively in Monaco for 1 month, eating a variety of food and drinking untreated water. Two days before the end of the trip, he had an acute episode of watery diarrhea, with four to five bowel movements a day, with low-grade fever, abdominal cramps and fatigue. He traveled to Germany where he continued to have relapsing diarrhea with high fever and general malaise. After 15 days, he returned to his home in Greece, and presented to the hospital after persistent diarrhea for 5 days. Fecal samples were sent to the laboratory for bacterial culture and parasitic examination. The cultures were negative but acid-fast coccidian parasites were observed and later identified as *C. cayetanensis*. Treatment was initiated with trimethoprim-sulfamethoxazole with prompt relief of symptoms and clearance of the parasite from stool specimens. Untreated water or contaminated food was the most likely source of infection for this patient, and the prolonged, relapsing course of infection is well-described. (Kansouzidou et al. *J Travel Med*. 2004;11:61–63.)

LISTERIA GASTROENTERITIS AND BACTEREMIA

A 53-year-old man who was receiving immunosuppressive therapy for Crohn disease presented to the hospital with diarrhea and fever. He had been in his usual state of health until 2 days before admission, when he woke with severe malaise and headache. Over the next 2 days, his symptoms included sharp, fluctuating abdominal pain, and episodes of urgent, uncontrollable nonbloody diarrhea. When his symptoms did not improve and he developed a temperature of 39.8°C, he went to the hospital. Blood cultures that were collected in the Emergency Department were positive within 24 h for small gram-positive rods. Although a variety of bacteria and viruses can produce clinical symptoms such as this patient's, the positive blood culture was highly suggestive of *L. monocytogènes*, which was confirmed by biochemical tests and mass spectrometry. Other gram-positive bacteria associated with gastrointestinal disease include *Bacillus cereus* (much larger than this organism) and *Clostridioides difficile*, both of which are much larger than this isolate and neither cause bacteremia. The patient reported a recent history of eating cantaloupe, which was provocative because cantaloupes were implicated in a multistate outbreak of *Listeria* gastroenteritis at the time of this patient's disease; however, the patient's strain was a different serotype from that implicated in the outbreak. This case illustrates the syndrome of fever and nonbloody diarrhea that is typical of *Listeria* infections, and the increased risk of bacteremia (as well as meningitis) for specific risk groups: immunocompromised patients such as in this case, as well as very young children, pregnant women, and the elderly. A careful food history (such as consumption of raw vegetables, unpasteurized mild soft cheeses, and delicatessen foods) is important because the individual case may be part of a broader outbreak of disease. (*N Engl J Med*. 2012;366:1039–1045.)

SHIGELLA INFECTIONS IN DAY-CARE CENTERS

In 2005, three states reported outbreaks of multidrug-resistant *Shigella* infections in day-care centers. A total of 532 infections were reported in the Kansas City area, with the patients' median age of 6 years old. The predominant pathogen was a multidrug-resistant strain of *S. sonnei*, with 89% of the isolates resistant to ampicillin and trimethoprim-sulfamethoxazole. Shigellosis spreads easily in day-care centers because of the increased risk of fecal contamination and the low infectious dose responsible for disease. Parents and teachers, as well as classmates, are at significant risk for disease so clusters of infections with this pathogen are common. (*MMWR*. 2006;5:1068–1071.)

SHIGA TOXIN *ESCHERICHIA COLI* (STEC) OUTBREAK

In 2006, *E. coli* O157 was responsible for a large, multi-state outbreak of gastroenteritis. The outbreak was linked to the contamination of spinach, with a total of 173 cases reported in 25 states, primarily over an 18-day period. The outbreak resulted in the hospitalization of more than 50% of the patients with documented disease, a 16% rate of hemolytic uremic syndrome, and one death. Despite the wide distribution of the contaminated spinach, publication of the outbreak and the rapid determination that spinach was responsible resulted in prompt removal of spinach from grocery stores and termination of the outbreak. This outbreak illustrates how contamination of a food product, even with small numbers of organisms, can lead to a widespread outbreak with a particularly virulent organism, such as strains of Shiga toxin-producing *E. coli* (STEC). Other food products associated with STEC infections include raw or under-cooked beef (most commonly hamburger), raw milk and cheeses, and contaminated vegetables.

SHIGELLA GASTROENTERITIS IN GAY MALES

Shigella infections are predominantly a disease in pediatric patients or their families. It is also well-documented that shigellosis occurs in gay male populations. Wilmer et al. described their experience with *Shigella* infections in the Vancouver, Canada gay male population (HIV infection, 86%). Over the 7-year study period, there was a more than 25-fold increase in infections and a shift from infection caused by *Shigella sonnei* to infections with *S. flexneri*. The prevalence of *S. flexneri* has been reported in other populations (Montreal, Toronto, London). More than 70% of the isolates were serogroup 1, consistent with person-to-person spread. Almost 60% of the patients visited the Emergency Department and two-thirds were hospitalized. Diarrhea was present in all patients, abdominal pain in most (80%), and blood in the stools of one-third of the patients. The average length of hospitalization was 3 days. Two-thirds of the infected patients were treated with ciprofloxacin, for which all isolates were susceptible. A careful medical and social history is important for the rapid etiologic diagnosis of gastroenteritis in adult male patients. (Wilmer et al. *HIV Med*. 2015;16:168–175.)

ENTEROHEMORRHAGIC *ESCHERICHIA COLI* HEMOLYTIC UREMIC SYNDROME

Enterohemorrhagic *Escherichia coli* (EHEC) is now more commonly referred to a Shiga toxin-producing *E. coli* (STEC) in recognition of the role of toxin in disease. A complication of disease produced by this organism is hemolytic uremic syndrome (HUS) as illustrated in the case of a 1-year-old girl who initially presented to the Children's Hospital in Bucharest, Romania. The onset of disease was 5 days before hospital admission with diarrhea and anorexia. On the second day of illness, a stool culture was performed and was positive for enteropathogenic *E. coli*. On the fourth day of illness, the patient produced two "dark colored" stools, so she was admitted to the pediatric hospital. On admission, she was found anemic, thrombocytopenic, increased serum urea, and normal serum creatinine. Based on her clinical symptoms and an ongoing outbreak of HUS in the community, a tentative diagnosis of HUS was made and she was transferred to the Nephrology Department. Physical examination revealed an alert but irritable and ill-appearing child with a normal body temperature, elevated heart rate, normal blood pressure, and oxygen saturation. Laboratory findings included microangiopathic hemolytic anemia, thrombocytopenia, increased serum urea, and elevated lactate dehydrogenase, hemolytic uremic syndrome was

Continued

ENTEROHEMORRHAGIC *ESCHERICHIA COLI* HEMOLYTIC UREMIC SYNDROME—cont'd

the diagnosis after additional testing ruled out alternative diagnoses. STEC was recovered in the patient's stool specimen. The patient was treated with ceftriaxone and meropenem for 7 days, and by hospital day 11, she was discharged from the hospital and followed as an outpatient. HUS as a complication of STEC infections occurs primarily in pediatric patients, and although this complication can severely compromise renal function, this patient has a relatively mild course. HUS has also been associated with Enteroinvasive *E. coli* (EIEC) and with *Shigella* infections in pediatric patients. (Costin et al. *Maedica J Clin Med*. 2019;14:298–300.)

SALMONELLA GASTROENTERITIS

On July 16, 2019, a 30-year-old man developed abdominal pain, vomiting, diarrhea, and fever up to 41°C a few hours after a kebab meal containing goat meat. The next day, he presented to the local hospital in Rome, Italy where fecal and blood specimens were collected for culture and a molecular test for enteric pathogens was performed on the fecal specimen. *Salmonella enterica* was isolated from the cultures and detected as positive on the molecular test. The patient was initially treated with intravenous rehydration, and the patient's diarrhea and fever rapidly subsided. Because the blood culture was positive, an 8-day course of ceftriaxone was started. Two friends of the patient who ate the same kebab meal were also admitted to the hospital 3 days after the meal with fever, diarrhea, and vomiting. Molecular tests with their fecal specimens were positive for *Salmonella* although the cultures of feces and blood remained negative. The rapid onset of symptoms in the initial patient was unusual for a *Salmonella* infection, with the 2–3 day delay observed in the other two patients more common. Although culture of stool specimens is usually positive because large numbers of organism are typically present, it is now recognized that the most sensitive diagnostic method is use of molecular tests. The tests are designed to detect a large variety of bacterial and viral enteric pathogens. (Chinello et al. *Pathogens*. 2020;9.doi:10.3390/pathogens9080656.)

CLOSTRIDIOIDES DIFFICILE COLITIS

Limaye and colleagues presented a classic presentation of *C. difficile* disease in a 60-year-old man. He had received a transplanted liver 5 years prior to his hospital admission for evaluation of crampy abdominal pain and severe diarrhea. Three weeks prior to admission, he received a 10-day course of oral trimethoprim-sulfamethoxazole for sinusitis. On physical examination, the patient was febrile and had moderate abdominal tenderness. Abdominal computed tomography scan revealed right-colon thickening but no abscess. Colonoscopy showed numerous whitish plaques and friable erythematous mucosa consistent with pseudomembranous colitis. Empiric therapy with oral metronidazole and intravenous levofloxacin was initiated. A stool immunoassay for *C. difficile* toxin A was negative, but *C. difficile* toxin was detected by both culture and cytotoxicity assay (demonstration stool filtrate causes cytotoxicity to cell cultures that is neutralized by specific antisera against *C. difficile* toxins). Therapy was changed to oral vancomycin, and the patient responded with resolution of diarrhea and abdominal pain. This is an example of severe *C. difficile* disease following antibiotic exposure in an immunocompromised patient, with a characteristic presentation of pseudomembranous colitis. The diagnostic problems with immunoassays are well known and have now been replaced by polymerase chain reaction assays that target the toxin genes. Treatment with metronidazole was the initial treatment of choice but the Infectious Disease Society of America (IDSA) now recommends the use of fidaxomicin. (Limaye et al. *J Clin Microbiol*. 2000;38:1696–1697).

HIV AND AMEBIC LIVER ABSCESS

Liu and colleagues described a 45-year-old homosexual man who developed intestinal and hepatic amebiasis. The patient initially presented with intermittent fever followed by right upper quadrant pain and diarrhea. On admission to the hospital, he was afebrile with an elevated white blood cell count and abnormal liver function tests. Stool examinations were positive for occult blood and white blood cells. He underwent colonoscopy, and multiple discrete ulcers were detected in the rectum and colon. The diagnosis of amebic colitis was confirmed by the demonstration of numerous trophozoites on histopathologic examination of colon biopsy specimens. Ultrasound examination of the abdomen revealed a large heterogeneous mass within the liver, consistent with an abscess. Percutaneous drainage of the abscess obtained chocolate-like pus, and examination of a biopsy from the margin of the abscess revealed only a necrotic material, without evidence of amebae. Polymerase chain reaction (PCR) amplification of amebic 16S ribosomal RNA from the aspirate was positive, indicating infection with *E. histolytica*. The patient was treated with metronidazole followed by iodoquinol to eradicate the luminal amebae. Subsequent history revealed he traveled to Thailand 2 months before the onset of the present illness. HIV serology was positive as well. The patient improved rapidly on anti-amebic therapy and was discharged on antiretroviral therapy.

Although amebic cysts are frequently detected in the stools of homosexual men, previous studies in Western countries suggested that almost all isolates belong to the nonpathogenic species *Entamoeba dispar*, and invasive amebiasis was considered rare in HIV-positive individuals. This case illustrates that invasive amebiasis, such as amebic liver abscess and colitis, can accompany HIV infection. The possible association of invasive amebiasis with HIV infection should be considered for patients living in or with a history of travel to areas where *E. histolytica* is endemic. (Liu et al. *J Clin Gastroenterol.* 2001;33:64–68.)

DIPHYLLOBOTHRIASIS

Lee and colleagues reported a case of diphyllobothriasis in a young girl. A 7-year-old girl was seen in an outpatient clinic after the discharge of a chain of tapeworm proglottids measuring 42 cm in length. She had no history of eating raw fish, except once when she ate raw salmon flesh along with the rest of her family approximately 7 months earlier. The salmon was caught in a local river. She did not complain of any gastrointestinal discomfort, and all blood chemistry and hematologic studies were normal. Examination of the stool specimen was positive for *D. latum* eggs. The worm was identified as *D. latum* based on the biological characteristics of the proglottids: broad narrow external morphology, coiling of uterus, number of uterine loops, and position of the genital opening. A single dose of praziquantel 400 mg was given, but stool examination remained positive 1 week later. Another dose of 600 mg was given and repeat stool examination 1 month later was negative. Among four family members who ate raw fish, just two—the girl and her mother—were identified as being infected. Consumption of raw salmon, especially those produced by aquaculture, is a risk for human diphyllobothriasis. (Lee et al. *Korean J Parasitol.* 2001;39:319–321).

HYMENOLEPIS NANA INFECTION IN A PREGNANT WOMAN

Kandi et al. described a *Hymenolepis nana* infection in 24-year-old pregnant woman living in India. The woman presented in her 35th week of gestation to an outpatient clinic with complaints of loose, nonbloody stools as frequent as 10 times per day over the last 2 days and two episodes of vomiting with associated abdominal pain. Stool examination for intestinal parasites was ordered and direct microscopic examination revealed eggs morphologically resembling *H. nana*. The patient was treated with a single dose of albendazole and repeat stool examination after 2 days showed no parasite eggs, but adult forms of the worm were observed. *H. nana* is the most common cestode causing human disease, with a worldwide distribution. Infections are most common in temperate regions. (Kandi et al. *Cureus.* 11(1):e3810.)

32

Genitourinary Tract Infections

Infections of the genitourinary tract should be subdivided into urinary tract infections and genital infections. Urinary tract infections include cystitis, pyelonephritis, and prostatitis. Infections of the genital tract include urethritis, vulvovaginitis, cervicitis, epididymitis, genital ulcerative disease, endometritis, and pelvic inflammatory disease.

Most urinary tract infections are ascending infections; that is, infections that originate outside the urinary tract, primarily in the intestinal tract, with the pathogens migrating through the urethra to the bladder and potentially to the kidneys or to the prostate. Disease by this route is caused by organisms that can adhere to the uroepithelium (via adhesins or colonizing factors) and produce localized damage by expression of toxins. Thus, even though *Lactobacillus* is the predominant organism in the urethra, it rarely is associated with disease because it lacks these virulence factors. Some organisms can also produce renal calculi, primarily by excess production of urease that results in an alkaline urine and struvite stone formation. Hematogenous urinary tract infections (i.e., bloodstream pathogens that produce kidney damage) are primarily restricted to *Staphylococcus aureus* and *Candida* species. Most urinary tract infections are caused by *Escherichia coli*, with other gram-negative uropathogens also observed including *Proteus mirabilis*, *Klebsiella pneumoniae*, *Pseudomonas aeruginosa*. Gram-positive pathogens are less common, although *Staphylococcus saprophyticus* is the second most common uropathogen in young, sexually active, adult women; *Enterococcus* is a common pathogen in hospitalized patients receiving antibiotic treatment; and coagulase-negative *Staphylococcus* in patients with indwelling urinary catheters. The most common pathogens associated with kidney stones are *S. saprophyticus*, *Proteus mirabilis*, and *Corynebacterium urealyticum*. Yeasts that are commonly associated with infections of the urinary tract are *Candida albicans* and *Candida glabrata*. Three viruses produce a hemorrhagic form of cystitis, primarily in immunocompromised patients: adenovirus, cytomegalovirus, and BK virus.

Genital infections are primarily transmitted by sexual contact, and the pathogens are well-known. Inflammation of the urethra with painful discharge is most commonly caused by *Neisseria gonorrhoeae* and *Chlamydia trachomatis*, and less frequently by *Mycoplasma genitalium* and *Trichomonas vaginalis*. Clinical symptoms and sexual history are not sufficient to differentiate these pathogens so diagnostic tests are required for specific guided therapy. Likewise, the specific pathogens responsible for vulvovaginitis cannot be identified reliably by clinical criteria, although this is frequently attempted. Three distinct forms of vulvovaginitis are recognized: bacterial vaginosis which is a disruption of normal vaginal bacterial flora (i.e., decrease in *Lactobacillus* and increase in mixed anaerobic bacteria); vaginal candidiasis with a proliferation of *Candida* species; and trichomoniasis caused by *T. vaginalis*. Comprehensive syndromic molecular tests are now becoming more widely available that allow identification of the specific pathogen in a single test. Infectious cervicitis, epididymitis, and pelvic inflammatory disease are primarily caused by *N. gonorrhoeae*, *C. trachomatis*, or *M. genitalium*. Genital ulcerative diseases can be separated into those with painful lesions (i.e., herpes simplex virus, *Haemophilus ducreyi* [disease called chancroid], *Klebsiella granulomatis* [granuloma inguinale]) and painless lesions (*Treponema pallidum* [syphilis], *C. trachomatis* serovars L1-3 [lymphogranuloma venereum]). Finally, it is important to include human papilloma virus (HPV) as a sexually transmitted genital pathogen, responsible for the majority cases of cervical, penile, and anal cancers.

The following case reports are examples of urinary tract infections and genital diseases caused by the most common sexually transmitted pathogens.

ESCHERICHIA COLI URINARY TRACT INFECTIONS

Urinary tract infections (UTIs) are one of the most common infectious diseases globally, with an estimated 150 million people worldwide developing infections annually. It is estimated that 40% of women develop at least one UTI during their lifetime and that 11% of women over 18 years have an episode of UTI per year. UTIs caused by *E. coli* are more common in women than men until about age 60, and then, they are more common in men, particularly males with prostatitis. Approximately 80% of community-acquired UTIs are caused by *E. coli* while a smaller proportion are documented in hospital-acquired infections. Specific strains of *E. coli* are uropathogenic, based on the presence of adhesive factors (fimbriae, pilae, colonization factors) that facilitate attachment to the uroepithelial cells and toxins that produce an inflammatory response to the bacteria. The clinical presentation of *E. coli* UTIs includes acute cystitis, acute or chronic pyelonephritis, and prostatitis, generally indistinguishable from other bacterial uropathogens. (Terlizzi et al. *Frontiers Microbiol.* 2017;doi:10.3389/fmicr.2017.01566.)

PROTEUS MIRABILIS URINARY TRACT INFECTION

Proteus mirabilis is a common pathogen responsible for complicated urinary tract infections (UTI), including those with urolithiasis, anatomic abnormalities, chronic indwelling catheters, and bacteremia. As with other urease-producing bacteria that cause urinary tract infections, ammonia is generated from the degradation of urea, leading to an alkaline pH of the urine and formation of urinary calculi. Additionally, isolation of P. *mirabilis* in the blood is almost always associated with UTIs. Chen et al. studied risk factors for bacteremia in patients with P. mirabilis UTIs. They found community-acquired infections, hydronephrosis, hyperthermia or hypothermia, and elevated serum C-reactive protein were independent risk factors for bacteremia. Bacteremic patients were also at increased risk for mortality. (Chen et al. *J Microbiol Immunol Infect.* 2012;45:228–236.)

STAPHYLOCOCCUS SAPROPHYTICUS URINARY TRACT INFECTION

A 60-year-old woman was admitted to the emergency department with chest pain, fever of 38.6°C, and left flank pain. For the purposed of this discussion, I will focus on the urinary tract symptoms and not her complicating cardiac problem. Left-sided costovertebral angle tenderness was noted, and laboratory data showed an elevated white cell count and glucose level. Urea nitrogen and creatinine were within normal limits, and urinalysis showed pH 7, negative nitrates, and pyuria. CT scan of the patient's abdomen revealed an obstructive left renal pelvic stone with left hydroureteronephrosis and proximal ureter wall thickening. Urine cultures and blood cultures upon admission grew *Staphylococcus saprophyticus* resistant to oxacillin and susceptible to vancomycin and ciprofloxacin. Treatment with ciprofloxacin resolved the infection. *S. saprophyticus* is the second most common cause of urinary tract infections in women, with only *Escherichia coli* more common. Typically, these infections are most frequently observed in young, sexually active women so this case is somewhat atypical. Urinary tract stone formation is common with this pathogen. Because this organism is coagulase-negative, it should not be discounted as a common contaminating coagulase-negative staphylococci, particularly in the presence of signs and symptoms of an infection with urinary stone formation. (Hur et al. *Infect Chemother.* 2016;doi:10.3947/ic.2016.48.2.136.)

NEISSERIA GONORRHOEAE URETHRITIS

A 26-year-old man came to the University Dermatology Clinic in Egypt with complaints of severe burning with urination and dysuria for 4 days. Additionally, he was suffering from penile discharge and testicular tenderness. On physical examination, mucopurulent urethral discharge, swollen testicles, and redness of one eye with copious discharge were observed. Urethral and ocular swabs of the exudates were collected and cultured on Thayer Martin and chocolate agar plates. After overnight incubation at 37°C in 5% CO_2, small grayish-white colonies were observed that were identified as *Neisseria gonorrhoeae*. Antimicrobial susceptibility tests were performed, and the organism was resistant to multiple antibiotics (i.e., ampicillin, ampicillin/clavulanic acid, cefotaxime, cefepime, cefuroxime, ceftriaxone, ciprofloxacin, tetracycline, and trimethoprim-sulfamethoxazole) and susceptible only to gentamicin, rifampicin, and azithromycin. This case is a classic presentation of *N. gonorrhoeae* genital infection with the complication of gonococcal conjunctivitis and broad antimicrobial resistance. It is recognized that *N. gonorrhoeae* isolates are becoming progressively more resistant to antimicrobials and challenging to treat. Additionally, because most infections are diagnosed by molecular methods, resistance is generally not recognized until patients fail treatment. (Al-Madboly, Gheida. *Frontiers Med.* 2017;4:194.)

GENITAL HERPES INFECTION IN PATIENT WITH DIABETES MELLITUS

Aounallah et al. described a 14-year-old girl with insulin-dependent diabetes mellitus who presented to their clinic with a 3-day history of burning vaginal pain. Examination revealed an erythematous and edematous perineal area with numerous painful vesicles extending over the entire genital area including clitoris, labia majora, and the anal area. Regional lymphadenopathy was present but no vaginal discharge. Blood gas analysis documented metabolic acidosis, and the urinalysis results were consistent with glycosuria and ketonuria. Diagnostic tests were positive for HSV-2. She was diagnosed with diabetic ketoacidosis induced by her genital herpes infection, and intravenous acyclovir and insulin therapy were initiated. The genital lesions began to respond after 2 days of antiviral treatment. The main differential diagnosis in this patient was vulvo-vaginal candidiasis, characterized by pruritus and a thick whitish discharge. The presence of painful vesicles and inguinal adenopathy in the absence of a discharge was consistent with HSV infection. Although HSV-2 was responsible for this infection and the majority of herpetic genital infections, HSV-1 genital infections are becoming increasingly more common. (Aounallah et al. *Ind. Pediatrics.* 2017;54:697–698.)

TREPONEMA PALLIDUM SYPHILIS

A 59-year-old man presented to the Emergency Department with a 1-month history of progressive submental swelling, subjective fevers, and chills. A review of systems was positive for dysphagia, sore throat, and significant weight loss. He reported a history of genital herpes simplex virus infection. He also admitted to multiple sexual partners in the past. Physical examination revealed marked swelling and tenderness under his mandible and a diffuse erythematous maculopapular rash across his chest with scattered hyperpigmented macular lesions involving his palms and lower extremities extending to the soles of his feet. All lesions were nonpruritic and nontender. Further examination revealed a 1 cm × 1 cm nontender ulcerative lesion on the hard palate of his oral cavity. A genital examination revealed no lesions. Serologic tests for syphilis (Rapid Plasma Reagin, RPR; Microhemagglutination Assay, MHA-TP) were positive. Syphilis is classified into three stages (primary, secondary, tertiary) that typically appear sequentially. In this patient, the primary stage painless ulcer appeared at the same time as the secondary stage rash. Although the painless ulcer is typically in the genital area, a small percentage of patients present with oral ulcers as observed in this patient. (Streight et al. *J Med Case Rep.* 2019;13:227–229.)

CHLAMYDIA TRACHOMATIS LYMPHOGRANULOMA VENEREUM (LGV)

In August 2015, a man in his 40s who had sex with men presented to the University Medical Center in Ljubljana with a one-week history of painful swelling in the left groin and sore throat. He reported no urethral discharge, genital ulcers, or symptoms. Fine needle aspiration tested negative for malignant cells, and no antibiotics were prescribed. One week later, he returned to the hospital with fever, malaise, and unilateral inguinal erythema and much increased swelling. Ultrasound of the left groin revealed two necrotic lymph nodes with abscess formation. Since LGV was suspect, a bubo aspirate was collected as well as urine, urethral, pharyngeal, and rectal specimens. The urine and urethral specimens for *Chlamydia trachomatis* PCR were positive, and treatment with doxycycline was initiated. Further testing confirmed this was a LGV serotype. Despite following European guidelines for treatment of LGV, this patient had continued problems requiring surgical drainage of the abscesses and prolonged antimicrobial treatment. LGV is caused by *C. trachomatis* serovars L1, L2, and L3, with some strains are more aggressive and difficult to treat. Infections have been widely reported in men who have sex with men, and this patient admitted to multiple partners where unprotected oral and anal sex was performed. LGV can present with mild or absent symptoms in the early stages of disease so transmission may be unrecognized. (Maticic et al. *Euro Surveill.* 2016;21:2–5.)

PELVIC ACTINOMYCOSIS

Quercia and associates described a classic presentation of pelvic actinomycosis associated with an intrauterine contraceptive device (IUD). The patient was a 41-year-old woman who presented with a 5-month history of abdominal and pelvic pain, weight loss, malaise, and a yellow vaginal discharge. She had used an IUD since 1994, and it was removed in June 2004. Her symptoms began soon after the removal of the IUD. A computed tomography scan revealed a large pelvic mass involving the fallopian tubes, as well as numerous hepatic abscesses. A surgical biopsy was performed, and *Actinomyces* was recovered in culture. She underwent surgical debridement and received oral therapy with a penicillin antibiotic for 1 year. The medical team thought the woman's pelvis was infected with *Actinomyces* at the time the IUD was removed. This episode illustrates the chronic nature of actinomycosis, and the need for surgical drainage and long-term antibiotic therapy. (Quercia et al. *Med Mal Infect.* 2006;36:393–395.)

CHLAMYDIA TRACHOMATIS PELVIC INFLAMMATORY DISEASE AND REITER SYNDROME

Serwin and associates described a 30-year-old man who presented to a university hospital with complaints of dysuria for a 3-year duration, penile inflammation, joint swelling, and fever. Skin lesions and nail changes were also noted. High levels of *Chlamydia* antibodies were present, but antigen tests and nucleic acid amplification tests of the urethral exudates and conjunctiva were negative for *C. trachomatis*. A diagnosis of Reiter syndrome was made, and treatment with ofloxacin was initiated. Complete remission of the skin lesions and urethral symptoms was achieved. The patient's wife was also admitted to the hospital with a history of 2 years of lower abdominal pain and vaginal bleeding and discharge. The diagnosis of pelvic inflammatory disease was made, and *C. trachomatis* infection was confirmed by positive cervical and urethral antigen tests (direct fluorescent antibody). The vaginal smear was also positive for *Trichomonas vaginalis*. These patients illustrate two complications of *C. trachomatis* urogenital infections: Reiter syndrome and pelvic inflammatory disease. (Serwin et al. *J Eur Acad Derm Vener.* 2006;20:735–736.)

SCHISTOSOMA HAEMATOBIUM INFECTION IN ITALIAN FAMILY

Raglio et al. reported an Italian family who acquired a *Schistosoma haematobium* infection when vacationing in Malawi for 3 weeks. During their holiday, they enjoyed swimming in Lake Malawi on two occasions. Two months after they returned home to Italy, the father and one son experienced a dull discomfort in the perianal region and increased urinary frequency with slight hematuria. Microbiology cultures of the urine were negative. The symptoms in both individuals became less annoying until approximately 8 months later when the father's symptoms became more acute, and he was admitted to the Urology division of the regional hospital. All imaging studies and laboratory tests were negative, so he was referred to another Urology Center. No etiologic cause of his symptoms could be determined so he was referred to the Infectious Disease service. After a careful clinical history of exposure to presumed schistosome-infected water, *S. haematobium* infection was suspected. Urine specimens were collected, concentrated by filtration, and examined microscopically. *S. haematobium* eggs were observed. Because the man's wife and two sons had also swam in the waters, urine was collected from each. The two sons also have eggs detected in their concentrated urine, but the wife was negative. This is consistent with the fact that unlike the other family members, she did not swim in the waters for an extended period. Treatment for the infected family members was with one dose of praziquantel. Follow-up at 3 and 6 months was negative for eggs. This case illustrates the difficulty in diagnosing *Schistosoma* infections unless a careful history is taken. (Raglio et al. *J Travel Med.* 1995;2:193–195.)

INVASIVE CERVICAL CARCINOMA MISSED BY COLPOSCOPY

Livingston and Papagiannakis described a 45-year-old woman who presented for gynecologic evaluation after experiencing heavy periods for the last 5 years with increasing pain. Her Pap test one year previously was interpreted as normal. Pelvic ultrasound showed a cyst in her right ovary and NAAT for human papillomavirus (HPV) was positive. Colposcopy was performed, and no significance findings were observed except for Nabothian cysts. The assessment was there were no lesions suspected for neoplasia, and biopsy was not warranted. However, adjunctive dynamic spectral imaging (DSI) highlighted an area of suspicion, so a punch biopsy was performed. Histopathological review of the biopsy showed an invasive squamous carcinoma. The patient elected to have radical hysterectomy with pelvic lymphadenectomy and bilateral salpingo-oophorectomy. Pathology review confirmed a poorly differentiated squamous cell carcinoma of the cervix. This case illustrates the limitations of the manually interpreted Pap test and the value of NAAT HPV testing. This patient is complex because colposcopy did not initially reveal the carcinoma and additional special imaging was required to identify the involved focus. (Livingston, Papagiannakis. *Case Reports Ob Gyn.* 2016;doi:10.1155.2016/5857370.)

HPV TYPE 16 PENILE CANCER

Nguyen et al. reported a morbidly obese 54-year-old man with penile cancer caused by HPV type 16. Initial physical examination showed a patient with morbid obesity, weighing 150 kg, with the tip of his penis barely visible. PET-CT scan showed a highly hypermetabolic 7-cm mass in the distal penis and lymphadenopathy. Biopsy of the mass showed squamous cell carcinoma, and the HPV type 16 stain was strongly positive. A radiotherapy treatment program was initiated, and a follow-up MRI and repeat biopsy at 24 months showed complete resolution of the tumor. HPV types 16 and 18 are the most common strains associated with cancers of the cervix, vulva, penis, anus, and oropharynx. (Nguyen et al. *Urology Case Rep.* 2019;doi:10.1016/j.eucr.2019.101009.)

33

Central Nervous System Infections

Infections of the central nervous system are subdivided into meningitis, encephalitis, focal CNS syndromes (i.e., brain abscess, subdural empyema, epidural abscess), and neurological manifestation of systemic infections. Meningitis, inflammation of the meninges or covering of the brain, is further subdivided into acute and subacute meningitis. Acute meningitis is characterized by fever, headache, meningismus, and altered mental status that develops with a rapid onset (5 days or less). A wide spectrum of pathogens can cause acute meningitis but the most common are enterovirus, West Nile virus, herpes simplex virus (HSV), and bacterial causes. The bacteria can be subdivided into those responsible for disease in newborns (group B *Streptococcus* [*Streptococcus agalactiae*], *Escherichia coli*), 3 months to 5 years of age (*Haemophilus influenzae* type b, *Streptococcus pneumoniae*), children and adults (*S. pneumoniae*, *Neisseria meningitidis*), and the extremes of age or immunocompromised patients (*Listeria monocytogenes*). Maternal screening and use of prophylactic antibiotics have significantly reduced the incidence of group B *Streptococcus* infection, and vaccination has essentially eliminated *H. influenzae* infections. Patients with head trauma or following neurosurgical procedures are susceptible to infections with *Staphylococcus aureus* and aerobic gram-negative rods such as *Klebsiella*, other Enterobacteriales, *Pseudomonas* and *Acinetobacter*. Subacute or chronic meningitis is characterized by more prolonged meningeal symptoms and is most commonly observed in immunocompromised patients. The most common pathogens include *Mycobacterium tuberculosis*, *Treponema pallidum* (syphilis), fungal pathogens (*Cryptococcus neoformans*, *Coccidioides immitis*), and parasitic pathogens (*Acanthamoeba*, *Balamuthia*), as well as noninfectious causes such as malignancy.

Encephalitis is an inflammatory process involving the brain parenchyma with altered mental status (altered level of consciousness, lethargy, or personality change) lasting 24 h or more. Additionally, the following minor criteria are considered for defining encephalitis: fever >38°C, seizures, new onset focal findings, CSF pleocytosis, new or acute onset of neuroimaging abnormalities consistent with encephalitis, and abnormalities on electroencephalography consistent with encephalitis. The presence of two of the six minor criteria is defined as possible encephalitis and three or more criteria as probably or confirmed encephalitis. The most common infectious causes of encephalitis are viruses: HSV and other members of the herpes group (VZV, CMV, HHV6, EBV), arbovirus (West Nile, eastern equine, St. Louis, LaCrosse, Japanese encephalitis viruses), rabies virus. Bacteria associated with encephalitis include *M. tuberculosis, Listeria, Rickettsia, Ehrlichia,* and *Bartonella*; parasites include *Toxoplasma, Naegleria, Acanthamoeba,* and *Balamuthia*.

Focal infections of the CNS such as brain abscess, subdual empyema, and epidural abscess are typically preceded by infection as a distal site (e.g., lungs, sinuses, endocardium, and skin). Abscess formation originating in the lungs or sinuses typically has *Streptococcus* as the primary pathogen associated with a mixture of aerobic and anaerobic bacteria. *S. aureus* endocarditis can be the source of staphylococcal brain abscess. Organisms such as *Nocardia* that can have a primary infection of the lungs or skin can disseminate to the brain or epidural space.

Finally, a variety of infections can present with neurological symptoms, such as *Clostridium botulinum, Clostridium tetani, Borrelia burgdorferi,* and HIV. The following case presentations illustrate some example of infectious CNS diseases.

STREPTOCOCCUS AGALACTIAE DISEASE IN A NEONATE

The following is a description of late-onset group B streptococcal disease in a neonate. A male infant weighing 3400 g was delivered spontaneously at term. Physical examinations of the infant were normal during the first week of life; however, the child started feeding irregularly during the second week. On day 13, the baby was admitted to the hospital with generalized seizures. A small amount of cloudy cerebrospinal fluid was collected by lumbar puncture, and *S. agalactiae* serotype III was isolated from culture. Despite the prompt initiation of therapy, the baby developed hydrocephalus, necessitating implantation of an atrioventricular shunt. The infant was discharged at age 3.5 months with retardation of psychomotor development. This patient illustrates neonatal meningitis caused by the most commonly implicated serotype of group B streptococci in late-onset disease and the complications associated with this infection. (*Eur J Pediatr.* 1977;126:189–197.)

ESCHERICHIA COLI MENINGITIS IN NEONATE

A 4-day-old female infant with a normal birth history and a birth weight of 3,250 g presented to an outlying hospital with a history of poor feeding, irritability, and fever (38.3°C). On presentation, cultures of blood, urine, and CSF were performed, and therapy with intravenous ampicillin and gentamicin was started. Examination of CSF revealed a WBC count of 227×10^6/L, and Gram stain revealed numerous gram-negative rods. A diagnosis of meningitis was made and all cultures yielded *Escherichia coli*. The child's clinical course was complicated by a left thalamic infarct resulting in quadriplegia that only partially resolved following recovery from the bacterial meningitis. Meningitis in neonates is primarily caused by either *Streptococcus agalactiae* (group B) or *E. coli*. Gram stain of CSF is critical for a rapid preliminary diagnosis and selection of appropriate empiric therapy. (Moffett, Berkowitz. *Clin Infect Dis.* 1997;25:211–214.)

HAEMOPHILUS INFLUENZAE MENINGITIS

A previously healthy 6-month-old boy presented in September 1984 with a 7-day history of rhinopharyngitis and two days of fever and irritability. On examination, he was found to be lethargic and to have neck rigidity and positive Kernig's sign consistent with meningitis. Lumbar puncture showed a white blood cell count of 4050 cells/mm^3 and a glucose concentration of 583 mmol/L. Gram stain of CSF showed small gram-negative coccobacilli and cultures of CSF and blood was positive for *Haemophilus influenzae* type b, resistant to ampicillin and chloramphenicol. Treatment was initiated with cefotaxime for 14 days and the patient underwent an uneventful recovery. Systemic disease (e.g., meningitis, epiglottis, and cellulitis) in children with *H. influenzae* type b (Hib) has been essentially eliminated with the introduction of Hib vaccination. The vaccine history in this child was not given but it is likely the child was not vaccination because vaccine failures are uncommon in immunocompetent children. (Guiscafre et al. *Arch Dis Childhood.* 1986;61:691–707.)

STREPTOCOCCUS PNEUMONIAE MENINGITIS

A 10-year-old child presented with complaints of high fever for 3 days with vomiting and altered mental status of 1 day duration. The patient was febrile, tachypneic, and had decreased consciousness and signs of meningeal irritation. He was diagnosed as community acquired acute bacterial meningitis, and CSF was collected. CSF was turbid in appearance with pleocytosis (80% neutrophils), decreased glucose (20 mg/dL), and elevated protein (136 mg/dL). Microscopy of the Gram stain smear showed gram-positive lancet-shaped diplococci with numerous leukocytes. Alpha-hemolytic colonies with depressed centers were observed on culture. The Gram stain and colony morphology were consistent with *Streptococcus pneumoniae* and were confirmed with biochemical tests (catalase-negative, bile soluble, optochin susceptible). The organism was resistant to penicillin and susceptible to ceftriaxone and multiple other antibiotics. The patient was treated with ceftriaxone and discharged from the hospital after 10 days. *S. pneumoniae* is one of the most common causes of meningitis in pediatric patients after the vaccine for *Haemophilus influenzae* B was introduced. The Gram stain of this organism and clinical presentation is sufficient to make a preliminary clinical diagnosis and resistance to penicillin is common so alternative empiric therapy such as used here is appropriate. (Srirangaraj, Kali. *Asian J Pharmaceut Clin Res.* 2014;7:101–102.)

LISTERIA MENINGITIS IN IMMUNOCOMPROMISED MAN

The following patient illustrates the clinical presentation of *Listeria* meningitis. A 73-year-old man with refractory rheumatoid arthritis was brought to the local hospital by his family because he had a decreased level of consciousness and a 3-day history of headache, nausea, and vomiting. His current medications were infliximab, methotrexate, and prednisone for his rheumatoid arthritis. On physical examination, the patient had a stiff neck and was febrile, with a pulse of 92 beats/minute, and blood pressure of 179/72 mmHg. Meningitis was suspected; therefore, blood and CSF were collected for culture. The Gram stain of the CSF was negative, but listeria grew from both blood and CSF. The patient was treated with vanco-

mycin, the infliximab was discontinued, and he made an uneventful recovery despite using less-than-optimal antimicrobial therapy. Ampicillin or penicillin G combined with an aminoglycoside is considered treatment of choice, while clinical failures are reported for vancomycin therapy. Infliximab has been associated with a dose-dependent monocytopenia. Monocytes are key effectors for clearance of *Listeria*, which meant this immunocompromised patient was specifically at risk for infection with this organism. Failure to detect *Listeria* in CSF by Gram stain is typical of this disease because the bacteria fail to multiply to detectable levels. (Bowie et al. *Ann Pharmacother.* 2004;38:58–61.)

DISSEMINATED NOCARDIOSIS

A 63-year-old man received a liver transplant for liver cirrhosis caused by hepatitis C. The patient was treated with immunosuppressive drugs, including tacrolimus and prednisone for 4 months, at which time he returned to the hospital with fever and lower leg pain. Although the chest radiograph was normal, ultrasound revealed an abscess in the soleus muscle. Poorly staining gram-positive rods were observed in the Gram stain of the pus aspirated from the abscess, and *Nocardia* grew after 3 days of incubation. Treatment with imipenem was started; however, the patient developed convulsions 10 days later and

partial left-sided paralysis. Brain imaging studies revealed three lesions. Treatment was switched to ceftriaxone and amikacin. The subcutaneous abscess and brain lesions gradually improved, and the patient was discharged after 55 days of hospitalization. This patient illustrates the propensity of *Nocardia* to infect immunocompromised patients, disseminate to the brain, and the slow rate of growth of the organism in culture and related need for prolonged treatment. (Shin et al. *Transplant Infect Dis* 2006;8:222–225.)

ASEPTIC MENINGITIS COMPLICATING ACUTE HSV-2 PROCTITIS

Atia and colleagues reported the clinical history of a male homosexual patient who developed aseptic meningitis during the course of acute proctitis due to HSV-2. The 23-year-old man was seen at a healthcare clinic 4 days after passive homosexual contact. On examination, the rectal tissue was inflamed and with purulent discharge. Bacteria consistent with *Neisseria gonorrhoeae* were observed on Gram stain, but the culture was negative. Ampicillin was administered but 2 days later the patient was readmitted with complaints of anal discomfort and pain on defecation. Multiple clusters of herpetiform vesicles were observed around the anus, and cultures were positive for HSV-2. Three days later, the patient returned to the hospital with symptoms of malaise, headache, photophobia, hesitancy of micturition, and pain radiating down

his legs. His temperature and pulse rate were elevated, and the patient had signs of meningitis. Cerebrospinal fluid was collected and was consistent with the diagnosis of aseptic lymphocytic meningitis. No viral cultures were performed with the cerebrospinal fluid, but the anorectal lesions were again positive for HSV-2. Even though specific antiviral therapy was not available (in the early 1980s), this patient had an uneventful recovery. This case illustrates the significant risk for sexually transmitted diseases in male homosexuals practicing unsafe sexual activities and the limited diagnostic and therapeutic options that were available in the 1980s during the early years of the AIDS epidemic. Currently, specific molecular tests and antiviral treatment are available for HSV CNS infections. (Atia et al. *Br J Vener Dis.* 1982;58:52–53.)

TOXOPLASMOSIS IN A WOMAN WITH HODGKIN DISEASE

Vincent and colleagues described a 67-year-old woman with a 3-year history of Hodgkin disease, who received chemotherapy followed by autologous stem-cell transplantation. Shortly afterward, she became febrile and neutropenic, and treatment with broad-spectrum antibiotics was started. The results of blood and urine cultures were negative. After resolution of neutropenia (1-month post transplantation), confusion and lethargy developed. Imaging studies of the brain revealed microinfarcts in both hemispheres and the midbrain. Findings from a lumbar puncture were unrevealing. Based on the suspicion of toxoplasmosis, pyrimethamine and sulfadiazine were added to the patient's regimen. When toxic epidermal necrolysis developed, the sulfadiazine was discontinued

and clindamycin was begun. Multiorgan failure ensued, and the patient died 1 week later. At autopsy, cyst forms with bradyzoites were detected in the woman's brain and heart. Histopathologic findings and immunohistochemical staining confirmed a diagnosis of disseminated toxoplasmosis.

Disseminated toxoplasmosis is rare, especially after autologous stem-cell transplantation. The likely cause of reactivation and dissemination of Toxoplasma in this patient was the cell-mediated immunosuppression associated with Hodgkin disease and its treatment. In addition to the brain, the heart, liver, and lungs are frequently involved in cases of disseminated toxoplasmosis. (Vincent. *Infect Med.* 2006;23:300.)

SHUNT INFECTED WITH *CUTIBACTERIUM* (*PROPIONIBACTERIUM*) ACNES

Chu and associates reported three patients with *Cutibacterium (Propionibacterium) acnes* infections of the central nervous system. The following patient illustrates the problems with this organism. A 38-year-old woman with congenital hydrocephalus presented with a 1-week history of decreased level of consciousness, headaches, and emesis. She had undergone numerous ventriculoperitoneal shunt placements in the past, with the last one placed 5 years before this presentation. The patient was afebrile and had no meningeal signs, but she was somnolent and arousable only by deep stimuli. Cerebrospinal fluid (CSF) collected from the shunt contained no erythrocytes but had 55 white blood cells; protein levels were

high and glucose slightly low. Pleomorphic gram-positive rods were observed on Gram stain and *C. acnes* grew in the anaerobic culture of the CSF. After 1 week of therapy with high-dose penicillin, the CSF remained positive by Gram stain and culture. The patient was taken to surgery where all foreign material was removed, and the patient was treated with penicillin for an additional 10 weeks. This patient illustrates the chronic, relatively asymptomatic nature of this disease, the need to remove the shunt and other foreign bodies, and the need to treat for a prolonged period. Note that *Propionibacterium acnes* has been renamed *Cutibacterium acnes*. (Chu et al. *Neurosurgery.* 2001;49:717–720.)

CRYPTOCOCCAL BRAIN ABSCESS IN HIV PATIENT

Kalinoski et al. reported the presentation of a 48-year-old man with HIV/AIDS and a history of recurrent *Cryptococcus neoformans* meningitis. His most recent episode of meningitis was 8 months previous to this hospital admission (CD4 <20 cells/μL at that time). He had been treated with amphotericin B and flucytosine for 2 weeks and then continued on fluconazole for consolidation therapy. Anti-retroviral therapy (ART) was started 24 days after antifungal initiation. At the time of presentation, antiviral therapy was reinitiated and his ART was continued. CSF studies revealed WBC count 72 cells, total protein 620 mg/dL, glucose 35 mg/dL, and Cryptococcal antigen titer >1:2560. Fungal culture and PCR tests were negative. MRI of the brain showed multiple microabscesses. Repeat studies 2 weeks later were unchanged although new abscess in the cerebellum were observed.

The differential diagnosis included treatment refractory cryptococcal disease, tuberculosis, bacterial meningitis with abscess formation, and immune reconstitution inflammatory syndrome (IRIS). All additional cultures were negative, and the patient did not respond to antibiotic treatment. The diagnosis of IRIS was confirmed when the patient's neurologic symptoms improved with treatment of prednisone. HIV/AIDS patients are predisposed to opportunistic infections with pathogens like *Cryptococcus neoformans* as was observed in this patient. When severely immunocompromised patients are started on ART, the reconstitution of their immune response can result in worsening symptoms of their opportunistic infection. It is important to differentiate between this immune response and progression of their infection. (Kalinoski et al. *Am J Trop Med Hyg.* 2020;103:713–718.)

EPSTEIN-BARR VIRUS (EBV) LYMPHOMA IN HIV PATIENT

Fallo et al. described a 30-month-old child with HIV-AIDS (diagnosed at 3 months) admitted to the hospital with mild encephalopathy, diarrhea, fever, oral thrush, mild hepatosplenomegaly, and weight loss. She had a complex medical course that included a history of *Pneumocystis* (*carinii*) *jiroveci* pneumonia, recurrent oral candidiasis, chronic diarrhea, and bacterial pneumonia. At 1 month of age, she was vaccinated with BCG (standard procedure for Argentina) and during her hospitalization, it was documented that she had disseminated BCG infection. Microsporidia diarrhea and urinary tract infection with *Klebsiella pneumoniae* were diagnosed that were managed with hydration and antibiotics. At day 10 of hospitalization, a behavioral change was noticed with features of increasing apathy and decreasing willingness to speak, walk or eat. A CT scan of the brain showed a mass lesion causing compression of the frontal horn and lateral ventricle with surrounding edema. The presumptive diagnosis of CNS tuberculosis was made. However, CSF examination was normal, and CSF acid-fast stains, Gram stains, and cultures for bacteria, mycobacteria, and fungi were negative. Blood cultures were also negative. Serologic tests for *Cryptococcus* and *Toxoplasma* were negative. The child continued to deteriorate and died at hospital day 71. At autopsy, a biopsy of the mass CNS lesion documented that this was an EBV lymphoma. Although the course of this infection likely would not have been altered, use of quantitative PCR test for EBV with blood or CSF could have been used to document this infection. This child illustrates the complexity of managing opportunistic infections in HIV/AIDS patients. Unless the HIV infection is adequately controlled with antiretroviral treatment (ART), the patient is susceptible to infections with bacterial, mycobacterial, fungal, and parasitic opportunistic pathogens. (Fallo et al. *Int J Infect Dis.* 2005;9:96–103.)

CONGENITAL CYTOMEGALOVIRUS (CMV) INFECTION

Kawai and Itoh described a 35-year-old woman who presented to the obstetrical clinic at 24 weeks of gestation for routine fetal ultrasound. Her pregnancy had been uneventful except for a febrile illness that occurred shortly after conception. The ultrasound images showed ventricular dilation, and MRI revealed ventriculomegaly and cerebellar hypoplasia. Serology for CMV was positive for IgG and IgM antibodies, consistent with a recent infection. At 38 weeks, the woman had a normal delivery, but the male baby weighed 2556 g (8th percentile) and had a head circumference of 30.5 cm (1st percentile). Petechiae were observed on the newborn's face and trunk. Imaging studies showed ventricular dilation, parenchymal hypoplasia, and periventricular calcifications. Immunohistochemical stains of the placenta and PCR of the baby's urine were positive for CMV, confirming the diagnosis of congenital CMV infection. The newborn was treated with ganciclovir and follow-up visit at 11 months revealed hearing loss, epilepsy, spastic quadriparesis, and developmental delay. This case illustrates the potential complications of a primary CMV infection in a pregnant woman. The infection occurred in the first trimester, increasing the risk for severe infection. Most congenital infections that occur later during pregnancy are either asymptomatic or associated with hearing loss or other mild developmental abnormalities. (Kawai, Itoh, *N Engl J Med.* 2018;379:e21.)

CENTRAL NERVOUS SYSTEM BLASTOMYCOSIS

Buhari reported a case of CNS blastomycosis. The patient was a 56-year-old homeless man from Detroit who presented with a 2-week history of left hemiparesis, aphasia, and generalized headache. There was no history of rash, respiratory symptoms, or fever. His medical history was significant for a left craniotomy 30 years previously for intracranial hemorrhage caused by trauma. He lived in an abandoned building and was not taking any medicines. On examination, he had expressive aphasia, new onset left hemiparesis, and bilateral carotid bruits. The rest of the physical examination was unremarkable, as were routine serum chemistries and hematologic parameters. He was negative for antibodies to HIV. A chest radiograph was unremarkable. A contrast-enhanced computed tomography (CT) scan of the head demonstrated multiple ring-enhancing lesions in the right cerebrum, with surrounding vasogenic edema and midline shift; significant encephalomalacia and generalized atrophy were present in the left cerebral hemisphere. Serum and urine tests were negative for *Cryptococcus* (serum) and *Histoplasma* (serum and urine) antigens. Tuberculin skin tests were nonreactive, and imaging studies of the sinuses, chest,

Continued

CENTRAL NERVOUS SYSTEM BLASTOMYCOSIS—cont'd

and abdomen were unremarkable. A brain biopsy was performed, and histopathologic examination revealed granulomatous inflammation and budding yeasts consistent with *B. dermatitidis*. Subsequent culture confirmed the diagnosis of CNS blastomycosis. The patient was treated with dexamethasone and amphotericin B but developed hypertension and bradycardia, with subsequent cardiopulmonary arrest and death.

This is an example of an unusual presentation of CNS blastomycosis without any other evidence of dissemi-nated disease. The clinical syndrome of hypertension, bradycardia, and cardiopulmonary arrest suggest that the patient died of increased intracranial pressure, either as a complication of the infection or the diagnostic brain biopsy. Although *Blastomyces* can disseminate to the brain as in this case, it is more typical that infection begins as a pulmonary infection and disseminates to the skin. *Cryptococcus* and *Histoplasma* are fungi that more commonly disseminate to the brain. (Buhari. *Infect Med.* 2007;24(suppl 8):12–14.)

SCHISTOSOMIASIS

Ferrari described a case of neuroschistosomiasis caused by *Schistosoma mansoni* in an 18-year-old Brazilian man. The patient was admitted to the hospital because of the recent onset of paraplegia. He was in good health until 33 days before admission, when he noted the onset of progressive low back pain with radiation to the lower limbs. During this period, he was evaluated three times in another institution, where radiographic films of the lower thoracic lumbar and sacral spine were normal. He received anti-inflammatory agents, with only transient relief in his symptoms. Four weeks after the pain began, the disease progressed acutely, with sexual impotence, fecal and urinary retention, and paraparesis progressing to paraplegia. At this time, the pain disappeared, replaced by a marked impairment of sensation in the lower limbs. On admission to the hospital, he gave a history of exposure to schistosomal infection. Neurologic examination revealed flaccid paraplegia, marked sensory loss, and absence of superficial and deep reflexes at and below the level T11. The cerebrospinal fluid contained 84 white blood cells/mL (98% lymphocytes, 2% eosinophils) and 1 red blood cell, 82 mg/dL total protein, and 61 mg/dL glucose. Myelography, computed tomography myelography, and magnetic resonance imaging showed a slight widening of the conus. The diagnosis of neuroschistosomiasis was confirmed by the demonstration of viable and dead eggs of *S. mansoni* on rectal mucosal biopsy. The concentration of cerebrospinal fluid immunoglobulin G against soluble egg antigen of *S. mansoni* quantitated by enzyme-linked immunosorbent assay was 1.53 µg/mL. He was treated with prednisone and praziquantel. Despite therapy, his condition remained unaltered at follow-up 7 months later. *S. mansoni* is the most frequently reported cause of schistosomal myeloradiculopathy worldwide. Schistosomal myeloradiculopathy is among the most severe forms of schistosomiasis, and prognosis depends largely on early diagnosis and treatment. (Ferrari TC. *Medicine.* 1999;78:176–190.)

NEUROCYSTICERCOSIS IN ITALIAN TRAVELLER

Chatel and colleagues described a case of neurocysticercosis in an Italian traveler to Latin America. The patient was a 49-year-old man with a history of a 30-day stay in Latin America (El Salvador, Colombia, and Guatemala) 3 months before presentation with fever and myalgia. The clinical examination and routine laboratory test results were normal except for elevated creatine phosphokinase levels and mild eosinophilia. He received symptomatic anti-inflammatory therapy, rapidly improved, and was discharged with a diagnosis of polymyositis. Two years later, he was admitted to the hospital with retroocular headache and recurrent right hemianopsia. A neurologic examination revealed a left Babinski reflex with no motor or sensory dysfunctions. Laboratory tests were unremarkable, including a negative stool examination for ova and para-sites. Cerebral magnetic resonance imaging showed the presence of several intraparenchymal, subarachnoid, and intraventricular cysts (4–15 mm in diameter) with perilesional focal edema and ring-like enhancement. A specific antibody response to cysticercosis was demonstrated by enzyme-linked immunosorbent assay and immunoblotting techniques. The patient was treated with albendazole for two cycles of 8 days each. One year later, he was in good health, and cerebral magnetic resonance imaging revealed significant reduction in the diameter of lesions. This case provides an interesting reminder of the minimal but real risks to travelers for acquiring *Taenia solium* infections during foreign travel. (Chatel et al. *Am J Trop Med Hyg.* 1999;60:255–256.)

CLOSTRIDIUM TETANI INFECTION

The following is a typical history of a patient with tetanus. An 86-year-old man saw a physician for care of a splinter wound in his right hand, acquired 3 days earlier while gardening. He was not treated with either a tetanus toxoid vaccine or tetanus immune globulin. Seven days later he developed pharyngitis, and after an additional 3 days, he presented to the local hospital with difficulty talking, swallowing, and breathing, and with chest pain and disorientation. He was admitted to the hospital with the diagnosis of stroke. On his 4th hospital day, he had developed neck rigidity and respiratory failure, requiring tracheostomy and mechanical ventilation. He was transferred to the medical intensive care unit, where the clinical diagnosis of tetanus was made. Despite treatment with tetanus toxoid and immune globulin, the patient died 1 month after admission to the hospital. This case illustrates that *C. tetani* is ubiquitous in soil and can contaminate relatively minor wounds. It also highlights the unrelenting progression of neurologic disease in untreated patients. Clinical improvement in survivors is slow because the toxin binds to nerve endings and is protected from the patient's antibody response. The toxic effects of this pathogen must be controlled symptomatically until normal regulation of synaptic transmission is restored. (*MMWR* 2002;51:613–615.)

CLOSTRIDIUM BOTULINUM INFECTION

The CDC reported an outbreak of foodborne botulism associated with contaminated carrot juice. On September 8, 2006, three patients went to a hospital in Washington County, GA, with cranial nerve palsies and progressive descending flaccid paralysis resulting in respiratory failure. The patients had shared meals on the previous day. They were treated with botulinum antitoxin because botulism was suspected. There was no progression of the patients' neurologic symptoms, but they remained hospitalized and on ventilators. An investigation determined that the patients had consumed contaminated carrot juice produced by a commercial vendor. Botulinum toxin type A was detected in the serum and stool of all three patients and in leftover carrot juice. An additional patient in Florida was also hospitalized with respiratory failure and descending paralysis after drinking carrot juice sold in Florida. Carrot juice has a low acid content (pH 6.0); therefore, *C. botulinum* spores can germinate and produce toxin if contaminated juice is left at room temperature. (*MMWR* 2006;55:1098–1099.)

INFANT BOTULISM

In January 2003, four children with infant botulism were reported by the CDC. The following is a description of one of the children. A 10-week-old infant with a history of constipation in the 1st month of life was admitted to a hospital after having difficulty in sucking and swallowing for 2 days. The infant was irritable and had loss of facial expression, generalized muscle weakness, and constipation. Mechanical ventilation was required for 10 days because of respiratory failure. A diagnosis of infant botulism was established 29 days after the onset of symptoms by detection of *C. botulinum* producing toxin type B in stool enrichment cultures. The patient was treated with botulism immune globulin intravenous (BIG-IV) and discharged fully recovered after 20 days. In contrast with foodborne botulism, diagnosis of infant botulism can be made by detecting the organism in the baby's stools. (*MMWR* 2003;52:21–24.)

TREPONEMA PALLIDUM NEUROSYPHILIS

A 42-year-old previously healthy man was hospitalized due to a 1-year history of progressive cognitive decline, confusion attacks, rare hallucinations, gait disturbances and involuntary movements. On neurological examination, he had predominantly left-sided bradykinesia and rigidity and tremor in his left hand and both legs. His gait was cautious and wide-based. According to neuropsychological testing, he had severe dementia with severe attention deficit. Blood tests were normal and HIV tests negative, but syphilis serology was highly positive in serum and CSF. The diagnosis of neurosyphilis was made and intravenous penicillin-G treatment was initiated for 14 days. On follow-up 6 months later, the patient had mild dementia but there were neither myoclonus nor parkinsonism. On subsequent follow-up visits (twice a year), no consistent changes have been found. Neurosyphilis has been referred to as the "great imitator" because clinical presentation lacks specificity. It is important to consider syphilis in the workup of neurological dysfunction. (Sabre et al. *BMC Res Notes*. 2016;9:372–375.)

34

Skin and Soft Tissue Infections

Skin and soft tissue infections can either be primary infections resulting from hematogenous dissemination or secondary manifestations of infections (e.g., rash). These infections can also vary from superficial presentations to rapidly progressing, life-threatening infections.

The infections can have an acute onset (e.g., characteristic of many *Staphylococcus aureus* infections) or a chronic, slowly progressive process (e.g., leprosy caused by *Mycobacterium leprae*). The following are examples of skin and soft tissue infections.

Impetigo	Superficial, vascular infection of the skin; most commonly caused by *S. aureus* or *Streptococcus pyogenes* (group A strep)
Folliculitis	Erythematous papules located within hair follicles; *S. aureus* is the most common cause; specific infections with *Pseudomonas aeruginosa*, rapidly growing *Mycobacterium* species, and *Aeromonas* are associated with immersion in contaminated water (e.g., whirlpools, hot tubs, and foot baths)
Furuncles, Carbuncles	Inflammatory nodule(s) extending into the subcutaneous tissues; *S. aureus* is the most common cause
Cellulitis	Rapidly spreading infection of the skin that can be superficial (erysipelas) or involve deeper tissues; most commonly associated with *S. pyogenes* or *S. aureus*; may also be a secondary manifestation of other in infections (e.g., animal or human bite wound caused by *Pasteurella multocida*, *Eikenella corrodens*, or mixed aerobic/anaerobic bacteria)
Necrotizing fasciitis	Rapidly progressive infection involving necrosis of subcutaneous tissues and the overlying skin; *S. pyogenes* ("flesh-eating bacteria") most widely recognized but other pathogens include *P. aeruginosa*, mixtures of aerobic and anaerobic bacteria (synergistic necrotizing cellulitis), *Rhizopus* or *Mucor* (necrotizing mucormycosis), and *Clostridium perfringens* and *Clostridium septicum* (clostridial gas gangrene)
Primary fungal infection	A variety of fungi can produce infections of the skin including dermatophytes (e.g., *Trichosporon*, *Microsporum*, and *Epidermophyton*), *Malassezia*, and *Candida*, as well as the subcutaneous tissues (e.g., *Sporothrix*, *Fusarium*, *Cladosporium*, *Alternaria*, and *Curvularia*)

Skin lesions, such as those caused by injuries, burns, or surgical procedures, can be secondarily infected with organisms normally on the skin surface (e.g., *Staphylococcus*, *Corynebacterium*, and *Cutibacterium*) or infected with specific organisms that cause infections in this setting (e.g., burn wound infections caused by *Enterobacter*, *Pseudomonas*, or *Enterococcus*). Caution must be exercised in interpreting culture results in this setting because insignificant, superficial colonization is not uncommon (e.g., colonization of diabetic skin ulcers).

Skin manifestations of infections at distal sites are also well-recognized. Examples include infections caused by *S. aureus*, *Neisseria meningitidis*, *Treponema pallidum*, *P. aeruginosa*, and rashes caused by many organisms including *Rickettsia* and many viruses. It is important to differentiate between skin manifestations of active replication of organisms at that site and those manifestations that result from the expression of toxins at a distal site, such as skin pathology caused by staphylococcal toxins in toxic shock syndrome.

The following clinical cases illustrate the presentation of a variety of skin and soft tissue infections.

STAPHYLOCOCCUS AUREUS SCALDED SKIN SYNDROME

Kouakou et al. reported a newborn with staphylococcal scalded skin syndrome (SSSS). The infant was hospitalized for erythroderma. The disease started with a sore throat and conjunctivitis. Within 48 hours, the newborn developed a fever and tender erythema that progressed to generalized erythematous skin lesions primarily seen in the axillary and groin. The lesions were associated with large superficial blisters that ruptured on slight pressures (Nikolski sign). The skin blistering spread to cover one-third of the infant and a skin biopsy showed superficial intraepidermal split into the granular layer with no inflammatory infiltrate or necrosis, essentially excluding drug-induced toxic epidermal necrosis and staphylococcal toxic shock. Cultures of urine, skin, and vagina were negative, but *Staphylococcus aureus* was recovered in conjunctiva, nasopharynx, and blood. The newborn was treated with ceftriaxone and an aminoglycoside, the erythroderma decreased within 7–10 days, and full recovery was observed after 3 weeks. (Kouakou et al. *Case Reports Dermatol Med.* 2015, doi:10.1155/2015/901968.)

STAPHYLOCOCCAL FURUNCLE AND SEPTIC SHOCK

Moellering and colleagues described a 30-year-old woman who presented to their hospital with hypotension and respiratory failure. One month earlier, the patient, who had previously been in good health, was seen at an urgent care clinic because of a red, hard, painful lump that had developed on her right lower leg 3 days earlier. The lesion was excised and drained, and she was treated with a 10-day course of cephalexin and trimethoprim-sulfamethoxazole. Culture of the lesion grew *S. aureus* that was resistant to oxacillin, penicillins, cephalosporins, levofloxacin, and erythromycin; it was susceptible to vancomycin, clindamycin, tetracycline, and trimethoprim-sulfamethoxazole. Upon arrival in the emergency department, the patient was agitated, had a temperature of 39.6°C, blood pressure 113/53 mmHg, pulse 156 beats/minute, and respiratory rate 46 breaths/minute. Small cutaneous vesicles were noted on her forehead and abdomen. She rapidly deteriorated and was transferred to the intensive care unit where she was managed for septic shock. Despite clinical efforts, her hypoxemia, hypercardia, acidosis, and hypotension worsened, and she died less than 12 hours after arrival at the hospital. Chest radiographs that were obtained upon admission to the hospital showed diffuse pulmonary infiltrates with small areas of cavitation in both lungs; a computed tomography (CT) scan of the abdomen and pelvis showed ascites and lymph node enlargement; and a CT scan of the brain showed multiple foci of hyperintensity in the frontal, temporal, parietal, and occipital lobes. *S. aureus*, with the same antibiotic susceptibility profile as the isolate from the leg furuncle, was cultured from blood and multiple tissue specimens. The clinical diagnosis was that this woman died of sepsis due to infection with community-acquired MRSA that progressed from a localized furuncle to necrotizing pneumonia and then overwhelming sepsis with multiple disseminated septic emboli. This infection illustrates the pathogenic potential of drug-resistant *S. aureus* in an otherwise healthy individual. (Moellering et al. *N Engl J Med.* 2011;364:266–275.)

MYCOBACTERIAL INFECTIONS ASSOCIATED WITH NAIL SALONS

In September 2000, a physician reported to the California Department of Health four females who developed lower extremity furunculosis. Each patient presented with small erythematous papules that became large, tender, fluctuant, violaceous boils over several weeks. Bacterial cultures of the lesions were negative, and the patients failed empiric antibacterial therapy. All the patients had visited the same nail salon before the furuncles developed. As a result of an investigation of the nail salon, a total of 110 patients with furunculosis were identified. *M. fortuitum* was cultured from the lesions of 32 patients, as well as from the footbaths used by the patients before their pedicures. Shaving the legs was identified as a risk factor for disease. Similar outbreaks have been reported in the literature, which illustrates the risks associated with contamination of water with rapidly growing acid-fast mycobacteria; the difficulties of confirming these infections by Gram stain and routine bacterial cultures, which are typically incubated for only 1 to 2 days; and the need for effective antibiotic therapy. (*N Engl J Med.* 2002;346:1366–1371.)

PSEUDOMONAS FOLLICULITIS

Ratnam and associates described an outbreak of folliculitis caused by *Pseudomonas aeruginosa* in guests at a Canadian hotel. A number of guests complained of a skin rash, which began as pruritic erythematous papules, and progressed to erythematous pustules distributed in the axilla and over the abdomen and buttocks. For most patients, the rash resolved spontaneously over a 5-day period. The local health department investigated the outbreak and determined the source was a whirlpool contaminated with a high concentration of *P. aeruginosa*. The outbreak was terminated when the whirlpool was drained, cleaned, and super chlorinated. Skin infections such as this are common in individuals with extensive exposure to contaminated water. (Ratnam et al. *J Clin Microbiol.* 1986;23:655–659.)

STREPTOCOCCUS PYOGENES NECROTIZING FASCIITIS AND SEPTIC SHOCK

Filbin and colleagues described the dramatic clinical course of disease caused by group A *Streptococcus* in a previously healthy 25-year-old man. Two days before admission to the hospital, he noticed a lesion on the dorsum of his right hand and thought it was an insect bite. The next day the hand became painfully swollen and he felt ill. The next morning, he had chills and a temperature of 38.6°C. That evening, his mother found him obtunded, vomiting, and incontinent, and he was rushed to the emergency department. At the time of admission, his blood pressure was 73/25 mmHg, temperature 37.9°C, pulse 145 beats/minute, and respiratory rate 30 breaths/minute. The right hand was mottled, with a 1-cm black eschar on the dorsum, and swollen up his forearm. Manipulations of the fingers resulted in extreme pain. A radiograph of the hand revealed prominent soft tissue swelling and chest radiograph showed findings consistent with interstitial edema. A diagnosis of severe sepsis was made, and intravenous vancomycin and clindamycin were administered. The patient was taken to surgery 4 h after arrival in the hospital, and complete debridement of the skin and fascia up to the elbow of the right arm was required. Pathologic examination of the tissues revealed liquefactive necrosis involving the fascial planes and superficial fat. Small blood vessel intraluminal thrombi and infiltration of mononuclear cells and neutrophils was also observed in the tissues, as well as abundant gram-positive cocci subsequently identified as group A streptococci. Over the course of this patient's hospitalization, he developed severe systemic manifestations of hypotension, coagulopathy, renal failure, and respiratory insufficiency. The patient was aggressively treated with penicillin G, clindamycin, vancomycin, and cefepime and slowly improved until his discharge 16 days after hospitalization. This case illustrates the rapid progression of disease from a relatively innocuous superficial skin lesion to necrotizing fasciitis, septic shock, and multiorgan involvement. Mortality with necrotizing fasciitis and severe sepsis approaches 50% and is only successfully managed with aggressive surgical debridement and antibiotic therapy. (Filbin et al. *N Engl J Med.* 2009;360:281–290.)

PASTEURELLA MULTOCIDA NECROTIZING FASCIITIS

Chang et al. described a fatal case of *Pasteurella multocida* bacteremia and necrotizing fasciitis. The 58-year-old man had a history of chronic renal insufficiency, gouty arthritis, and Cushing syndrome treated with steroids. Upon admission to the hospital, his left hand was erythematous, warm, and tender with reddish to purplish macules over the surface. Over a 2-day period, bullae developed and extended rapidly to the left arm, left calf, and right foot, and the patient had systemic signs of shock and gastrointestinal bleeding. Blood cultures collected at the time of admission were positive for *P. multocida*. Despite aggressive antibiotic and surgical treatment, the lesions progressed rapidly and the patient eventually expired. A careful history at the time of admission revealed that the patient allowed his pet dog to lick his open wounds. This was the likely source of the bacteria because it is part of the resident oral flora of dogs and the steroid treatments allowed the organism to invade the wound and rapidly spread in the tissues. (Chang et al. *Scand J Infect Dis.* 2007;39:167–192.)

BACTEROIDES FRAGILIS NECROTIZING FASCIITIS

Pryor and associates described an unfortunate patient with a polycrotic fasciitis. A 38-year-old man with a 10-year history of human immunodeficiency virus infection underwent an uncomplicated hemorrhoidectomy. Over the next 5 days, thigh and buttock pain developed with nausea and vomiting. The man presented to the hospital with a heart rate of 120 beats/minute, blood pressure of 120/60 mmHg, respiratory rate of 22 respirations/minute, and temperature of 38.5°C. Physical examination revealed extensive erythema around the surgical site, flank, thighs, and abdominal wall. Gas was observed in the tissues underlying the areas of erythema and extended to his upper chest. At surgery, extensive areas of tissue necrosis and foul-smelling brownish exudates were found. Multiple surgeries to aggressively debride the involved tissues were necessary. Cultures obtained at surgery grew a mixture of aerobic and anaerobic organisms, with *Escherichia coli*, β-hemolytic streptococci, and *B. fragilis* predominating. This clinical case illustrates the potential complications of rectal surgery—aggressive destruction of tissue, polymicrobic etiology with *B. fragilis* as a prominent organism, and foul-smelling necrotic tissue with gas production. Resolution of this disease requires aggressive and repeated surgical intervention and prolonged antimicrobial therapy. (Pryor et al. *Crit Care Med.* 2001;29:1071–1073.)

LYME DISEASE IN LYME, CONNECTICUT

In 1977, Steere and associates reported an epidemic of arthritis in eastern Connecticut. The authors studied a group of 39 children and 12 adults who developed an illness characterized by recurrent attacks of swelling and pain in a few large joints. Most attacks were for a week or less, but some attacks lasted for months. Twenty-five percent of the patients remembered they had an erythematous cutaneous lesion 4 weeks before the onset of their arthritis. This was the first report of Lyme disease, named after the town in Connecticut, where the disease was first recognized. We now know the erythematous lesion (erythema migrans) is the characteristic presentation of early Lyme disease. A few years after this report, the *Borrelia* responsible for Lyme disease, *B. burgdorferi*, was isolated. (Steere et al. *Arthritis Rheum.* 1977;20:7–17.)

ROCKY MOUNTAIN SPOTTED FEVER

Oster and associates described a series of patients who acquired Rocky Mountain spotted fever after working with *R. rickettsii* in the laboratory. One patient, a 21-year-old veterinary technician, presented to a clinic with complaints of myalgia and a nonproductive cough. He was treated with penicillin and discharged. Over the next few days, he developed chills and a headache. When he returned to the hospital, he had a temperature of 40.0°C and a macular rash on his extremities and trunk. Intramuscular tetracycline was started but he remained febrile, and the rash evolved to petechiae on his truck, extremities, and soles of his feet. Bilateral pleural effusions developed, and intravenous tetracycline was begun. Over the next 2 weeks, the effusions resolved and the patient made a slow but uneventful recovery. Although this patient was not working directly with *R. rickettsii*, he had visited a laboratory that was processing the bacterium. This patient illustrates the characteristic presentation of Rocky Mountain spotted fever—headache, fever, myalgias, and a macular rash that can evolve into a petechial or spotted rash. (Oster et al. *N Engl J Med.* 1977;297:859–863.)

RICKETTSIALPOX IN NEW YORK CITY

Koss and associates described 18 patients with rickettsialpox who were diagnosed at Columbia Presbyterian Medical Center in New York City during a 20-month period after the anthrax bioterrorism attack in the fall of 2001. The patients presented to the hospital because they had a necrotic eschar and were thought to have cutaneous anthrax. The patients also had fever, headache, and a papulovesicular rash. Many patients also complained of myalgias, sore throat, arthralgias, and gastrointestinal symptoms. Immunohistochemical staining of eschar and skin biopsies confirmed the diagnosis of rickettsialpox and not cutaneous anthrax. The etiologic agent of rickettsialpox is *Rickettsia akari*, and the disease is transmitted from rodents to human by mites ("chiggers"). These patients illustrate the diagnostic difficulties of recognizing uncommon diseases, even when the clinical presentation is characteristic. (Koss et al. *Arch Dermatol.* 2003;139:1545–1554.)

ORIENTIA SCRUB TYPHUS

An 8-year-old boy presented to a hospital in India with fever, abdominal pain, and vomiting for 6 days. He had tachycardia, tachypnea, left cervical lymphadenopathy, hepatosplenomegaly and an escar hidden behind his left ear. Laboratory work-up was noncontributory except for thrombocytopenia and elevated hepatic transaminases. The child was started on doxycycline, and serology for scrub typhus was subsequently reported as positive. The child became afebrile with 36 hours and was discharged after 7 days following normalization of the laboratory and clinical parameters. Eschar formation at the site of the mite bite is a present in one-third of the pediatric cases. (Kumar Bhat et al. *Indian Pediat.* 2020;57:93.)

RICKETTSIA PROWAZEKII EPIDEMIC TYPHUS

A 65-year-old man came to a hospital in Marseilles, France for evaluation of fever, nausea, vomiting, myalgias, and diarrhea. He was a native Algerian who lived in France but had visited a small town in east central Algeria for 3 months. The patient recalled pruritus and scratching during his stay, but no lice or other insects were found on his clothing. Upon physical examination, he had a discrete rash (few rose spots on the trunk) and splenomegaly. Laboratory results revealed elevated liver enzymes. A presumptive diagnosis of typhoid fever was made, and empiric treatment with intravenous ceftriaxone was initiated as blood, urine and stools specimens were collected for culture. After 3 days, the cultures remained negative and the patient's condition worsened with fever, semicomatose, and severe dyspnea and diffuse purpuric rash. Laboratory tests now showed severe thrombocytopenia, elevated liver enzymes, and coagulation studies suggestive of disseminated intravascular coagulation and acute renal failure. Chest X-ray demonstrated bilateral interstitial pneumonia. Diagnosis was now suspected to be typhus (murine or epidemic) so the patient was transferred to the ICU and started on intravenous doxycycline. His clinical condition improved rapidly. The diagnosis of epidemic typhus was confirmed by positive serology for *Rickettsia prowazekii* and isolation of the *Rickettsia* in cell culture. The persistent negative blood cultures by conventional culture methods, lack of response to ceftriaxone, and rash are consistent with the diagnosis of typhus. *R. prowazekii* is a human pathogen that is spread person-to-person by body lice. (Niang et al. *Emerg Infect Dis.* 1999;5:716–718.)

RICKETTSIA TYPHI MURINE TYPHUS

During the COVID-19 pandemic, a 25-year-old man from Southern California presented virtually by telephone appointment with a 4-day history of headaches, myalgia, chills, and fevers. He was tested for SARS-CoV-2 by PCR and found negative. One day later (day 5 of his illness), he presented to the Emergency Department for persistent symptoms of fever, body aches, and headache. He also had vomiting, diarrhea, cough, congestion, chills, and fatigue. There was no evidence of rash, chest pain, or congestion. PCR testing was again negative for SARS-CoV-2. He was given ibuprofen and told to report back to the hospital if his symptoms worsened. He returned to the hospital 3 days later with worsening symptoms. Blood cultures were collected and remained negative after 5 days, and he was treated empirically with intramuscular ceftriaxone and discharged with recommendation for azithromycin for 5 days. On day 14 of illness, he reported persistent fevers, cough, chills, body aches, headache, dizziness, fatigue, and diarrhea. During the interview, it was elicited he was a dog trainer. Because of his occupation and potential exposure to fleas, murine typhus was included in the differential diagnosis, which was confirmed by serology. Treatment was changed to doxycycline for 2 weeks to which he promptly responded. His illness occurred during the COVID-19 pandemic, and his nonspecific presentation overlapped with COVID 10 symptoms. Additionally the classic triad of murine typhus symptoms—fever, headache, and rash—appear in only one-third of patients. Doxycycline is the treatment of choice, to which the patient promptly responded. (Patel. *BMJ Case Rep.* 2020;13:e23971.)

OUTBREAK OF TICK-BORNE BORRELIA RELAPSING FEVER

In August 2002, the New Mexico Department of Health was notified of an outbreak of tick-borne relapsing fever. Approximately 40 people attended a family gathering held in a cabin in the mountains of northern New Mexico. Half of the family members slept overnight in the cabin. Some of the family arrived 3 days before the event to clean the unoccupied cabin. Four days after the event, one of the individuals who arrived early sought care at a local hospital with a 2-day history of fever, chills, myalgia, and a raised pruritic rash on the forearms. Spirochetes were observed on a peripheral blood smear. As many as 14 individuals who attended the family gathering developed symptoms consistent with relapsing fever and had either positive serology or spirochetes observed in blood smears. The majority had a history of fever, headache, arthralgia, and myalgia. Rodent nesting material was found inside the interior walls of the cabin. This outbreak of endemic relapsing fever illustrates the risks associated with exposure to ticks that feed on infected rodents. The tick bites are generally not remembered because the feeding is for a short duration at night. Diagnosis is also complicated by the relapsing nature of this febrile illness caused by *Borrelia* species. (*MMWR*. 2003;52:809–812.)

CONGENITAL SYPHILIS

A 22-year-old second gravida primipara woman, who had not undergone clinical evaluation during pregnancy, delivered a female neonate weighing 2780 after 35 weeks of gestation. Immediately after delivery, the neonate was found to have a rash on her body (nonelevated pink maculae with uneven margins) located on her hands, legs, chest, abdomen, and back; ruptured bullous lesions were observed on her feet and hands. Laboratory tests revealed hypoglycemia, thrombocytopenia, and elevated C-reactive protein; CSF revealed an elevated count of leukocytes, with 86.5% lymphocytes, and elevated protein. Cultures of blood and CSF were negative. Treponemal and nontreponemal serological tests were positive in both the mother and neonate, and the diagnosis of congenital syphilis was made. X-rays of the neonate's long bones revealed signs of syphilitic osteochondritis in all bones. A 14-day course of penicillin G was administered. Clinical diagnosis of congenital syphilis can be challenging. *Treponema pallidum* cannot be grown in culture, so diagnosis is dependent on serologic testing as was done for this patient.

HUMAN HERPES VIRUS 6 (HHV-6) EXANTHEM SUBITUM

Miyake et al. described a 7-month-old girl who developed Guillain-Barre syndrome 20 days after HHV-6 exanthem subitum. The baby was healthy post-delivery until she developed a high-grade fever (39.0°C) that persisted for 5 days. On the 6th day, her temperature returned to normal, but a fine maculopapular, pinkish rash appeared on her trunk and face. Her family physician diagnosed this as typical HHV-6 exanthem subitum. Twenty days after the diagnosis, her mother noted the baby was irritable and loss lower limb movement. On admission to the hospital, the infant was normal except an absence of the deep tendon reflexes in the lower extremities. CSF was culture negative and normal for chemistry and cell counts. Nerve conduction studies showed a reduced motor conduction velocity and amplitude suggesting axonal damage. The diagnosis of Guillain-Barre syndrome (GBS) was made. Stool cultures were negative for *Campylobacter jejuni*, a common cause of GBS. Serologic tests confirmed the diagnosis of HHV-6 infection. Immunoglobulin therapy was administered for 5 days, and the symptoms promptly disappeared. On follow-up at 10 months of age, the baby's growth and development were normal. Major complications of HHV-6 commonly involve the central nervous system, including seizures, meningitis, or encephalitis. GBS is a rare complication. (Miyake et al. *Ped Infect Dis J*. 2002;21:569–570.)

ONCHOCERCIASIS

Choudhary and Choudhary described the case of a 21-year-old man who emigrated from Sudan to the United States 1 year before presenting with a maculopapular rash that was associated with severe pruritus. The rash and pruritus had been present for the past 3–4 years. In the past, the patient had undergone multiple treatments for this condition, including corticosteroids, without relief. The patient denied any systemic symptoms but did complain of blurred vision. On physical examination, his skin was somewhat thickened over different parts of the body, and he had scattered maculopapular lesions with increased pigmentation; some lesions had keloid nodules as well as wrinkling. There was no lymphadenopathy. The remainder of his evaluation was unremarkable. Because of the presence of intense pruritus unresponsive to treatment, blurred vision, and the prevalence of onchocerciasis in his native country, skin snips were taken from the scapular area. Microfilariae of *Onchocerca* volvulus were revealed on microscopic examination. Ivermectin was prescribed, to which the patient's condition responded. Onchocerciasis, although not common in the United States, should be considered in immigrants and expatriates with suggestive symptoms if they came from areas in which the disease is endemic. (Choudhary IA, Choudhary SA. *Infect Med* 2005;22:187–189.)

TINEA VERSICOLOR IN IMMUNOCOMPETENT WOMAN

Holliday and Grider reported a typical case of tinea versicolor in a 24-year-old woman. She presented with a 12-year history of a depigmenting rash over her neck, torso, and upper arms. It was most notable in the summer months, with spontaneous remission during the cooler seasons. Previous therapies with multiple topical antifungal agents had not regenerated the skin pigmentation. Scrapings of the skin and staining with periodic acid-Schiff stain revealed the presence of abundant fungi described as a "spaghetti and meatball" pattern. This is the classic description of *Malassezia* in these lesions, with the presence of spherical and rod-like forms. It is likely that this diagnosis was previously suspected because she had been treated with antifungals, but recurrent infections are common and repigmentation may take months once the fungus is eliminated. Mild cases may be treated with 1% selenium sulfate (the active ingredient in dandruff shampoos), and more severe infections such as in this woman are treated with a course of oral fluconazole and topical ketoconazole. (Holliday, Grider. *N Engl J Med.* 2016;374:e11.)

MALASSEZIA INFECTIONS IN PATIENTS RECEIVING HYPERALIMENTATION

Malassezia furfur is a yeast-like organism that commonly colonizes the skin of infants and adults. Colonization may be asymptomatic or cause localized hypopigmented or hyperpigmented macules on the colonized surfaces. *M. furfur* has also been associated with catheter-related sepsis in patients, particularly low-birth weight infants, receiving hyperalimentation fluids through central venous catheters. The organism requires lipids for growth (lipophilic) and can colonize the catheter and grow to high concentrations. Recovery in blood cultures requires supplementation of the media with lipids such as mineral oil so cultures are frequently negative in these patients. (Marcon, Powell. *Clin Microbiol Rev.* 1992;5:101–119.)

MYCOBACTERIUM LEPRAE INFECTION

A 35-year-old Brazilian man immigrated to the United States in 2006 and soon after reported nodules developing where he reported mosquito bites. The nodules continued to enlarge over several months and became diffuse. He sought help from the internet and a Brazilian "doctor" prescribed treatment with daily prednisone that he took sporadically over an 18-month period. Because his condition continued to worsen, he was brought to the local hospital where physical examination revealed diffuse infiltration of the skin, nasal mucosa, and soft palate with thick papules and plaques, some of which exhibited crusting and ulceration. Histopathologic findings of a skin biopsy showed numerous foamy histiocytes without epithelioid granuloma formation.

Mycobacterial organisms were seen within histiocytes with an acid-fast stain, confirming the clinical diagnosis of leprosy. A 2-year multidrug treatment consisting of dapsone, rifampin, ofloxacin, and minocycline with prednisone was initiated, but dapsone was discontinued because of low levels of glucose-6-phosphate dehydrogenase. Follow-up visits have shown a steady decrease in the size of the mucocutaneous plaques and nodules. This is a classic presentation of leprosy, with a slow, insidious onset, widespread lesions, and the need for prolonged treatment. *Mycobacterium leprae* does not grow in culture so laboratory diagnosis requires observation of acid-fast organisms in the skin lesions. (Hall et al. *Head Neck Pathol.* 2010;4:226–229.)

HUMAN GRANULOCYTIC ANAPLASMOSIS

Heller and associates described a 73-year-old man who presented to their hospital with fever, weakness, and leg myalgias. Six days before his admission, he had traveled to South Carolina, and 3 days later, he developed intense leg pains, a high fever, and generalized weakness. Upon admission, he was febrile, tachycardic, and hypertensive; the liver and spleen could not be palpated and no cutaneous rash was noted. Cultures for bacteria, fungi, and viruses were negative. A peripheral blood smear showed rare intracytoplasmic inclusions in the granulocytes ("morulae"). Polymerase chain reaction (PCR) analysis of blood samples collected on the second and third hospital days was positive for *Anaplasma*

phagocytophilum DNA, confirming the diagnosis of anaplasmosis. The patient was treated successfully with a 14-day course of doxycycline, although residual muscle weakness and pain persisted. Serum collected during the convalescent period was positive for *Anaplasma*. In contrast with *Rickettsia* infections, the presence of a rash is uncommon in *Ehrlichia* and *Anaplasma* infections (35% and <10%, respectively). It is noteworthy that the patient did not remember a tick bite during his South Carolina trip, consistent with the observation that the early tick stages (larva and nymphs) are commonly associated with human disease. (Heller et al. *N Engl J Med.* 2005;352:1358–1364.)

NEONATAL HSV INFECTION

Parvey and Ch'ien reported a case of neonatal herpes simplex virus (HSV) infection contracted during birth. During a breech presentation, a fetal monitor was placed on the buttocks of the baby, and because of the greatly prolonged labor, the baby was delivered by cesarean section. The 5-lb boy had minor difficulties that were successfully treated, but on the 6th day, vesicles with an erythematous base appeared at the site where the fetal monitor had been placed. HSV was grown from the vesicle fluid and from spinal fluid, corneal scraping, saliva, and blood. The baby became moribund, with frequent apneic episodes and seizures. Intravenous treatment with adenosine arabinoside (ara-A; vidarabine) was initiated. The baby also developed bradycardia and occasional vomiting. The vesicles spread to cover the lower extremities and were also

on the back, palm, nares, and right eyelid. Within 72 h of ara-A treatment, the baby's condition started to improve. Treatment was continued for 11 days but discontinued because of a low platelet count. The baby was discharged on the 45th day after his birth, and normal development was reported at 1 and 2 years of age. At 6 weeks after birth, a herpes lesion was found on the mother's vulva. The baby was successfully treated with ara-A and was able to overcome the damage caused by infection. The virus, most likely HSV-2, was probably acquired through an abrasion caused by the fetal monitor while the neonate was in the birth canal. Ara-A has since been replaced with antiviral drugs that are more effective, less toxic, and easier to administer: acyclovir, valacyclovir, and famciclovir. (Pavey, Ch'ien. 1980;65:1150–1153.)

CONCURRENT PRESENTATION OF VARICELLA AND ZOSTER

Xie et al. described a 44-year-old man who presented to the hospital with a 5-day history of painful vesicles surrounded by erythema on his left ear. The patient reported no history of varicella or drug allergies and denied taking any immunosuppressive medicines. Physical examination revealed numerous small painful vesicles (1–2 mm diameter) surrounded by erythema on his back, chest, and neck. The clinical diagnosis of varicella was made. Vesicles in the area of the left ear had a dermatomal distribution, consistent with the diagnosis of zoster. Vesicular fluid from both the back and ear was positive for varicella-zoster virus by PCR, negative for all other herpes viruses, and identified as identical by genome sequencing. This is an unusual presentation of concurrent varicella (chickenpox) and zoster in a primary infection. Although vesicles have the same clinical appearance, they are widely disseminated in varicella and distributed along 1 or more dermatomes in zoster. Genome sequencing confirmed the same virus was responsible for both clinical presentations in this man. (Xie et al. *BMC Infect Dis.* 2020;20:454–458.)

DERMATOPHYTOSIS IN AN IMMUNOCOMPROMISED MAN

Squeo and associates described a case of a 55-year-old renal transplant recipient with onychomycosis and chronic tinea pedis, who presented with tender nodules on his left medial heel. He then developed papules and nodules on his right foot and calf. A skin biopsy demonstrated periodic acid-Schiff-positive, thick-walled, round cells, 2–6 µm in diameter in the dermis. Skin biopsy culture grew *Trichophyton rubrum*. *T. rubrum* has been described as an invasive pathogen in immunocompromised hosts. The clinical presentation, histopathology, and early fungal culture growth suggested *Blastomyces dermatitidis* in the differential diagnosis before the final identification of *T. rubrum*. (Squeo et al. *J Am Acad Dermatol.* 1998;39:379–380.)

TALAROMYCES MARNEFFEI INFECTION IN HIV/AIDS PATIENT

Si and Qiao reported a 29-year-old man presented to an outpatient clinic in China with a 2-month history of fever, cough, dyspnea, and weight loss, as well as skin lesions that developed on his face, neck, trunk, arms, and legs over a period of 2 weeks. Physical examination demonstrated extensive umbilicated papules and a biopsy of the papules revealed numerous round fungal structures in histiocytes. Culture grew *Talaromyces* (*Penicillium*) *marneffei*. Serologic tests were positive for human immunodeficiency virus (HIV) and the CD4+ count was 25 cells per mm^3. Treatment with amphotericin B was initiated and 2 weeks later antiretroviral therapy was started. After 4 months, the cutaneous papules had diminished substantially. *T. marneffei* is endemic in Southeast Asia, responsible for infections in immunocompetent and immunocompromised patients, although the majority of infections are reported in HIV/AIDS patients. Yeast-like cells are observed in biopsied skin lesions and filamentous mold grow in cultures held at 30°C, characteristic of dimorphic fungi. Response to antifungal treatment is typically effective. (Zixiang, Ziao. *N Engl J Med.* 2017;377:2580).

TINEA CAPITIS IN AN ADULT WOMAN

Martin and Elewski described a 87-year-old woman with a 2-year history of pruritic, painful, scaling scalp eruption and hair loss. Her previous treatment for this condition included numerous courses of systematic antibiotics and prednisone, without success. Of interest in her social history was that she had recently acquired several stray cats that she kept inside her home. On physical examination, there were numerous pustules throughout the scalp, with diffuse erythema, crusting, and scale extending to the neck. There was extremely sparse scalp hair and prominent posterior cervical lymphadenopathy. She had no nail pitting. A Wood light examination of the scalp produced negative findings. A skin biopsy specimen and fungal, bacterial, and viral cultures were obtained. Bacterial culture grew rare *Enterococcus* species, whereas viral cultures showed no growth. The scalp biopsy specimen revealed an endothrix dermatophyte infection. Fungal culture grew *Trichophyton tonsurans*. The patient was treated with griseofulvin and Selsun shampoo (active ingredient 1% selenium sulfide). When seen at a 2-week

Continued

TINEA CAPITIS IN AN ADULT WOMAN—cont'd

follow-up visit, the patient demonstrated new hair growth and a resolution of her pustular eruption. With the brisk clinical response and culture growth of *T. tonsurans*, treatment with griseofulvin was continued for 8 weeks. The

scalp hair grew back normally without permanent alopecia. Adults with alopecia require an evaluation for tinea capitis, including fungal cultures. (Martin et al. *J Am Acad Dermatol*. 2003;49:S177–S179.)

CAT-ASSOCIATED *FRANCISELLA TULARENSIS* ULCEROGLANDULAR TULAREMIA

Capellan and Fong described a 63-year-old man who developed ulceroglandular tularemia complicated by pneumonia after a cat bite. He initially presented with pain and localized swelling of his thumb 5 days after the bite. Oral penicillins were prescribed, but the patient's condition worsened, with increased local pain, swelling, and erythema at the wound site, and systemic signs (fever, malaise, and vomiting). Incision of the wound was performed, but no abscess was found; culture of the wound was positive for a light growth of coagulase-negative staphylococci. Intravenous penicillins were prescribed, but the patient continued to deteriorate, with the development of tender axillary lymphadenopathy and pulmonary symptoms.

A chest radiograph revealed pneumonic infiltrates in the right middle and lower lobes of the lung. The patient's therapy was changed to clindamycin and gentamicin, which was followed by defervescence and improvement of his clinical status. After 3 days of incubation, tiny colonies of faintly staining gram-negative coccobacilli were observed on the original wound culture. The organism was referred to a national reference laboratory, where it was identified as *F. tularensis*. A more complete history revealed the patient's cat lived outdoors and fed on wild rodents. This case illustrates the difficulty in making the diagnosis of tularemia and the lack of responsiveness to penicillins. (Capellan, Fong. *Clin Infect Dis*. 1992;16:472–475.)

FRANCISELLA TULARENSIS ULCEROGLANDULAR TULAREMIA

A 5-year-old girl presented to the Pediatric Emergency Department with a 4-week history of painful swelling on both sides of her lower abdomen. Pets that she had regular contact with included a cat and a dog. Six weeks before presentation, her parents had noticed a tick buried in her umbilicus and had removed it with tweezers. Five days later, the patient had fever, loss of appetite, fatigue, and redness around the umbilicus. These symptoms abated after 4 days. At the time of this presentation, examination showed marked inguinal lymphadenopathy on both sides. Treatment with oral ciprofloxacin was initiated

for suspected ulceroglandular tularemia. Serologic testing supported the diagnosis, with the *Francisella tularensis* antibody titer 1:1280. Two weeks after the completion of treatment, there was a reduction in the lymphadenopathy. After an additional 2 weeks, the swelling had completely resolved. In some ways, this is an unusual presentation of tularemia because embedded ticks are typically found on the extremities with enlargement of the draining regional lymph nodes. Diagnosis was made by serology although *F. tularensis* can also be recovered in blood cultures. (Buettcher and Imbimbo. *N Engl J Med*. 2021;384:1349.)

SPOROTRICHOSIS IN A FISHERMAN

Haddad and colleagues described a case of lymphangitic sporotrichosis after injury with a fish spine. The patient was an 18-year-old male fisherman, resident in a rural town of São Paulo state in Brazil, who wounded his third left finger on the dorsal spines of a fish netted during his work. Subsequently, the area around the injury developed edema, ulceration, pain, and purulent secretion. The pri-

mary care physician interpreted the lesion as a pyogenic bacterial process and prescribed a 7-day course of oral tetracycline. No improvement was noted, and the therapy was charged to cephalexin, with similar results.

At examination 15 days after the accident, the patient presented with an oozing ulcer and nodules on the dorsum of the left hand and arm, forming an ascending

SPOROTRICHOSIS IN A FISHERMAN—cont'd

nodular lymphangitic pattern. The diagnostic hypotheses considered were localized lymphangitic sporotrichosis, sporotrichoid leishmaniasis, and atypical mycobacteriosis (*Mycobacterium marinum*). A histopathologic examination of material from the lesion revealed a chronic ulcerated granulomatous pattern of inflammation with intraepidermal microabscesses. No acid-fast bacilli or fungal elements were found. Culture of biopsy material on Sabouraud agar grew a mold characterized by thin septate hyphae, with conidia arranged in a rosette at the end of the conidiophores, consistent with *Sporothrix schenckii*.

An intradermal reaction to the sporotrichin was positive as well. The patient was treated with oral potassium iodide, with clinical resolution at 2 months of therapy.

The clinical presentation in this case was typical sporotrichosis; however, the source of the infection (fish spine) was unusual. Despite the greater incidence of infection by *M. marinum* among fisherman and aquarists, sporotrichosis must be remembered when these workers show lesions in an ascending lymphangitic pattern after being injured by contact with fish. (Haddad et al. *Med Mycol.* 2002;40:425–427.)

PARACOCCIDIOIDES BRASILIENSIS INFECTION IN BRAZILIAN MAN

Araujo et al. described a 46-year-old man, living in Brazil, who presented with disseminated plaque-like, ulcerated skin lesions. Laryngoscopy showed additional lesions on the pharyngeal, nasal, and laryngeal mucosa. The man was a heavy smoker and drank heavily but had no immunocompromising diseases. The differential diagnosis included secondary syphilis, sporotrichosis, histoplasmosis, tuberculosis, and leishmaniasis. Biopsy of the skin lesions showed granulomatous inflammation and yeasts, with a morphology characteristic of paracoccidioidomycosis (a "mother" cell surrounded by multiple budding cells). Serology was strongly positive for paracoccidioidomyco-

sis. Cultures were not reported in this case but *P. brasiliensis* is a dimorphic fungus with yeast cells observed in clinical material and a mold form growing at room temperature in laboratory fungal cultures. Prolonged treatment with antifungal is generally successful. The fungus is endemic in Latin America with the largest number of infections reported in Brazil. Acute disease typically involves dissemination to multiple organs and skin manifestations as observed in this man. Chronic disease is more common in older individuals with prominent lung involvement and lesions in the mucosae, skin, adrenal glands, and other organs. (Araujo et al. *Am J Trop Med Hyg.* 2012;86:2012.)

CUTANEOUS BLASTOMYCOSIS

Gray and Baddour presented an unusual case of cutaneous blastomycosis. The patient was a 28-year-old previously healthy man who was struck on the right cheek by a rock thrown from a lawn mower 3 weeks before he presented to the hospital. The initial lesion was discolored and then developed a scab surrounded by an area of redness. Approximately 1 week after the accident, the patient noted painful swelling on the right side of his neck, and he sought care from his primary physician who prescribed oral cephalexin. The patient noticed no improvements in his symptoms and sought further medical care. At the time of physical examination, the patient was afebrile and abnormalities were limited to his face and neck, where he had a raised verrucous lesion with an erythematous

base. An area of induration was noted on the right neck that was tender, but no crepitus or fluctuation was noted. A fine needle aspirate of the neck mass was obtained that was positive for fungus on microscopy and culture positive for *Blastomyces dermatitidis*. The patient was treated for 6 months with itraconazole with resolution of the right facial and neck abnormalities. This case is unusual because infection with *B. dermatitidis* is primarily an initial pulmonary infection that can then disseminate to the skin or central nervous system. It is rare that the primary infection is due to inoculation of the fungus directly into the skin. The patient had no evidence of pulmonary infection, so it is believe this is a case of primary cutaneous blastomycosis. (Gray, Baddour. *Clin Infect Dis.* 2002;34:e44–e449.)

KAPOSI'S SARCOMA IN HIV PATIENTS

Hymes et al. described the first reports of Kaposi's sarcoma in young, sexually active homosexual men living in New York. The eight patients presented with unusual manifestations of the sarcoma. They were younger than traditional patients (4th decade rather than the 7th decade), the skin lesions were disseminated rather than localized on the lower limbs, and the disease progressed more rapidly. Because all the men had evidence of other sexually transmitted diseases, it was believed that sexual exposure contributed to the observed syndrome. It was unknown at the time of this report that these patients were infected with human immunodeficiency virus (HIV) and susceptible to opportunistic infections. Later, it was determined that Kaposi's syndrome was caused by human herpes virus 8 (HHV-8). (Hymes et al. *Lancet* 1981;318(8247):598–600.)

CRYPTOCOCCOSIS IN HEART TRANSPLANT PATIENT

Pappas and colleagues describe a case of cryptococcosis in a heart transplant recipient. The 56-year-old patient, who underwent heart transplant surgery 3 years earlier, presented with new-onset cellulitis of his left leg and a mild headache of 2 weeks' duration. The patient was on chronic immunosuppressive therapy with cyclosporine, azathioprine, and prednisone and was admitted for intravenous antibiotics. Despite 5 days of intravenous nafcillin, the patient failed to improve, and a skin biopsy of the cellulitis area was obtained for histopathologic studies and culture. Laboratory results revealed the presence of a yeast consistent with *C. neoformans*. A lumbar puncture was also performed, and an examination of the cerebrospinal fluid (CSF) disclosed cloudy fluid and an elevated opening pressure of 420 mm H_2O. Microscopic examination revealed encapsulated budding yeast forms. Cryptococcal antigen titers of CSF and blood were markedly elevated. Blood, CSF, and skin biopsy cultures grew *C. neoformans*. Systematic antifungal therapy with amphotericin B and flucytosine was initiated. Unfortunately, the patient suffered progressive mental status decline despite aggressive management of intracranial pressure and maximal doses of antifungals. He experienced slow, progressive decline, leading to death 13 days after initiation of antifungal therapy. CSF cultures obtained 2 days before death remained positive for *C. neoformans*.

The patient in this case was highly immunocompromised and presented with cellulitis and headache. Such presentations should arouse suspicion of atypical pathogens such as *C. neoformans*. Given the high mortality associated with cryptococcal infection, rapid and accurate diagnosis is important. Unfortunately, despite these efforts and the use of aggressive therapy, many such patients succumb to infection. (Pappas. www.frontlinefungus.org.)

MYCOBACTERIUM AND *PNEUMOCYSTIS* LYMPHADENITIS

Khawcharoenporn et al. described a 30-year-old woman admitted to the hospital with a 1-week history of intermittent high-grade fevers, night sweats, and generalized abdominal pain. Her diagnosis of HIV was originally made 1 month previously when her CD4 count was 61 cells/mm^3 and the HIV RNA was 150,000 copies/mL. She was started on antiretroviral therapy (ART) and trimethoprim-sulfamethoxazole (TMP-SXT) for *Pneumocystis* prophylaxis. At the time of her current admission, she reported compliance with her medications as confirmed by her pharmacy records. She presented with a temperature of 40°C, heart rate 90 beats/min, respiratory rate 20 breaths/min, and blood pressure 110/70 mm Hg. She had generalized abdominal tenderness without rebound tenderness and a normal chest radiograph. CT scan of the abdomen showed matted mesenteric and retroperitoneal lymphadenopathy. A fine needle aspiration of the retroperitoneal lymph nodes was performed, and aspirates were submitted for histopathology and bacterial, mycobacterial and fungal stains and cultures. The initial acid-fast stains were positive for numerous acid-fast bacilli so antimycobacterial treatment (isoniazid, rifampicin, pyrazinamide, ethambutol, azithromycin) was started and her ART regimen was modified. Two weeks into treatment, she continued to have high fevers, nights sweats, and abdominal pain. The result of silver stains from the original biopsies became available and were remarkable for abundant *Pneumocystis* cystic forms. TMP-SXT was reinitiated and within 4 days the patient showed remarkable response. The patient was discharged on her anti-mycobacterial antibiotics and TMP-SXT. When the culture results of the lymph node were reported positive for *Mycobacterium tuberculosis*, the azithromycin (added for treatment of *Mycobacterium avium intracellulare*) was discontinued. Follow-up at 6 months showed resolution of the infection. This patient illustrates lymphadenitis caused by a dual infection with *M. tuberculosis* and *Pneumocystis jiroveci*. (Khawcharoenporn et al. *AIDS Patient Care STDs*. 2006:201–205.)

DISSEMINATED HISTOPLASMOSIS IN HIV/AIDS PATIENT

Mariani described a case of disseminated histoplasmosis in a patient with AIDS. The patient was a 42-year-old El Salvadoran woman who was admitted to the hospital for evaluation of progressive dermatitis involving the right nostril, cheek, and lip, despite antibiotic therapy. She was positive for HIV (CD4 lymphocyte count 21/µL) and had lived in Miami for the past 18 years. The lesion first appeared on the right nostril 3 months before admission. The patient sought medical attention and was treated unsuccessfully with oral antibiotics. Over the following 2 months, the lesion increased in size, involving the right nares and malar region, and was accompanied by fever, malaise, and a 50-lb weight loss. A necrotic area developed on the superior aspect of the right nostril, extending to the upper lip. A presumptive diagnosis of leishmaniasis was entertained, based in part on the patient's country of origin and possible exposure to a sandfly bite.

Laboratory studies revealed anemia and lymphopenia. A chest radiograph was normal, and a CT scan of the head showed a soft-tissue mass in the right nasal cavity. Histopathologic evaluation of a skin biopsy showed chronic inflammation, with intracytoplasmic budding yeasts. Culture of the biopsy grew *H. capsulatum*, and the results of a urine *Histoplasma* antigen test were positive. The patient was treated with amphotericin B followed by itraconazole with good results.

This case underscores the ability of *H. capsulatum* to remain clinically latent for many years, only to reactivate upon immunosuppression of the host. Cutaneous manifestations of histoplasmosis are usually a consequence of progression from primary (latent) to disseminated disease. Histoplasmosis is not endemic to southern Florida but is endemic to much of Latin America, where the patient had lived before moving to Miami. A high index of suspicion and conformation with skin biopsies, cultures, and testing for urinary antigen are crucial for timely and appropriate treatment of disseminated histoplasmosis. (Mariani. *Infect Med.* 2007;24(suppl 8):17–19.)

MUCORMYCOSIS IN COVID-19 PATIENT

Mohammadi et al. reported a 59-year-old man was admitted to their hospital with cough, shortness of breath, and oxygen saturation of 76%. SARS-CoV-2 infection (COVID-19) was documented with PCR. Because the patient had severe lung involvement, he was treated with methylprednisolone. The patient was successfully managed for COVID-19 and after 10 days was discharged from the hospital. However, four days after discharge, the patient was readmitted to the hospital with nasal obstruction and left side facial and orbital swelling. Involvement of the ethmoid, sphenoid, and maxillary sinuses by observed by CT scan, and sinus endoscopic surgery was performed, with debridement of the involved tissues. Specimens sent to the pathology and mycology laboratories demonstrated wide hyphae without septa in the tissues and *Rhizopus* was obtained in culture. Despite treatment with amphotericin B and daily paranasal sinus debridement, the patient rapidly deteriorated and died after 7 days of hospitalization. *Rhizopus, Mucor,* and related genera are opportunistic molds primarily responsible for diabetic patients with uncontrolled disease and immunocompromised patients. Paranasal infections as observed in this patient are the most common infections, and rapidly fatal progression occurs despite aggressive therapy. Infections in SARS-CoV-2 patients are most frequently observed when aggressive steroid treatment is used to manage their pulmonary disease. (Mohammadi et al. *BMC Infect Dis.* 2021;21:906–912.)

STREPTOCOCCUS ANGINOSUS ABSCESSES

A previously healthy 56-year-old man presented to the Emergency Department with a week history of generalized abdominal pain associated with nausea and anorexia. Physical examination revealed generalized peritonitis and chest radiograph showed extensive free air under both hemidiaphragms suggesting a perforated viscus. He underwent emergency surgery where multiple intraperitoneal abscess cavities were present and an inflamed and thickened sigmoid colon. The abscesses were drained, an aspirate cultured, and the peritoneum lavaged. Despite empiric treatment with amoxicillin/clavulanic acid and metronidazole, the patient had a slow postoperative response. The cultures were reported positive for *Streptococcus milleri* (current name *Streptococcus anginosus*) and *Escherichia coli,* and histopathology was consistent with a perforated diverticulum. Treatment was

Continued

STREPTOCOCCUS ANGINOSUS ABSCESSES—cont'd

changed to piperacillin/tazobactam and gentamicin. On the fifth postoperative day, CT scan revealed extensive multiloculated gas and fluid collection in the abdomen from the diaphragm to the pelvis, which was relieved with percutaneous drains. The patient made good clinical improvement over the subsequent 2-week period.

S. anginosus, a member of the viridans group of streptococci, is characteristically associated with abscess formation. The older nomenclature, S. milleri, is still in common use so it is important to recognize S. milleri and S. anginosus are the same organisms. (Gana et al. Case Reports Surg. 2016; doi:10.1155/2016/6297953.)

EIKENELLA CORRODENS BITE WOUND INFECTIONS

Bite wound infections are typically caused by the organisms colonizing the oropharynx of the biting animal or human. Infections due to human bites or clenched fist injuries sustained during fighting have a different etiology compared with animal bites, with the most common pathogens Staphylococcus aureus, Streptococcus species, mixed anaerobes, and Eikenella corrodens. E. corrodens is particularly problematic because the organism grows slowly, is susceptible to penicillin (unusual for gram-negative bacteria), and is resistant to dicloxacillin and

clindamycin (commonly used to treat S. aureus). Critical for the management of human bite wounds is wound management and radiograph imaging of the wound to be sure no foreign bodies (i.e., tooth fragments) are present. I remember the presentation of a man who was involved in a bar fight. The man's lacerated fist was cleaned and sutured, but he returned to the Emergency Department with swelling and erythema of the hand. When images of the hand were taken (not done during the initial presentation), a tooth was observed deep in the tissues.

35

Sepsis and Cardiovascular Infections

Sepsis is defined as life-threatening organ dysfunction caused by dysregulated host response to infection. If multiple organs are involved, then this is referred to as **Severe Sepsis**. A key for this definition is infection. Although bacteria and fungi are typically documented as the cause of sepsis, it should be remembered that all microbes including viruses may be responsible for sepsis. I mention this because the cause of infection is not documented in many septic patients, either because the pathogen is not detected by traditional diagnostic tests or the appropriate test was not selected or performed properly. The most common infections associated with sepsis are (in descending order) pneumonia, peritonitis, urinary tract infections, soft tissue infections, and intravascular infections. Because a wide spectrum of pathogens can cause sepsis, the differential diagnosis for a suspected septic patient should initially focus on the most likely source of infection and the pathogens associated with these infections. For that purpose, it is useful to consider the discussions in the other chapters of this book section, which should be useful for narrowing the list of potential pathogens. To further refine documentation of the cause of sepsis, cultures should be collected from the most likely source of infection and from the blood stream. Because relatively few organisms circulate in blood, even in a patient with severe sepsis, a large volume of blood must be cultured to maximize the value of blood cultures (recommendation: 2 to 3 cultures within 24 h, each with 20 mL of blood divided equally between two culture bottles). Although the distribution of organisms recovered in blood cultures will vary with different patient populations (e.g., pediatric vs adult, inpatient vs outpatient, immunocompetent vs immunodeficient, patients with specific underlying disease, presence of intravenous catheters or foreign bodies such as shunts), the most common organisms are gram-negative rods followed by gram-positive cocci and then yeasts.

Cardiovascular infections are a specific subset of infections involving the endocardial surface of the heart (endocarditis), myocardium (myocarditis), or pericardium (pericarditis). *Staphylococcus aureus* is the leading cause of acute onset endocarditis, and associated with cardiac surgery, bacteremia from a distal infection, or intravascular injection of contaminated material (e.g., medication and drugs). Subacute endocarditis is more commonly associated with coagulase-negative staphylococci, viridans streptococci (primarily *Streptococcus mutans*), and fastidious organisms resident in the oropharynx (e.g., *Aggregatibacter*, *Cardiobacterium*, *Eikenella*, and *Kingella*). Also, several organisms not readily cultured from blood have been associated with subacute endocarditis include *Bartonella*, *Coxiella*, and *Brucella*. Myocarditis is clinically characterized by chest pain, arrhythmias, and congestive heart failure. The most common causes of this disease are viruses including enterovirus, adenovirus, human herpesvirus 6, and dengue virus. Bacteria are an uncommon pathogen in this setting. Pericarditis is characterized by chest pain with pericardial effusions and friction rub. As with myocarditis, viruses such as the enteroviruses are the most common cause of pericarditis. One subset of patients where bacteria are an important consideration is AIDS patients in regions endemic for *Mycobacterium tuberculosis* such as Africa. Pericarditis is a well-recognized complication of pulmonary tuberculosis in this population.

The following are clinical cases illustrating the spectrum of sepsis and cardiovascular infections.

STAPHYLOCOCCUS AUREUS ENDOCARDITIS

A 21-year-old woman with a history of intravenous drug abuse, HIV, and a CD4 count of 400 cells/mm³ developed acute endocarditis with a 1-week history of fever, chest pain, and hemoptysis. Physical examination revealed a 3/6 pansystolic murmur and rhonchi in both lung fields. Multiple bilateral, cavitary lesions were observed by chest radiography, and cultures of blood and sputum were positive for MSSA. The patient was treated with oxacillin for 6 weeks with resolution of the endocarditis and the pulmonary abscesses. This case illustrated the acute onset of *S. aureus* endocarditis in an immunocompromised intravenous drug abuser and the frequency of complications caused by septic emboli. (Chen, Li. *N Engl J Med.* 2006;355:e27.)

STAPHYLOCOCCUS LUGDUNENSIS ENDOCARDITIS

A 44-year-old man in Abu Dhabi presented to the hospital with a 10-day history of fever associated with a left-side headache, dry cough, and night sweats. He also reported impaired sensation of the left side of his face and facial droop, and left-sided weakness was observed. Blood cultures on the day of admission and day 3 of hospitalization grew *Staphylococcus lugdunensis*, and transthoracic echo and transesophageal echo identified vegetations on the aortic and mitral valves, with moderate mitral regurgitation. He was started on vancomycin for treatment of endocarditis, and his neurological deficits were attributed to secondary embolic stroke. On the third day of hospitalization, the patient complained of worsening headache. Lumbar puncture was performed, and CSF analysis showed leukocytosis with neutrophil predominance, high protein, and low glucose levels. CSF cultures also grew *S. lugdunensis*. Flucloxacillin was added to the vancomycin treatment, and the patient received the combination therapy for 17 days and the flucloxacillin alone for an additional 1 month. This case illustrates the ability of *S. lugdunensis* to cause endocarditis on native heart valves, a somewhat unique feature for a coagulase-negative *Staphylococcus* attributed to the ability of the bacterium to form biofilms on the surface of the valve. Septic emboli are a recognized complication with this organism but meningitis is less common. (AlDhaleei et al. *Case Reports Infect Dis.* 2019; doi:10.1155/2019/7910262.)

STAPHYLOCOCCUS EPIDERMIDIS ENDOCARDITIS

Elegino-Steffens et al. described a 72-year-old man with a history significant for hypertension and congestive heart failure who underwent a prosthetic aortic valve replacement secondary to acute onset of aortic insufficiency. Cultures of the native valve were positive for *Staphylococcus epidermidis* sensitive to nafcillin, and intravenous cefazolin was initiated. On postoperative day 24, he developed acute decompensated heart failure. A transesophageal echocardiogram demonstrated a structurally abnormal mitral valve with severe regurgitation, anterior and posterior leaflet vegetations, and scallop prolapse. Blood cultures were positive for methicillin-resistant *S. epidermidis*. He underwent a prosthetic mitral valve replacement, and antibiotic treatment was changed from cefazolin to vancomycin for a total of 6 weeks. This case illustrates the risk of endocarditis with relatively avirulent bacteria for patients with an artificial heart valve. Treatment generally requires replacement of the valve and prolonged antibiotic treatment. (Elegino-Steffens et al. *Case Reports Cardiol.* 2012; doi:10.1155/2012/467210.)

ENTEROCOCCUS FAECALIS ENDOCARDITIS

Zimmer and associates described the epidemiology of enterococcal infections and the difficulties in treating a patient with endocarditis. The patient was a 40-year-old man with hepatitis C, hypertension, and end-stage renal disease who developed fevers and chills during hemodialysis. In the 2 months before this episode, he was treated with ampicillin, levofloxacin, and gentamicin for group B streptococcal endocarditis. Cultures performed during the hemodialysis grew *E. faecalis* resistant to levofloxacin and gentamicin. Because the patient had an allergic reaction to ampicillin, he was treated with linezolid. Echocardiography showed vegetation on the mitral and tricuspid valves. Over a 3-week period, the patient's cardiac output deteriorated so that the patient was desensitized to ampicillin, and therapy was switched to ampicillin and streptomycin. After 25 days

ENTEROCOCCUS FAECALIS ENDOCARDITIS—cont'd

of hospitalization, the patient's damaged heart valves were replaced, and therapy was extended for an additional 6 weeks. Thus, the use of broad-spectrum antibiotics predisposed this patient with previously damaged heart valves to endocarditis caused by *Enterococcus*, and treatment was complicated by resistance of the isolate to many commonly used antibiotics. (Zimmer et al. *Clin Infect Dis*. 2003;37:e29–e30.)

KINGELLA KINGAE ENDOCARDITIS

A previously well 16-month-old girl had been mildly ill for one week with a febrile illness, mouth ulcers and diarrhea. One hour before she was seen in the pediatric Emergency Department, she had suddenly become unresponsive. On arrival, she was unconscious with no response to pain. Her eyes were deviated to the left, and the fundi were normal. Her airway was patent, and although she was making poor respiratory effort, she was maintaining oxygen saturation at 94% in high flow oxygen. Blood pressure was 80/45 mm Hg, and peripheral perfusion was poor. The only other significant findings were a pansystolic murmur not previously heard and hepatomegaly. An emergency computerized tomography brain scan showed a right parietal infarction. Imaging demonstrated a large mass attached to the mitral valve resulting in obstruction and incompetence of the valve. She underwent emergency surgery to remove the large vegetation from the posterior leaflet of the mitral valve, and no congenital abnormality of the valve was noted. All blood cultures collected before surgery were positive with a gram-negative rod, subsequently identified as *Kingella kingae*. She was successfully treated with a combination of cefotaxime, flucloxacillin, and gentamicin for 2 weeks and cefotaxime for an additional 4 weeks. *K. kingae* is a member of a group of gram-negative organisms associated with subacute endocarditis collectively referred to as HACEK organisms—*Haemophilus* (*Aggregatibacter*) *aphrophilus*, *Aggregatibacter actinomycetermcomitans*, *Cardiobacterium hominis*, *Eikenella corrodens*, *Kingella kingae*. *K. kingae* is noteworthy for causing endocarditis in young children with associated complications as observed in this patient. (Wells et al. 2001;20:454–455.)

LACTOBACILLUS ENDOCARDITIS

The following is a classical description of endocarditis caused by *Lactobacillus*. A 62-year-old woman was admitted for atrial fibrillation and a 2-week history of flulike symptoms. The patient had dental treatment 4 weeks before this admission and did not take antibiotic prophylaxis despite a history of rheumatic fever in childhood, with resultant mitral valve prolapse and regurgitation. On examination, the patient was afebrile, tachycardic, and mildly tachypneic. Cardiac examination was significant for a systolic murmur. Three blood cultures were collected, all of which yielded *Lactobacillus acidophilus* upon culture. The patient was treated with the combination of penicillin and gentamicin for a total of 6 weeks, resulting in complete recovery. This case illustrates the need for antibiotic prophylaxis during dental procedures for patients with underlying damaged heart valves, and the requirement for combined antibiotic therapy for successful treatment of serious infections caused by lactobacilli. *Lactobacillus* as a cause of endocarditis in this setting is unusual, with members of the viridans group (e.g., *Streptococcus mutans and S. mitis*) a more common cause. This illustrates the importance of blood cultures and accurate bacterial identification for optimum patient management. (Maurice et al. *J Infect*. 2006;53:e5–e10.)

COXIELLA BURNETII ENDOCARDITIS

Karakousis and associates described a 31-year-old man from West Virginia who developed chronic endocarditis caused by *C. burnetii*. At the time the patient was admitted to the hospital, he described an 11-month history of fevers, night sweats, paroxysmal coughing, fatigue, and weight loss. He had received various antibiotic treatments for bronchitis, with no relief. His past medical history was significant for congenital heart disease, with placement of a shunt as an infant. He lived on a farm and participated in birthing his calves. His cardiac examination upon

Continued

COXIELLA BURNETII ENDOCARDITIS—cont'd

admission revealed a murmur, no hepatosplenomegaly or peripheral stigmata of endocarditis were noted, and his liver enzymes were elevated. All bacterial and fungal blood cultures were negative; however, serology for *Coxiella* phase I and phase II antibodies was markedly elevated. Treatment with doxycycline and rifampin was initiated, and the patient rapidly defervesced. Although prolonged treatment was recommended, the patient was unreliable, and he rapidly became symptomatic every time he discontinued one or both antibiotics. He also refused to take hydroxychloroquine because of his concerns about retinal toxicity. This patient typifies the risk for patients with underlying heart disease and the difficulties in treating this infection. Patients with bacterial or fungal subacute endocarditis consistently have positive blood cultures unless they were pretreated with antibiotics, so the negative cultures should dictate consideration of alternative pathogens that require alternative diagnostics, such as serology for *Coxiella*. (Karakousis et al. *J Clin Microbiol*. 2006;44:2283–2287.)

STAPHYLOCOCCAL TOXIC SHOCK SYNDROME

Todd and colleagues were the first investigators to describe a pediatric disease they called "toxic shock syndrome." This patient illustrates the clinical course of this disease. A 15-year-old girl was admitted to the hospital with a 2-day history of pharyngitis and vaginitis associated with vomiting and watery diarrhea. She was febrile and hypotensive on admission, with a diffuse erythematous rash over her entire body. Laboratory tests were consistent with acidosis, oliguria, and disseminated intravascular coagulation with severe thrombocytopenia. Her chest radiograph showed bilateral infiltrates suggestive of "shock lung." She was admitted to the hospital intensive care unit where she was stabilized and improved gradually over a 17-day period. On the 3rd day, fine desquamation started on her face, trunk, and extremities and progressed to peeling of the palms and soles by the 14th day. All cultures were negative except from the throat and vagina, from which *S. aureus* was isolated. This case illustrates the initial presentation of toxic shock syndrome, the multiorgan toxicity, and the protracted period of recovery. It is noteworthy that despite the systemic signs of this infection, cultures from patients with toxic shock syndrome are consistently positive only from the focus of infection, in this case the vagina and throat and today most cases are associated with staphylococcal wound infections. (Todd et al. *Lancet* 1978;2:1116–1118.)

STREPTOCOCCUS PYOGENES ACUTE RHEUMATIC FEVER

Acute rheumatic fever is relatively rare in the United States, which can complicate the diagnosis. Casey and colleagues described a 28-year-old woman who presented with a history of joint pain and swelling, initially in her right foot and ankle that resolved after a few days and then pain and swelling in other joints. Upon physical examination, diffuse tenderness of the joints was noted on palpation but no swelling or erythema. Cardiovascular examination was notable for tachycardia, but no murmurs were detected. The diagnosis of a "viral infection" was made, and she was discharged with a course of nonsteroidal anti-inflammatory drugs. After 5 days, the patient returned with progressive shortness of breath and persistent pain in her knee. Physical examination revealed a low-grade temperature, tachycardia, and a new heart murmur with mitral valve regurgitation. The left knee was warm to the touch, the range of motion was limited, and it was painful on flexion. The diagnosis of bacterial endocarditis was considered but all blood cultures were negative. Medical history revealed that as a child she became short of breath easily and was unable to play with other children. The patient's history of dyspnea is consistent with rheumatic heart disease, as is the combination of fever, mitral regurgitation, and migratory arthritis. Recent evidence of infection with group A *Streptococcus* is required to confirm the diagnosis, but throat culture is insensitive because symptoms of acute rheumatic fever appear 2–3 weeks after the infection. The diagnosis was confirmed by demonstrating elevated antistreptolysin and anti-DNase B antibodies. (Casey et al. *N Engl J Med*. 2013;369:75–80.)

STREPTOCOCCUS PNEUMONIAE FULMINANT SEPTICEMIA

Chironna et al. reported a fatal case of overwhelming pneumococcal infection in an asplenic young adult. A male in his early thirties with a history of post-traumatic splenectomy presented with symptoms of hyperpyrexia, nausea, vomiting, and diarrhea. He was transferred from the Emergency Department to the intensive care unit where he rapidly became cyanotic, tachypneic, and progressed to shock. The patient died within a few hours of presentation despite ventilatory support, administration of intravenous fluid, antibiotics, and vasopressor agents.

Initial blood cultures were positive within the first few hours of incubation for *Streptococcus pneumoniae*. Asplenic patients are highly susceptible to overwhelming sepsis caused by encapsulated organisms such as *S. pneumoniae*. This is one of the few organisms where the level of bacteremia is so high that the organisms can be detected by a Gram stain of blood. Mortality is high because the infection progresses rapidly. (Chironna et al. *Euro Surveil*. 2010;15(23):doi:10.2807/ese.15.23.19585-en.)

VIBRIO VULNIFICUS SEPSIS

Septicemia and wound infections are well-known complications following exposure to *V. vulnificus*. The following clinical case, published in *Morbidity and Mortality Weekly Report*, illustrates typical features of these diseases. A 38-year-old man with a history of alcoholism and insulin-dependent diabetes developed fever, chills, nausea, and myalgia 3 days after eating raw oysters. He was admitted to the local hospital the next day with high fevers and two necrotic lesions on his left leg. The clinical diagnosis of sepsis was made, and the patient was transferred to the intensive care unit. Antibiotic therapy was

initiated, and on the second hospital day, *Vibrio vulnificus* was isolated from blood specimens collected at the time of admission. Despite aggressive medical management, the patient continued to deteriorate and died on the third day of hospitalization. This case illustrates the rapid, often fatal progression of *V. vulnificus* disease, and the risk factor of eating raw shellfish, particularly for individuals with liver disease. A similar progression of disease could have been observed if this individual had been exposed to *V. vulnificus* through a contaminated, superficial wound. (*MMWR*. 1996;45:621–624.)

CLOSTRIDIUM PERFRINGENS SEPSIS

A 69-year-old man presented to the hospital with fever (40.6°C) and altered consciousness. He had been undergoing chemotherapy for prostate cancer for the last 7 years. On physical examination, the patient's conjunctivae were pale and no icterus was observed. Blood tests showed a highly elevated white blood cell count and anemia. The peripheral blood smear showed cytoplasmic vacuolation of white blood cells, anisocytosis, and spherocytes. Severe hemolysis was suspected. A redrawn blood sample also showed findings of severe hemolysis as well as a specimen drawn 6h later. Comparison of the blood and biochemistry test results between the time of arrival and six hours later also showed progressive anemia, hemolysis, and disseminated intravascular coagulation. Chest X-ray showed no abnormalities and computed tomography of the chest and abdomen showed no indication of a clear source of the fever. Treatment for sepsis with piperacillin/tazobactam was started immediately, and blood, sputum, and urinary cultures were obtained. The patient's blood pressure dropped suddenly after arrival in

the hospital, and the patient went into cardiopulmonary arrest. After immediate cardiopulmonary resuscitation, circulation recovered spontaneously. Although blood cell transfusion, vasopressors, and hypothermia treatment were initiated, the hemolysis worsened, and the patient died 30h after arrival at the hospital. *Clostridium perfringens* susceptible to piperacillin-tazobactam was recovered from all blood cultures and when the peripheral blood smears were re-examined, the organism was observed. An autopsy was not performed so the source of this infection was not determined. This patient presented with rapidly developing hemolysis and large numbers of organisms in the blood. It is highly unusual to observe bacteria in a peripheral blood smear since most patients in severe septic shock have fewer than 1 organism per ml of blood. In my experience, I have only seen this with three organisms—*Neisseria meningitidis*, *Streptococcus pneumoniae*, and *Clostridium perfringens*. When this is observed, the prognosis is poor. (Fukui et al. ID Cases 2021;24. doi:10.1016/j.idcr.2021.e01112.)

STENOTROPHOMONAS INFECTION IN A NEUTROPENIC PATIENT

Teo and associates described an 8-year-old Chinese girl with acute myeloid leukemia and a complex history of recurrent fungal and bacterial infections during treatment of her leukemia. Infections included pulmonary aspergillosis and septicemia with *Klebsiella*, *Enterobacter*, *Staphylococcus*, *Streptococcus*, and *Bacillus*. While receiving treatment with meropenem (a carbapenem antibiotic) and amikacin (an aminoglycoside) and during a period of severe neutropenia, she became bacteremic with *Stenotrophomonas maltophilia* that was sensitive to trimethoprim-sulfamethoxazole (TMP-SMX). Over the next few days, she developed painful, erythematous, and nodular skin lesions. *S. maltophilia* was isolated from a biopsy of one of the lesions. Treatment with intravenous TMP-SMX led to gradual resolution of the skin lesions. This case illustrates the predilection for *Stenotrophomonas* to cause disease in immunocompromised patients receiving a carbapenem antibiotic. Characteristically, *Stenotrophomonas* is one of the few gram-negative bacteria that are inherently resistant to carbapenems and susceptible to TMP-SMX. Morphologically, this organism looks identical to *Pseudomonas aeruginosa* on Gram stain and differentiation is important because *P. aeruginosa* is inherently resistant to TMP-SXT and frequently susceptible to carbapenem antibiotics. (Teo et al. *Ann Acad Med Singapore*. 2006;35:897–900.)

LACTOBACILLUS BACTEREMIA

Yelin et al. reported a significant increase in *Lactobacillus* bacteremia in ICU patients treated with supplemental probiotics. They found that ICU patients at Boston Children's Hospital receiving *Lactobacillus rhamnosus* probiotics had an increased risk of developing *Lactobacillus* bacteremia. Over a period of 5.5 years, a total of 22,174 patients were treated in an ICU, with 522 of the patients receiving the probiotic. Six of the 522 patients developed bacteremia with *L. rhamnosus* identical to the strain used in the probiotic while only 2 out of the 21,652 patients not receiving the probiotic developed bacteremia, both with *Lactobacillus* species unrelated to the probiotic strain. They were not able to specifically identify risk factors that would be predictive of increased risk for infection, although other studies have correlated probiotic-related *Lactobacillus* infections in patients whose bowel integrity was compromised by disease or medical management. Immunocompromised patients also appear at increased risk for these infections. (Yelin et al. *Nat Med*. 2019;25(11):1728–1732.)

CAMPYLOBACTER FETUS SEPTICEMIA

A 33-year-old woman, who was on maintenance chemotherapy for acute lymphoblastic leukemia (ALL), presented with the chief complaints of severe headache and nausea. Her headache and nausea started after receiving an intrathecal chemotherapy (methotrexate, cytarabine, and prednisolone) 2 weeks before. She also complained at presentation of photosensitivity, loss of appetite, left temporal and eye pain, and tinnitus. Notably, she had eaten undercooked beef 2 days prior to admission. On admission, the patient experienced acute distress but did not have neck stiffness, any neurologic deficits, or abdominal tenderness. Computed tomography of the brain did not reveal any abnormalities. On day 2, her temperature rose to 38.0°C, and CSF analysis showed a cell count of 71 (PMNs 59.2%), protein level of 87 mg/dL, and glucose level of 82 mg/dL (serum glucose 124 mg/dL); CSF Gram stain was negative. Blood cultures were collected, and empiric antibiotics (ampicillin, ceftriaxone) were initiated. On day 6, blood and CSF cultures were positive for spiral shaped gram-negative rods that were subsequently identified as *Campylobacter fetus*, susceptible to meropenem. Therapy was changed to meropenem for 3 weeks. After her treatment, the patient was discharged without neurological sequelae. Although *C. fetus* infection most likely originated from consumption of the undercooked beef, diarrheal disease is relatively uncommon and *C. fetus* has a propensity to cause disseminated infections including endocarditis, pericarditis, mycotic aneurysms of the abdominal aorta, and meningoencephalitis. (Nakatani et al. *BMC Infect Dis*. 2021.doi:10.1186/s12879-021-06364-5.)

INHALATION ANTHRAX

Bush and associates reported the first case of inhalation anthrax in the 2001 bioterrorism attack in the United States. The patient was a 63-year-old man living in Florida who had a 4-day history of fever, myalgias, and malaise without localizing symptoms. His wife brought him to the regional hospital because he awoke from sleep with fever, emesis, and confusion. On physical examination, he had a temperature of 39°C, blood pressure of 150/80 mmHg, pulse of 110 beats/minute, and respiration of 18 breaths/minute. No respiratory distress was noted. Treatment was initiated for presumed bacterial meningitis. Basilar infiltrates and a widened mediastinum were noted on the initial chest radiograph. Gram stain of cerebrospinal fluid (CSF) revealed many neutrophils and large gram-positive rods. Anthrax was suspected, and penicillin treatment was initiated. Within 24 h of admission, CSF and blood cultures were positive for *Bacillus anthracis*. During the 1st day of hospitalization, the patient had a grand mal seizure and was intubated. On the 2nd hospital day, hypotension and azotemia developed, with subsequent renal failure. On the 3rd hospital day, refractory hypotension developed and the patient had a fatal cardiac arrest. This patient illustrates the rapidity with which patients with inhalation anthrax can deteriorate, despite a rapid diagnosis and appropriate antimicrobial therapy. Although the route of exposure is via the respiratory tract, patients do not develop pneumonia; rather, the abnormal chest radiograph characteristic of this disease is caused by hemorrhagic mediastinitis. (Bush et al. *N Engl J Med.* 2001;345:1607–1610.)

BACILLUS ANTHRACIS DISEASE WITH SEPSIS

Klempner and colleagues described an unusual presentation of anthrax. The patient was a 24-year-old woman who was transferred to their hospital because of severe abdominal pain, vomiting, ascites, and shock. The patient had been healthy until 9 days before admission, when she developed fatigue, fevers, headache, and diffuse body aches. She subsequently developed a progressive cough, and 3 days before admission, nausea, and vomiting. Upon admission, blood cultures were collected and intravenous fluids and ertapenem were administered. Exploratory laparotomy revealed ascites, hemorrhagic lesions in the mesentery, and necrotic small bowel. Although cultures of the ascites were negative, gram-positive rods were recovered in multiple blood cultures. These were initially dismissed as contaminants but subsequently identified as *Bacillus anthracis*. Treatment was adjusted to include ciprofloxacin. Her clinical course was stormy, requiring hospitalization for nearly 2 months, followed by 3 weeks in a rehabilitation facility. She continued to have ascites, nausea, vomiting, and abdominal pain that resolved very slowly. This patient was a resident of Massachusetts and had not traveled outside the area, so the discovery of *B. anthracis* infection was alarming. Exposure was traced to imported drums made of animal hides. The most common forms of anthrax in this setting would either be cutaneous exposure (development of wound anthrax) or inhalation anthrax (aerosolization of anthrax spores). The patient's disease is attributed to ingestion of spores, presumably when the aerosolized spores contaminated either her food or drink. It should be noted that *Bacillus* species are an uncommon contaminant in blood cultures, so any isolate should be carefully examined. In my experience, if the isolate is not associated with a patient's disease, commercial contamination of the blood culture bottles should be considered. (Klempner et al. *N Engl J Med.* 2021;363:766–777.)

NEISSERIA MENINGITIDIS SEPSIS

A previously healthy 18-year-old man presented to a local emergency department with the acute onset of fever and headache. His temperature was elevated (40°C), and he was tachycardic (pulse of 140 beats/minute) and hypotensive (blood pressure at 70/40 mmHg). Petechiae were noted over his chest. Although the result of a cerebrospinal fluid (CSF) culture was not reported, *N. meningitidis* was recovered in the patient's blood cultures. Despite the prompt administration of antibiotics and other support measures, the patient's condition rapidly deteriorated, and he died 12 h after arrival in the hospital. This patient illustrates the rapid progression of meningococcal disease, even in healthy young adults. The presence of petechiae is consistent with *N. meningitidis* infection and the presence of gram-negative diplococci the CSF should be observed in untreated patients for a rapid preliminary diagnosis (Gardner. *N Engl J Med.* 2006;355:1466–1473.)

BRUCELLA MELITENSIS SEPSIS

Lee and Fung described a 34-year-old woman who developed brucellosis caused by *B. melitensis*. The woman presented with recurrent headaches, fever, and malaise that developed after she had handled goat placenta in China. Blood cultures were positive for *B. melitensis* after extended incubation. She was treated for 6 weeks with doxycycline and rifampicin and had a successful response. The case was a classical description of exposure to contaminated tissues high in erythritol where *Brucella* is concentrated, a presentation of recurrent fevers and headaches, and response to the combination of doxycycline and rifampicin. (Lee, Fung. *Hong Kong Med J.* 2005;11:403–406.)

SALMONELLA TYPHI INFECTION

Scully and associates described a 25-year-old woman who was admitted to a Boston hospital with a history of persistent fever that did not respond to amoxicillin, acetaminophen, or ibuprofen. She was a resident of the Philippines who had been traveling in the United States for the previous 11 days. On physical examination, she was febrile, had an enlarged liver, abdominal pain, and an abnormal urinalysis. Blood cultures were collected upon admission to the hospital and were positive the next day with *Salmonella typhi*. The organism was susceptible to fluoroquinolones; therefore, this therapy was selected. Within 4 days, she had defervesced and was discharged to return home to the Philippines. Although typhoid fever can be a very serious, life-threatening illness, it can initially present with nonspecific symptoms, as was seen in this woman. Specific identification of this organism is important because infection is only acquired through human-to-human transmission. (Scully et al. *N Engl J Med.* 2007;345:201–205.)

YERSINIA PESTIS SEPSIS

In 2006, a total of 13 human plague cases caused by *Yersinia pestis* were reported in the United States—7 in New Mexico, 3 in Colorado, 2 in California, and 1 in Texas. The following is a description of a 30-year-old man with a classic presentation of bubonic plague. On July 9, the man presented to his local hospital with a 3-day history of fever, nausea, vomiting, and right inguinal lymphadenopathy. He was discharged without treatment. Three days later, he returned to the hospital and was admitted with sepsis and bilateral pulmonary infiltrates. He was placed on respiratory isolation and treated with gentamicin, to which he responded. Cultures of his blood and enlarged lymph node were positive for *Y. pestis*. The bacteria were also recovered in fleas collected near the patient's home. The reservoirs for sylvatic plaque are small mammals, and the vectors are fleas. When the mammals die off, the fleas will seek human hosts. Typically, the disease is manifested as an inflammatory swelling of the lymph nodes. Pulmonary manifestations are more commonly associated with person-to-person transmission through infectious aerosols. (*MMWR.* 2006;55:940–943.)

ESCHERICHIA COLI BACTEREMIA

Escherichia coli is the most common cause of bacteremia in high-income countries. Bonten et al. performed a systematic review of the literature over a 12-year period to better understand the epidemiology of invasive *E. coli* infections. Overall, *E. coli* accounted for 27% of documented bacteremia episodes with 18% if acquired in the hospital and 33% if acquired in the community. Although not specifically called out in this review, *E. coli* strains in hospital-acquired infections were more resistant to antibiotics than the strains recovered in the community although the overall rate of antimicrobial resistance increased over time. The incidence of *E. coli* infections increased with age with threefold more infections in 75- to 85-year-olds compared with 55- to 75-year-olds. Urinary tract infections were the primary source in greater than 50% of the septic episodes. Biliary infections and intraabdominal infections were other common sources. The overall estimated case fatality rate was 12%. (Bonten et al. *Clin Infect Dis.* 2021;72:1211–1219.)

HUMAN MONOCYTIC EHRLICHIOSIS (HME)

A 72-year-old man with a history of hypertension, aortic stenosis, and prostatic hyperplasia was admitted to the hospital with a 2-day history of fever, chills, headache, myalgias, diarrhea, and confusion. After admission, he had respiratory failure requiring intubation and rapid atrial fibrillation. Laboratory studies revealed leukopenia and thrombocytopenia. Blood and urine cultures were negative. The patient was started on empiric treatment with cefepime, vancomycin and doxycycline. Blood smears for *Babesia* were ordered as well as serologic tests for *Rickettsia typhi*, Rocky Mountain spotted fever, Lyme PCR,

Anaplasma PCR and *Ehrlichia* PCR. All tests were negative except the *Ehrlichia* PCR. The diagnosis of HME was confirmed when typical intracytoplasmic inclusions were observed in monocytes. His fever abated after 3 days of doxycycline, and he continued to gradually improve until her was discharged after 10 days of treatment. The diagnosis of *Ehrlichia* HME is a serologic diagnosis supported by observation of typical mononuclear inclusion. This pathogen must be considered in the differential diagnosis or the patient can rapidly progress to multiorgan failure. (Yachoui. *BMJ Case Report.* 2013. doi:10.1136/bcr-2013-008716.)

CANDIDEMIA IN IMMUNOCOMPETENT WOMAN

Posteraro and associates describe a case of recurrent fungemia in a 35-year-old woman. The patient was seen at 5 weeks' gestation after intrauterine insemination. She presented with fever, tachycardia, and hypotension. The white blood cell count was 23,500/μL with 78% neutrophils. She experienced a spontaneous abortion. Severe chorioamnionitis was diagnosed, placental and fetal tissues were cultured, and blood cultures and vaginal swabs were obtained. The patient was treated with broad-spectrum antibacterial agents. Five days later, no clinical improvement was seen. The cultured blood and placental samples grew the yeast *Candida glabrata*, which was also isolated from the patient's vaginal cultures. Based on fluconazole minimal inhibitory concentrations, which indicated that the organism was susceptible, the patient was placed on fluconazole. Four weeks later, she experienced complete resolution of her symptoms, with eradication of the fungus from her bloodstream. Antifungal treatment was discontinued, and the patient was sent home where she did well. Six months later, she was readmitted to the

hospital with fever, chills, and fatigue. The white blood cell count was elevated at 21,500/μL with 73% neutrophils. Consecutive blood cultures were again positive for *C. glabrata*, which was also found in cultures of vaginal fluid. All isolates were found to be resistant to fluconazole, so the patient was treated with amphotericin B. Within 1 week, that patient's clinical condition was improved. After 1 month of amphotericin B treatment, blood cultures were sterile, and she was discharged from the hospital. Three years later, she remained free of any evidence of infection.

This was an unusual case in that the patient was not immunocompromised yet experienced recurrent candidemia with *C. glabrata*. The use of fluconazole as initial therapy, although apparently successful, induced upregulation of drug efflux pumps in the organism and allowed later isolates to become resistant to fluconazole and other azoles. *C. glabrata* infections typically originate in the genitourinary tract as was observed in this patient. (Posteraro et al. *J Clin Microbiol.* 2006;44:3046–3047.)

MALARIA

Mohin and Gupta described a case of severe malaria caused by *P. vivax*. The patent was a 59-year-old man who presented with a 1-day history of high-grade fever after recently returning from Guyana in South America. He did not take any medications before, during, or after the trip. He noted that his symptoms were like those of a malaria infection 5 years previously, also acquired in Guyana. A peripheral blood smear as a part of the initial workup showed numerous red blood cells with schizonts consistent with *Plasmodium* infection, with more than 5% parasitemia.

Several blood tests, including a DNA PCR, were sent for parasite species determination. The patient was started on quinine and doxycycline oral therapy because of the concerns regarding chloroquine-resistant malaria. During the next 4 days, the patient developed more severe thrombocytopenia and nonoliguric renal failure, acute respiratory failure, and circulatory failure, despite a decrease in parasitemia to less than 0.5%. He received intravenous quinidine and an exchange transfusion to treat *P. falciparum* infection, suspected at the time because of the severity of

Continued

MALARIA—cont'd

his symptoms. The next day, however, the PCR results of the blood revealed the parasite was *P. vivax* and not *P. falciparum*. The patient gradually improved and was treated with primaquine to prevent relapse.

This case shows that although it is unusual, severe respiratory and circulatory compromise may complicate *P. vivax* malaria. *P. vivax* should be considered if the patient's condition deteriorates despite the presence of relatively low parasite levels. As opposed to *P. falciparum*, *P. vivax* infections carry the additional risk of relapse, which warrants appropriate and adequate treatment. This case also emphasizes the importance of chemoprophylaxis and personal protective measures for anyone planning a trip to a malaria-infested region. (Mohin et al. *Infect Dis Clin Pract.* 2007;15:209–212.)

TRYPANOSOMIASIS IN AN 18-MONTH-OLD BOY

Herwaldt and colleagues described a case in which the mother of an 18-month-old boy in Tennessee found a triatomine (reduviid) bug in his crib, which she saved because it resembled a bug shown on a television program about insects that prey on mammals. An entomologist identified the bug as *Triatoma sanguisuga*, a vector of Chagas disease. The bug was found to be engorged with blood and infected with *T. cruzi*. The child had been intermittently febrile for the preceding 2 to 3 weeks but was otherwise healthy except for pharyngeal edema and multiple insect bites of unknown type on his legs. Whole-blood specimens obtained from the child were negative by buffy coat examination and hemoculture, but positive for *T. cruzi* by PCR and DNA hybridization, suggesting that he had low-level parasitemia. Specimens obtained after treatment with benznidazole were negative. He did not develop anti–*T. cruzi* antibody; 19 relatives and neighbors were also negative. Two of three raccoons trapped in the vicinity had positive hemocultures for *T. cruzi*. The child's case of *T. cruzi* infection—the fifth reported US autochthonous case—would have been missed without his mother's attentiveness and the availability of sensitive molecular techniques. Given that infected triatomine bugs and mammalian hosts exist in the southern United States, it is not surprising that humans could become infected with *T. cruzi*. Furthermore, given the nonspecific clinical manifestations of the infection, it is likely that other cases have been overlooked. (Herwaldt et al. *J Infect Dis.* 2000;181:395–399.)

TSUKAMURELLA BACTEREMIA

A 48-year-old Japanese man presented with symptoms of right-sided facial asymmetry and right hand palsy that had lasted for 10 days. He had a past medical history of syphilis, gonorrhea, varicella, and hepatitis B viral infection. Laboratory tests revealed the man was HIV-positive with a CD4 lymphocyte count of 84 cells/µL, and an HIV-1 RNA viral load of 180,000 copies/mL. Imaging of the head showed three mass lesions in the brain and biopsy from these lesions revealed diffused large B cell lymphoma. Antiretroviral therapy was started, and azithromycin was also used for prophylaxis of *Pneumocystis* pneumonia. A PICC line (peripheral inserted central catheter) was inserted, and R-CHOP chemotherapy was initiated (rituximab, cyclophosphamide, doxorubicin hydrochloride, vincristine, prednisone). Five days after the last R-CHOP chemotherapy course, he suddenly developed a fever with shivering chills. His white blood cell count was 4300/µL, CD4 lymphocyte cell count was 228 cells/µL, and HIV-1 RNA viral load was 20 copies/µL. A broad-spectrum cephalosporin and vancomycin were administered and the PICC line was removed. Blood cultures obtained before the removal of the PICC line were positive for weakly staining acid-fast rods that were identified as *Tsukamurella pulmonis*. The patient was treated for a total of 2 weeks and subsequent blood cultures remained negative. *T. pulmonis* is an opportunistic pathogen associated with infection of central intravenous catheters. Because only a few bacteria are acid-fast (i.e., *Mycobacterium, Nocardia, Rhodococcus, Tsukamurella, and Gordonia*), the staining properties and microscopic morphology are useful for making a preliminary diagnosis. (Suzuki et al. *BMC Infect Dis.* 2017;17:677.)

MYCOBACTERIUM CATHETER ASSOCIATED BACTEREMIA

A 49-year-old woman with non-Hodgkin's lymphoma treated for the previous 3 months with cycles of R-CHOP chemotherapy (rituximab, cyclophosphamide, doxorubicin hydrochloric, vincristine, prednisone) was admitted to the hospital with fever for several hours. Physical examination revealed a temperature of 39.8°C and the presence of a Hickman catheter with no evidence of inflammation at the exit site. Laboratory data and chest radiograph were within normal limits. Three sets of blood cultures were drawn (2 from the catheter and 1 from a peripheral vein). Two days later, all blood cultures were positive with a weakly staining acid-fast organism that grew slowly when subcultured onto blood agar and chocolate agar plates. The organism was eventually identified as *Mycobacterium senegalense* by DNA sequencing and was susceptible to most antibacterial agents except vancomycin. Despite treatment with imipenem-cilastatin and amikacin, she remained febrile. On the sixth day of hospitalization, the Hickman catheter was removed, and treatment was changed to ciprofloxacin and doxycycline. After removal of the catheter, the patient became afebrile, and all subsequent cultures were negative. This is an example of mycobacterial contamination of a central line. Mycobacterial species are subdivided into rapidly growing species (growth detected in less than 7 days) and slow-growing species (growth detected after 7 days). Most mycobacterial infections of this type are caused by rapidly growing species that are present in water and other environmental sources. This particular species is unusual, with most infections caused by *M. chelonae*, *M. fortuitum*, and *M. mucogenicum*. Detection of these infections may be delayed because the bacteria typically require 3–7 days of incubation for growth and may not be detected by Gram stain. (Oh et al. *BMC Infect Dis.* 2005;5:107.)

CATHETER-RELATED *CANDIDA AURIS* SEPSIS

Dewaele et al. reported a patient from Kuwait was transferred to their hospital after complicated gastric bypass surgery for weight loss. A few days after transfer, she developed fever and signs of sepsis and blood cultures obtained through an intravenous catheter were positive for yeasts. Initial identification with mass spectrometry (MALDI-TOF-MS) gave a low confidence identification of *Candida auris*, while biochemical identification reported *Candida haemulonii*. Definitive identification of *C. auris* was obtained by gene sequencing. The isolate was determined to be resistant to fluconazole so the patient was treated with anidulafungin and catheter removal. Persistence of *C. auris* clones with acquired echinocandin resistance was documented for up to 18 months after the infection. *C. auris* is a recently discovered fungal pathogen, frequently colonizing the skin surface, and associated with catheter-related sepsis. This case illustrates the difficulties in identifying this organism and the challenges in treatment because the yeast is resistant to many antifungal agents. Control of hospital infections is also problematic once the organism is established in a hospital population. (Dewaele et al. *Intl J Clin Lab Med.* 2020;75:221–228.)

FUSARIOSIS IN NEUTROPENIC LEUKEMIA PATIENT

Badley and associates describe a 38-year-old man, undergoing chemotherapy for recently diagnosed acute myeloid leukemia, who developed neutropenia and fever. He was placed on broad-spectrum antibacterial agents but remained febrile for 96 h. A left internal jugular catheter was in place. Blood and urine cultures showed no growth. To combat a potential fungal infection, voriconazole was added to the therapeutic regimen. After 1 week of treatment, the patient was still febrile and neutropenic, and his antifungal therapy was changed to caspofungin. Four days later, the patient developed a mildly painful rash. Initially the rash developed on the upper extremities and consisted of papular, erythematous, plaque-like lesions with centers that became necrotic. Blood cultures and skin biopsy specimens were sent to the laboratory for analysis. The laboratory report indicated that the blood cultures were positive for "yeast," based on the presence of budding cells and *pseudohyphae*. The skin biopsy showed "mold" consistent with *Aspergillus*. However, serum galactomannan testing was negative. All cultures grew *Fusarium solani*. The patient's caspofungin was discontinued, and he was switched to a lipid preparation of amphotericin B and voriconazole. Despite the antifungal therapy, the lesions increased in number over the next 2 weeks and spread throughout the extremities, trunk, and face. The neutropenia and fever persisted, and he died approximately 3 weeks after the initial diagnosis.

Continued

FUSARIOSIS IN NEUTROPENIC LEUKEMIA PATIENT—cont'd

The combination of skin lesions and positive blood cultures are typical findings in fusariosis. Although "yeast" was reported from the blood cultures, closer examination revealed the microconidia and hyphae of *Fusarium*. Likewise, the appearance of septate hyphae in the skin biopsy could represent several different hyaline molds, including *Fusarium*. *Fusarium* is one of the few molds that can be recovered in blood cultures. (Badley. www.frontlinefungus.org.)

CONTAMINATED BLOOD CULTURES WITH *CUTIBACTERIUM* (*PROPIONIBACTERIUM*)

Contamination of blood cultures with bacteria resident on the skin surface can occur if the phlebotomy site is not properly disinfected prior to collection of the blood specimen. The most common contaminating organisms are coagulase-negative *Staphylococcus* (e.g., *S. epidermidis*), *Corynebacterium* species, and the anaerobic counterpart *Cutibacterium* (formerly *Propionibacterium*) *acnes*. If multiple blood cultures are collected, these contaminants are typically found in a single blood culture unless the collection techniques are consistently poor, or the patient is truly bacteremic due to an intravascular infection such as a contaminated intravenous catheter. It is recommended that the skin disinfectant (i.e., Chlorhexidine, tincture of iodine) be applied for a minimum of 1–2 min before venipuncture.

STREPTOCOCCUS GALLOLYTICUS SEPSIS

53-year-old woman presented to the hospital with a history of 2 weeks of fever, nausea, and weight loss. On physical examination, she was febrile (39.1°C), blood pressure was 147/80, and pulse rate 89 beat/min. Laboratory values showed elevated WBC counts with 89% neutrophils and severe anemia. Transesophageal and transthoracic echocardiography was performed and revealed vegetations in the mitral and aortic valves. Blood cultures that were collected were positive for *Streptococcus gallolyticus*, and treatment with ceftriaxone and gentamicin was initiated. An infectious disease consult was requested and, because of the identity of the organism, imaging studies were performed to determine the source of the infection. Colonoscopy revealed ulcerovegetative tumor of the ascending colon and polyp in the rectosigmoid. This patient illustrates an important association with *S. gallolyticus* and occult colon cancer. Although this organism was responsible for endocarditis in this patient, it is always important to pose the question—what is the source of this organism? *S. gallolyticus* was previously named *Streptococcus bovis*. (Berevoescu et al. *J Clin Invest Surg*. 2018;3:105–109.)

STREPTOCOCCUS MUTANS SUBACUTE ENDOCARDITIS

A 50-year-old man was admitted to the hospital complaining of acute left flank pain that developed while bicycling. The patient's medical history included the diagnosis of Hodgkin disease 15 years previously that was treated with chemotherapy, radiation therapy, and splenectomy. On examination, the patient had a temperature of 37.3°C, blood pressure 158/72 mmHg, pulse 76 beats/minute, and respiratory rate 20 breaths/minute. A holosystolic soft murmur, grade 2/6 was heard at the apex, with radiation to the axilla (consistent with mitral regurgitation), and a crescendo-decrescendo systolic murmur, grade 2/6 also was heard at the border (consistent with aortic stenosis). Seven hours after the presentation, the patient's temperature rose to 37.8°C and he was admitted to the hospital. Urinalysis was performed, and blood and urine cultures were collected. The urinalysis was negative, which is inconsistent with flank pain related to pyelonephritis. Renal ischemia is consistent with the acute onset and severe pain and imaging studies revealed a hypodense renal area. The presence of fever, new heart murmurs, and renal infarction are strongly suggestive of an infectious process, specifically endocarditis. This was confirmed by the isolation of *S. mutans* from multiple blood cultures collected during the first week of the patient's hospitalization. *S. mutans*, a well-recognized cause of bacterial endocarditis, is able to spread from the mouth to the heart valve, adhere to the valve and grow, leading to vegetations that can shed microcolonies resulting in emboli. This patient was at particular risk for this because he was asplenic and unable to effectively clear the organisms when they were initially introduced into the blood. Consistent with an intravascular infection, multiple blood cultures were positive. The patient was treated successfully with a 4-week course of ceftriaxone. (Greka et al. *N Engl J Med*. 2013;368:46672.)

CLOSTRIDIUM SEPTICUM SEPSIS WITH OCCULT MALIGNANCY

A 71-year-old woman with comorbidities hypertension and end-stage renal disease presented to the Emergency Department with complaints of severe back pain. The patient had a low-grade fever, tachycardia, and blood pressure 160/78 mm Hg. Complete blood count on admission was significant for macrocytic anemia, and a significant left shift was noted on differential with 96.2% neutrophils. Comprehensive metabolic panel showed elevated renal function blood urea nitrogen 40 mg/dL and creatinine. Two blood cultures were sent for sepsis workup, and vancomycin and meropenem were started empirically. Computed tomography chest/abdomen/pelvis was done and was negative for any pulmonary or intraabdominal focus of infection. However, imaging showed the presence of spinal canal stenosis in the lumbar area. The blood cultures were positive for *Clostridium septicum*, necessitating a change in antibiotics to piperacillin/tazobactam. Due to the known association of *C. septicum* with GI malignancy, upper GI endoscopy and colonoscopy was performed and demonstrated a nonobstructive mass in the ascending colon. Biopsy was taken and reported positive for well-differentiated adenocarcinoma. This illustrates the important association of *C. septicum* with malignancy and the need to investigate the potential for an occult malignancy as was found in this woman. (Sidhu et al. *J Invest Med Case Reports.* 2019;7:1–3.)

36

Miscellaneous Infections

This last chapter is a collection of clinical cases that do not fit logically with the previous chapters that focused on infections of specific organ systems. Rather than create a series of additional chapters with a small number of clinical cases, I organized these cases under the appropriate term of "miscellaneous infections." Within the chapter, I have clustered the cases into similar presentations (e.g., eye infections and hepatitis), systemic infections of immunocompromised patients, and parasitic infections with nonspecific presentations. It is my belief that these clinical cases will be as informative as those in the previous chapters.

BACILLUS CEREUS TRAUMATIC ENDOPHTHALMITIS

Endophthalmitis caused by the traumatic introduction of *B. cereus* into the eye is unfortunately not uncommon. This is a typical presentation. A 44-year-old man suffered a traumatic eye injury while working in a vegetable garden, when a piece of metal was deflected into his left eye, damaging the cornea and anterior and posterior lens capsule. Over the next 12 h, he developed increasing pain and purulence in his eye. He underwent surgery to relieve the ocular pressure, drain the purulence, and introduce intravitreal antibiotics (vancomycin, ceftazidime) and dexamethasone. The culture of the aspirated fluid was positive for *Bacillus cereus*. Ciprofloxacin was added to his therapeutic regimen postoperatively. Despite the prompt surgical and medical intervention, and subsequent intravitreal antibiotic injections, the intraocular inflammation persisted, and evisceration was required. This patient illustrates the risks involved with penetrating eye injuries and the need to intervene aggressively if the eye is to be saved. Prompt diagnosis including Gram stain of the aspirated fluid is critical for preliminary diagnosis (i.e., gram-positive bacteria vs gram-negative bacteria vs fungal) and selection of appropriate antibiotics.

PSEUDOMONAS AERUGINOSA EYE INFECTION

The most common predisposing conditions of *Pseudomonas* infection of the eye are use of improperly cleaned extended-wear contact lenses or ocular trauma. Ultraviolet rays in individuals exposed to sun lamps or welders who do not wear protective goggles can also produce keratitis. Yilmaz et al. describe a patient who had the unusual presentation of keratitis following exposure to both ultraviolet light and *Pseudomonas*. The patient was an 18-year-old male who presented to their clinic with bilateral acute mucopurulent ulcerative keratitis. He gave a history of a 3-h exposure to a welding arc 7 days before the presentation. His eyes were red and painful after the initial exposure and was prescribed tobramycin eyedrops; however, the symptoms progressed and when he presented to the clinic, his eyelids were swollen and erythematous. The conjunctivae were markedly injected, and corneal infiltrates with mucopurulent discharge were observed in both eyes. Corneal scrapings were obtained for culture from both eyes and were positive 24 h later for *Pseudomonas aeruginosa*. Fortified gentamicin and ofloxacin eyedrops were administered and adjunctive IV vancomycin and ceftriaxone were begun. The patient significantly improved beginning at day 3 and was discharged from the hospital at day 15 with topical eyedrops. Both ulcers were reduced in size. This patient was fortunate because the diagnosis of *Pseudomonas* keratitis

PSEUDOMONAS AERUGINOSA EYE INFECTION—cont'd

is frequently delayed to the point where complete vision loss occur. *P. aeruginosa* produces a number of cytotoxin toxins, including exotoxin A, that essentially dissolves the eye before medical intervention can occur. Particularly in the case of eye trauma, Gram stain of the eye exudate can be critical in differentiating gram-positive organisms such as *Bacillus cereus* and gram-negative organisms like *P. aeruginosa*, leading to the most appropriate antimicrobial therapy. (Yilmaz et al. *Ophthalmology*. 2006;113:883–884.)

CHLAMYDIA TRACHOMATIS TRACHOMA

Noya-Alarcon et al. described four patients in the Venezuelan Amazon where trachoma, caused by *Chlamydia trachomatis*, is common. The first patient was a 38-year-old woman with a 5-month history of trachomatous trichiasis (TT), pain, madarosis, blepharitis, and conjunctivitis in both eyes. The second patient was a 35-year-old woman with a 6-month history of TT, pain, madarosis, blepharitis, and conjunctivitis in both eyes; corneal opacity in the right eye; and full blindness in the left eye. The third patient was a 45-year-old man with a 5-year history of TT, madarosis, blepharitis, conjunctivitis, and corneal opacity in both eyes. The fourth patient was a 22-year-old man with a 1-year history of TT, madarosis, blepharitis, and keratitis in both eyes; full blindness in the left eye and decreased vision in the right eye. The remote location of their community limited access to healthcare, which allowed this chronic disease to progress to blindness or decreased visual acuity in all four patients. (Noya-Alarcon et al. *Emerging Infect Dis*. 2019;25:182–183.)

CANDIDA KERATITIS FOLLOWING CATARACT SURGERY

Araki-Sasaki et al. described a 74-year-old man who developed *Candida albicans* keratitis 3 months after cataract surgery. The man underwent pterygium excision and cataract surgery on his right eye. At the time of the surgery, the posterior capsule was ruptured, and anterior vitrectomy was performed before the intraocular implant. A topical antibiotic (levofloxacin) and steroid (fluorometholone) were applied for one month. His corrected visual acuity was 0.5. Three months post-surgery, he complained of the sudden onset of redness and the sensation of a foreign body in his eye. His primary can doctor reinstituted levofloxacin and fluorometholone eye drops with only partial relief after 3 days. He was referred to an ophthalmologist who, upon slit lamp examination, did not observe stromal infiltration or edema, and the corneal epithelium was not eroded. Additional steroid treatment was initiated with the working diagnosis of uveitis; however, after 1 week with no improvement, the steroids were discontinued, and levofloxacin continued. The next day, the eye had the typical appearance of fungal keratitis, with stromal fluffy abscess with infiltration and edema. The corneal epithelium appeared eroded, and endothelial plaque enlarged with accumulation of hypopyon. The plaque was surgically removed, and fungal organisms typical of yeast were observed on microscopy. *Candida albicans* was recovered in culture. Topical treatment with fluconazole, micafungin, and pimaricin was started with oral itraconazole. This treatment was effective in resolving the infection. The clinical presentation in the case was compromised by the steroid treatment so it is important for the management of a patient to consider the impact of treatment on diagnostic findings. (Araki-Sasaki et al. *Clin Ophthalmol*. 2009;3:231–233.)

LOA LOA INFECTION IS A U.S. COLLEGE STUDENT

Burd et al. described a 18-year-old college student who sought medical attention because of eye complaints. She described feeling something moving in her right eye and observed a worm when she looked in the mirror. She had had similar symptoms 2 years previously but the abated after 2 h. She also described painless swelling at the base of her right thumb and the dorsum of her right hand that lasted for a few days and had waxed and waned over the past year. Her past history included living in Nigeria and attending a boarding school in a rural area. She moved to the United States to attend college and had not returned to Nigeria in the past 3 years. On physical examination, her sclera was clear and there was no evidence of a worm, but she had taken photographs of the subconjunctival parasite. Blood was collected for examination, and although no parasites were observed with the thin smear specimen, microfilariae were observed in the Giemsa-stained thick smear that were identified morphologically as adult *Loa loa*. The patient was treated with diethylcarbamazine for 21 days, and her symptoms resolved. This presentation is classic for *Loa loa*, the African Eye Worm. (Burd et al. *J Clin Microbiol*. 2020;59(1):e01587–e01520.)

NEISSERIA GONORRHOEAE ARTHRITIS

An 18-year-old previously healthy female presented to the hospital for evaluation of polyarticular arthritis. Two weeks prior, she presented to an outside hospital with body aches and onset of acute pain in the left arm and leg. She was discharged on naproxen and prednisone but returned 5 days later without improvement and now pain and swelling in her left knee, right thumb, right wrist, and bilateral ankles. She had markedly elevated erythrocyte sedimentation rate, C-reactive protein (CRP), and WBC count. Workup for autoimmune disease was negative as was Lyme disease serology. Arthrocentesis of the left knee was performed, revealing elevated synovial fluid WBC count but culture of the fluid on sheep blood agar and chocolate agar was negative. She was continued on prednisone and received opioid pain medication. After one week of no improvement, she left to seek a second opinion. When she presented to the Emergency Department she was afebrile and had swelling and limited range of motion of her left knee and right thumb. Urine specimen was collected for nucleic acid amplification test (NAAT) for *Chlamydia* and *Neisseria gonorrhoeae*. Her synovial fluid WBC count remained elevated and Gram stain revealed gram-negative diplococci. The fluid was cultured and after 24 h, the chocolate agar was positive for what was identified as *N. gonorrhoeae*. The patient was treated with 1 dose of azithromycin for the *Chlamydia* infection and 1 week of parenteral ceftriaxone for disseminated *N. gonorrhoeae* infection. Disseminated infections occur in <3% of genital infections and are more common in women than men. This is the most common cause of septic arthritis in sexually active women with no predisposing conditions and commonly presents as migratory arthritis. Involvement of the distal joint and polyarticular arthritis are specific to disseminated *N. gonorrhoeae* infections and are useful for refining the differential diagnosis. (Burns, Graf. *J Clin Microbiol.* 2018;56:e00932–e00917.)

NEISSERIA GONORRHOEAE ARTHRITIS

Gonococcal arthritis is a common presentation of disseminated *Neisseria gonorrhoeae* infection. Fam and associates described six patients with this disease, including the following patient, who has a typical presentation. A 17-year-old girl was admitted to the hospital with a 4-day history of fever, chills, malaise, sore throat, skin rash, and polyarthralgia. She reported being sexually active and having a 5-week history of a profuse yellowish vaginal discharge that was untreated. Upon presentation, she had erythematous maculopapular skin lesions over her forearm, thigh, and ankle, and acute inflammation of her metacarpophalangeal joint, wrist, knee, ankle, and midtarsal joints. She had an elevated leukocyte count and sedimentation rate. Cultures of her cervix were positive for *N. gonorrhoeae*, but blood specimens, exudates from the skin lesions, and synovial fluid were all sterile. The diagnosis of disseminated gonorrhea with polyarthritis was made, and she was successfully treated with penicillin G for 2 weeks. This case illustrates the limitations of culture in disseminated infections and the value of a careful history. *N. gonorrhoeae* does not grow on blood agar and recovery frequently requires the use of selective media such as Thayer-Martin agar, so it is important to inform the laboratory when this organism is suspected in a nongenital specimen. (Fam et al. *Can Med Assoc J.* 1973;108:319–325.)

LEPTOSPIROSIS IN TRIATHLON PARTICIPANTS

There are several reports of leptospirosis in athletes participating in water sports events. In 1998, public health officials reported leptospirosis in triathlon participants in Illinois and Wisconsin. A total of 866 athletes participated in the Illinois event on June 21, 1998, and 648 participated in the Wisconsin event on July 5, 1998. The case definition of leptospirosis used for this investigation was onset of fever, followed by at least two of the following symptoms or signs: chills, headache, myalgia, diarrhea, eye pain, or red eyes. Nine percent of the participants met this case definition, two-thirds sought medical care, including one-third who were hospitalized. Leptospirosis was confirmed in a portion of these patients by serologic tests. These outbreaks illustrate the potential danger of swimming in contaminated water, the presentation of leptospirosis in a previously healthy population, and the severity of disease that can be experienced. Presence of uveitis in leptospirosis patients can be highly variable, with more common causes associated with infections caused by *Toxoplasma*, herpes simplex virus, and varicella-zoster virus. (*MMWR.* 1998;47:673–676.)

DISSEMINATED *MYCOBACTERIUM AVIUM*-INTRACELLULAR (MAI) INFECTION IN HIV PATIENT

Viehman et al. described a 20-year-old woman with a documented history of HIV/AIDS who presented to the hospital with ear pain, weight loss, malaise, and night sweats. The patient had been homeless and a history of noncompliance with her medications. Prior to the presentation, she had been treated for pulmonary MAI infection as well as *Pneumocystis* pneumonia. In August 2009, the patient was diagnosed with pulmonary MAI and later with disseminated cutaneous MAI when a rash on her upper arms and thighs was biopsied and the culture was MAI positive. A bone biopsy of the thumb was also MAI culture positive. She was started on HAART (highly active antiretroviral treatment) and a MAI treatment regimen (azithromycin, dapsone, levofloxacin) but did not remain compliant for her treatments. When she presented in the Emergency Department, she complained of ear pain and was started on empiric broad-spectrum antibiotics. The left ear was painful on manipulation, and purulent discharge was noted. Her thighs and upper arms were notable for an annular erythematous lesion, and biopsy confirmed cutaneous MAI infection. HIV serologies and HIV PCR test were positive, with HIV RNA at >200,000 viral copies/mL. Imaging studies of the head showed left otomastoiditis and culture of biopsy material confirmed MAI involvement. Her course remained complicated by a lack of response to multidrug MAI treatment and further follow-up was not reported. This report illustrates the difficulties in treating *M. avium-intracellulare* infections in patients not compliant with their HAART or antimycobacterial treatments. (Viehman et al. *HIV/AIDS Res Palliative Care* 2013;5:61–66.)

EBV INFECTIOUS MONONUCLEOSIS ASSOCIATED WITH AGRANULOCYTOSIS

Hammond and colleagues described a series of patients with unusually severe infections with EBV. One patient was a 32-year-old man who developed sore throat, malaise, myalgias, and headaches. The symptoms persisted for 3 months before the patient saw a physician, who documented tender regional lymph nodes and an injected pharynx but no hepatosplenomegaly. The leukocyte count was 6600 cells/mm^3, with 2000 atypical lymphocytes and 660 monocytes. A monospot test was positive. The patient's symptoms persisted, and he returned to his physician 1 month later. He appeared acutely ill with an elevated temperature, severe exudative pharyngitis, and tender cervical and submandibular adenopathy. Hematology tests demonstrated severe leukocytopenia and thrombocytopenia. The monospot test was positive, as was specific EBV serology; CMV serology was negative. For the first 4 days of hospitalization, fever and agranulocytosis persisted, with the total leukocyte count remaining less than 2000 cells/mm^3 and no polymorphonuclear cells seen on smear. Thereafter, the total leukocyte count slowly increased (patient was discharged after hospitalization for 1 week), and although the malaise and fatigue persisted over the next 3 months, the adenopathy gradually resolved. This case illustrates the potential severity of primary EBV infection in an adult patient. (Hammond et al. *West J Med.* 1979;131:92–97.)

STRONGYLOIDES HYPERINFECTION

Gorman and colleagues described a case of necrotizing myositis complicated by diffuse alveolar hemorrhage and sepsis after corticosteroid therapy. The patient was a 46-year-old Cambodian man with a history of Raynaud phenomenon. He presented to the rheumatology clinic with worsening symptoms of Raynaud syndrome and diffuse muscle aches. He was employed as a truck driver and had emigrated from Cambodia 30 years earlier. Pertinent laboratory studies showed markedly elevated creatine kinase and aldolase levels. Pulmonary function studies showed decreased forced vital capacity, forced expiratory volume, and carbon monoxide diffusing capacity. A high-resolution CT scan of the chest showed mid ground-glass changes in both lung bases and interlobular septate thickenings. Muscle biopsy showed myocyte necrosis and random atrophy but no inflammatory cells. Bronchoscopy was unremarkable, and all cultures were negative. The patient was started on prednisone for presumed necrotizing myopathy secondary to undifferentiated connective tissue disease. He was admitted to the hospital 1 month later with profound muscle weakness and dyspnea, which improved with the administration of methylprednisolone and intravenous immunoglobulin. Three weeks later, the patient was readmitted with

Continued

STRONGYLOIDES HYPERINFECTION—cont'd

fever, nausea, vomiting, abdominal pain, and diffuse joint pain. A CT scan of the abdomen suggested small bowel intussusception and colitis, but his symptoms improved without treatment. Another high-resolution CT scan of the chest showed early honeycombing and worsening interstitial infiltrates. The patient was scheduled for a lung biopsy; however, while awaiting the biopsy he suffered an abrupt fulminant deterioration with hemoptysis and hypoxemic respiratory failure that required intubation and mechanical ventilation. A chest radiograph showed new, diffuse, and bilateral infiltrates. The patient developed an acute abdomen accompanied by purpura on the lower trunk. An abdominal CT showed pancolitis. Refractory septic shock caused by *Escherichia coli* bacteremia and lactic acidosis ensued. Bronchoscopy showed

diffuse alveolar hemorrhage, and numerous larvae of *S. stercoralis* were demonstrated on staining of an aspirate of endotracheal secretions. Serology was positive for anti-*Strongyloides* antibodies. Despite treatment with ivermectin, albendazole, cefepime, vancomycin, vasopressors, steroids, and dialysis, the patient died. This case of *Strongyloides* hyperinfection syndrome emphasizes the importance of screening and treating persons at risk for latent *S. stercoralis* infection (endemic in tropical and subtropical areas) before the initiation of immunosuppressive therapy. Contact precautions should be taken in patients with hyperinfection syndrome because of the risk of infection to healthcare workers and visitors upon exposure to infectious larvae in the patient's stool and secretions. (Gorman et al. *Infect Med.* 2006;23:480–484.)

SEVERE HEPATITIS A VIRUS INFECTION IN A FAMILY

Yoshida et al. described a cluster of Hepatitis A infections in a family of five adults. One adult had an asymptomatic infection, four infected members were hospitalized, two developed acute liver failure, and one patient died. The first patient was a 60-year-old woman who presented to the hospital with jaundice and general fatigue. She received steroid pulse therapy due to acute hepatitis and successfully recovered. Ten days after the first patient was seen, her 30-year-old son presented to the hospital with vomiting and anorexia. He was also successfully treated with steroid therapy. Patient 3, the husband of Patient 1, presented 15 days after Patient 2 with jaundice and evidence of acute liver failure. He was also successfully treated with steroids. Patient 4, brother of Patient 3, presented to the hospital with complaints of general fatigue, anorexia, diarrhea, and brown-colored urine. He had elevated liver enzyme levels and renal dysfunction.

He was treated with steroid pulse therapy, recombinant thrombomodulin, antithrombin II, platelet concentrates, and fresh frozen plasma because of complications including hepatorenal dysfunction and disseminated intravascular coagulation. Continuous hemodiafiltration treatment was started because of the development of hepatic encephalopathy. Complication including uncontrollable bleeding developed and he died 3 days after admission. Anti-HAV IgM antibody was detected in all four patients and the daughter of Patient 1 who was asymptomatic. The infections were believed due to consumption of raw shellfish and person-to-person spread of the virus. Although most Hepatitis A infections are either asymptomatic or acute self-limited hepatitis, fulminant infections as described here are reported. (Yoshida et al. *Medicine* 2017;96:35(e7847).)

HEPATITIS B VIRUS INFECTION IN AN IMMUNIZED MAN

Boot et al. described the medical history of 50-year-old homosexual man who developed Hepatitis B virus infection despite successful immunization 14 years previously. The patient was a hospital worker who received his first HBV-vaccinations (2 primary and 1 booster) in 1985–1986. Although he had a moderate response initially, he did not have detectable anti-HBs antibodies (antibodies against the HBV surface antigen) after 10 months. A booster was administered, and he had a moderate response; and, 6 years later, he was given a booster with recombinant HBV vaccine, resulting in a high level of anti-HBs

antibodies that was confirmed 6 month later. At the time of illness onset, the patient developed nausea, anorexia, mild upper-abdominal pain, and jaundice with yellow-brown feces. On physical examination, he was jaundiced, had a tender but not enlarged liver, and no signs of chronic liver disease or encephalopathy. At admission, his liver enzymes and total bilirubin were marked elevated. After 6 weeks, the liver transaminases were normal and the patient asymptomatic. Serologic tests at admission were positive for HBV surface antigen, e antigen, and anti-HBc IgM and IgG antibodies. Based on these results, the diagnosis of

HEPATITIS B VIRUS INFECTION IN AN IMMUNIZED MAN—cont'd

acute hepatitis B infection was made. The patient did not take any immunosuppressive drug, was HIV-negative, and had no recognized immunodeficiencies. The strain of virus was consistent with strains circulating in the community and should have been susceptible to vaccine-induced

immunity. I think the important lesson here is that although vaccines have proven remarkably effective in the control of infectious diseases, breakthrough infections can occur, and healthcare workers should consider this in the evaluation of a patient. (Boot et al. *J Hepat.* 2009;50:426–431.)

HEPATITIS C VIRUS INFECTION IN PREVIOUSLY HEALTHY WOMAN

In a case reported by Morsica and associates, a 35-year-old woman was admitted with malaise and jaundice. Elevated blood levels of bilirubin (71.8 µmol/L; normal value <17 µmol/L) and alanine aminotransferase (410 IU/L; normal value <30 IU/L) indicated liver damage. Serology was negative for antibodies to HAV, HBV, HCV, Epstein-Barr virus, cytomegalovirus, and HIV-1. However, HCV genomic RNA sequences were detected by RT-PCR (reverse transcriptase polymerase chain reaction analysis). Alanine aminotransferase levels peaked on the 3rd week after admission and returned to normal by the 8th week. Anti-HCV antibody was also detected by the 8th week. It was suspected that she was infected by her sexual partner, and this was confirmed by genotyping virus obtained from both individuals.

Confirmation was provided by partial sequence analysis of the *E2* gene from the two viral isolations. The 5% genetic divergence detected between the isolates was less than the 20% divergence expected from unrelated strains. Before analysis, the sexual partner was unaware of his chronic HCV infection. Even more than HBV, which is also transmitted by sexual and parenteral means, HCV causes inapparent and chronic infections. Inapparent transmission of the virus, as in this case, enhances spread of the virus. The molecular analysis demonstrates the genetic instability of the HCV genome, a possible mechanism for facilitating its chronic infection by changing its antigenic appearance to promote escape from the immune response. (Morica et al. *Scan J Infect Dis.* 2001;33:116–120.)

HEPATIC ASCARIASIS

Hurtado and colleagues described a case of a 36-year-old woman who presented with recurrent right upper quadrant (RUQ) abdominal pain. One year earlier, she also presented with RUQ abdominal pain, abnormal liver function tests, and positive serology for hepatitis C. An abdominal ultrasonography examination showed biliary dilation and endoscopic retrograde cholangiopancreatography (ERCP) showed multiple stones in the common bile duct, left hepatic duct and left intrahepatic duct. The majority of the stones were removed. Examination of the bile-duct aspirate was negative for ova and parasites. One month before the more recent admission, the patient experienced recurrent RUQ pain and jaundice. Repeat ERCP again showed multiple stones in the common and left main hepatic ducts; partial removal was accomplished. One month later, the patient was admitted with severe epigastric pain and fever. The patient was born in Vietnam and had immigrated to the United States when she was in her early 20s. She had no history of recent travel. An abdominal computed tomography (CT) scan contrast showed abnormal perfusion of the left hepatic lobe and dilation of the left biliary radicles with multiple filing defects. ERCP showed partial obstruction of the left main hepatic duct, a few small stones, and purulent bile. Magnetic resonance imaging

showed diffuse enhancement of the left lobe and left portal vein, suggestive of inflammation. Cultures of blood grew *Klebsiella pneumoniae*, and examination of a stool sample revealed a few *Strongyloides stercoralis* rhabditiform larvae. Biliary stents were placed, and the patient was treated with levofloxacin. Two weeks later, the patient was admitted to the hospital, where a partial hepatectomy was performed for treatment of recurrent pyogenic cholangitis. Gross examination of the left hepatic lobe showed bile-stained calculi in the bile ducts. Microscopic examination of the calculous material revealed collections of parasite eggs and a degenerated and fragmented nematode. *Klebsiella* spp. were identified in cultures by the microbiology laboratory. The findings were consistent with recurrent pyogenic cholangiohepatitis with infection by *Ascaris lumbricoides* and *Klebsiella* spp. In addition to antibiotics for the bacterial infection, the patient was treated with ivermectin for the *Strongyloides* infection and albendazole for the *Ascaris* organisms. This illustrates the importance of collecting a careful history. Specifically, the fact the woman had lived in Vietnam before this presentation is relevant because it is likely she had been an asymptomatic carrier for many years before her current disease developed. (Hurtado et al. *N Engl J Med.* 2006;354:1295–1301.)

FASCIOLIASIS

Echenique-Elizondo and colleagues described a case of acute pancreatitis caused by the liver fluke *F. hepatica*. The patient was a 31-year-old woman who was admitted to the hospital because of a sudden onset of nausea and upper abdominal pain. She was otherwise healthy and gave a negative history of drug abuse, alcohol ingestion, gallstone disease, abdominal trauma, or surgery. On physical examination, she was markedly tender in the epigastric region and had hypoactive bowel sounds. Serum chemistries showed elevated pancreatic enzymes (amylase, lipase, pancreatic phospholipase A2, and elastase). Her white blood cell count was elevated, as were tests for alkaline phosphatase and bilirubin. Serum blood urea nitrogen, creatinine, lactate dehydrogenase, and calcium were normal. Abdominal ultrasonography and computed tomographic scan showed diffuse enlargement of the pancreas, and a cholangiogram demonstrated dilation and numerous filing defects in the common bile duct. An endoscopic sphincterotomy was performed, with extraction of numerous large flukes that were identified as *F. hepatica*. The patient was treated with a single oral dose of triclabendazole (10 mg/kg). Follow-up demonstrated normal blood chemistries and no evidence of disease 2 years post-procedure. (Echenique-Elizondo et al. *JOP*.2005;6:36–39.)

CHOLANGITIS CAUSED BY *CLONORCHIS SINENSIS*

Stunell and colleagues described a 34-year-old Asian woman who presented to a local emergency department with a 2-day history of right upper quadrant abdominal pain, fever, and rigors. She had emigrated from Asia to Ireland 18 months earlier and gave a history of intermittent upper abdominal pain occurring over a 3-year period. On examination, she appeared acutely ill and was clammy to the touch. She was febrile, tachycardic, and had mild scleral icterus. Her abdomen was tender, with guarding in the upper right quadrant. Routine hematologic and biochemical studies revealed a marked leukocytosis and obstructive liver function tests. Contrast-enhanced computed tomography of the abdomen demonstrated evidence of multiple ovoid opacities within dilated intrahepatic bile ducts in the right lobe of the liver. The remainder of the liver parenchyma appeared normal. Upon stabilization of the patient, an endoscopic retrograde cholangiopancreatography was performed for biliary decompression. This demonstrated intrahepatic and extrahepatic bile duct dilation, with multiple filing defects and strictures. A stool sample sent for analysis confirmed the presence of ova and adult flukes of *C. sinensis*. The patient recovered with medical management (praziquantel) and had negative stool samples 30 days after treatment. This case, as well as the previous clinical case, demonstrates the various complications of liver fluke infestation. Of note, praziquantel is the drug of choice for treating the Oriental liver fluke (*C. sinensis*), whereas triclabendazole is used to treat fascioliasis, thus emphasizing the importance of an epidemiologic history and identification of the fluke. (Stunell et al. *Eur Radiol*. 2006;16:2612–2614.)

LIVER CIRRHOSIS AND SPLENOMEGALY IN SUDANESE WOMAN

Rajoo et al. described a 52-year-old woman who presented to their hospital in Malaysia with a complaint of left hypochondrium pain. She denied fever, jaundice, vomiting, bleeding, diarrhea, and dysuria. Systemic review was unremarkable. On abdominal examination, there was massive splenomegaly. Her admission blood showed pancytopenia. Abdominal ultrasound scan demonstrated appearances of liver cirrhosis with splenomegaly, gastric, and splenic varices. Upon questioning, the woman said she lives in a rural area of Sudan, and her drinking water is collected from snail infected canal and well water. Sanitation in the region is poor, and the canals are used as toilets. Blood samples were collected for serology, which was negative for leishmaniasis but positive for schistosomiasis. The diagnosis was confirmed by detection of *Schistosoma mansoni* eggs in fecal specimens. This woman presented with a chronic form of schistosomiasis were eggs deposited in the tissues led to hepatic disease with splenomegaly. (Rajoo Y, et al. *Asian Pacific J Trop Med*. 2015;334–336.)

SECTION VII Review Questions

QUESTIONS

1. One week after returning from a vacation in Mexico, a 24-year-old man developed a high fever for 3 days and then became jaundiced and fatigued for 1 week. Laboratory tests revealed the following: white blood cell count, 3200/mm³; hemoglobin, 11.6 gm/dL; platelets, 112,000/mm³; elevated liver function tests (aspartate aminotransferase, 2600 U/L; alanine aminotransferase, 3100 U/L); bilirubin, 12.6 mg/dL; creatinine, 1.3 mg/dL. Malaria smear was negative, and his hepatitis serology results were: hepatitis A, immunoglobulin M positive and immunoglobulin G negative; hepatitis B surface antigen negative, hepatitis B core antibody negative; hepatitis C antibody negative. The patient's roommate remained in excellent health, with normal liver function tests and was seronegative for hepatitis A, B, and C. Which of the following would best protect the roommate from being infected by the patient?
   A. Immune serum globulin
   B. Hepatitis A vaccine
   C. Hepatitis B hyperimmune globulin
   D. Hepatitis B vaccine
   E. Nothing is required

2. Collection of specimens for the diagnosis of which of the following diseases poses significant risks for physicians?
   A. Histoplasmosis
   B. Coccidiodomycosis
   C. Lyme disease borreliosis
   D. Tularemia
   E. Amebiasis

3. A 72-year-old diabetic man from Chicago, recently on etanercept for psoriasis, developed a fever on day 7 postresection of an adenocarcinoma of the descending colon. He is currently intubated and has a central venous line for hyperalimentation in his internal jugular vein. Two blood cultures were collected and after 2 days of incubation, yeast grew from the aerobic bottles of both cultures. What is the most likely identification of this fungus?

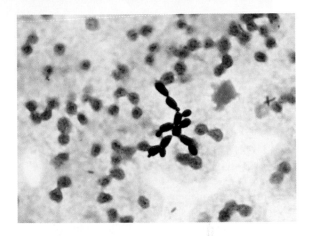

   A. *Blastomyces dermatitidis*
   B. *Candida parapsilosis*
   C. *Cryptococcus neoformans*
   D. *Histoplasma capsulatum*
   E. *Malassezia furfur*

4. A patient with lupus treated with prednisone (60 mg/day for 6 weeks) developed bilateral pulmonary infiltrates. The organism was observed in the modified acid-fast stain of the bronchoalveolar lavage as long, branching, partially staining rods. Which one of the following is the most likely pathogen?

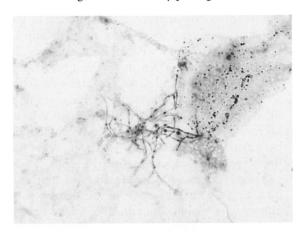

   A. *Actinomyces israelii*
   B. *Aspergillus fumigatus*

C. *Histoplasma capsulatum*
D. *Mycobacterium avium*
E. *Nocardia farcinica*

5. A wrestler developed a vesicular lesion on his shoulder. One of his teammates developed a similar lesion on his wrist, and another had a crusted lesion at the border of his lips. Which of the following viruses is most likely responsible for these lesions?
   A. Adenovirus
   B. Coxsackievirus
   C. Cytomegalovirus
   D. Herpes simplex virus
   E. Vaccinia virus

6. In July, a previously healthy 65-year-old man with a 40-year history of smoking developed severe bilateral pneumonia. He lived in Philadelphia his entire life and had no significant travel history. Sputum was collected and many neutrophils, but no organisms, were observed on Gram stain and acid-fast stain, and no growth was observed on routine bacterial or fungal culture. Which one of the following organisms is most likely responsible for this man's infection?
   A. *Klebsiella pneumoniae*
   B. *Legionella pneumophila*
   C. *Mycobacterium tuberculosis*
   D. *Histoplasma capsulatum*
   E. Influenza A virus

7. A 6-year-old boy arrives with his mother at the pediatric emergency room complaining of pain in his right hand where a stray cat had bitten him the previous day. The mother had washed the wound with soap and water but noticed the area around the wound was red by that evening. The next morning, the boy awoke crying and complaining of pain in his hand. The physical examination reveals that he has an oral temperature of 39°C. The skin over the wound is erythematous. A serosanguineous drop is expressed from the puncture wound and submitted for a culture and Gram stain. The microbiology laboratory reports abundant growth of gram-negative coccobacilli. Which of the following organisms is most likely responsible for this infection?
   A. *Capnocytophaga*
   B. *Eikenella*

C. *Escherichia*
D. *Fusobacterium*
E. *Pasteurella*

8. A 32-year-old woman farmer in Wisconsin presented to her family physician in June with a 3-week complaint of a low-grade fever, myalgias, a productive cough, and a skin lesion that developed during the previous week. The physician found an infiltrate on chest X-ray and collected sputum and a biopsy of the lesion for culture and microscopic stains (Gram, acid-fast). Faint-staining, large round cells, some with budding cells, were observed on the Gram stain and silver stain of the biopsy material (see figure) and the etiologic agent grew in culture after 2 weeks. The most likely diagnosis is:

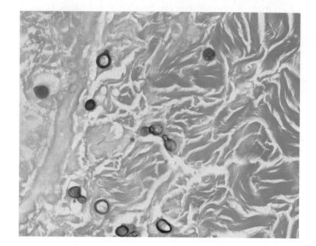

   A. *Blastomyces dermatitidis*
   B. *Candida albicans*
   C. *Histoplasma capsulatum*
   D. *Mycobacterium marinum*
   E. *Sporothrix schenckii*

9. A 14-day-old baby is admitted to the hospital with a fever, hyperactivity, and a stiff neck. At the time of giving birth to the baby, the mother complained of flu-like symptoms. Blood and cerebrospinal fluid were collected for culture. No organisms were seen on Gram stain but small, weakly beta-hemolytic colonies grew on the blood agar plates after 48 h. The Gram stain of the colonies reveals small,

gram-positive coccobacilli. The organism most likely responsible for this infection is:

A. *Escherichia coli*
B. *Listeria monocytogenes*
C. *Neisseria meningitidis*
D. Group B *Streptococcus*
E. *Streptococcus pneumoniae*

10. When waking her 6-year-old son for school, a mother observes that the boy is limping. She notices that his left knee is swollen, red, warm to the touch, and movement is painful. He states that he fell on the knee 2 days ago while playing with friends. The mother brings her son to see their pediatrician, who removes 15 mL of cloudy fluid from the knee. A Gram stain and culture of the fluid shows gram-positive cocci arranged in clusters (see figure). Which organism is most likely the cause of the boy's symptoms?

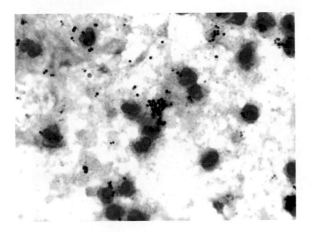

A. *Bacillus cereus*
B. *Enterococcus faecalis*
C. *Staphylococcus epidermidis*
D. *Staphylococcus aureus*
E. *Streptococcus pyogenes*

11. A 28-year-old sexually active woman presented to her gynecologist with a 3-day history of vaginal inflammation and a thick, whitish discharge. The discharge was examined microscopically and cultured on bacterial and fungal media. After 2 days, the organisms in the picture were observed. Based on this observation, what is the most likely diagnosis for this infection?

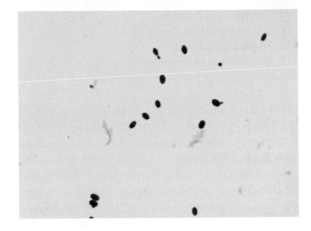

A. Gonorrhea
B. Chlamydial infection
C. Trichomoniasis
D. Bacterial vaginosis
E. Candidiasis

12. After an automobile accident, a 23-year-old woman requires an emergency splenectomy. Her subsequent recovery is uneventful. However, 4 weeks after the surgery, she is brought to the emergency department unconscious and nonresponsive. The physicians are unable to stabilize her, and she expires 1 h after she arrived. Blood is collected for culture, chemistry tests, and hematology tests. The technologist examining the peripheral blood smear observes abundant bacteria (see figure). Within 6 h, the blood cultures are also reported to be positive. Which organism is most likely responsible for this overwhelming infection?

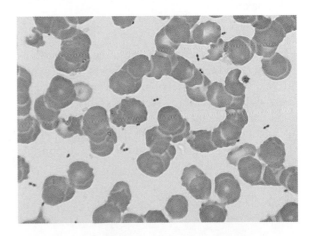

A. *Enterococcus faecium*
B. *Peptostreptococcus anaerobius*
C. *Staphylococcus aureus*
D. *Streptococcus pneumoniae*
E. *Streptococcus pyogenes* (group A)

13. For 4 days after returning from a fishing trip in Colorado, a 36-year-old man suffered with watery diarrhea, crampy epigastric pain, foul-smelling stools, and flatulence. When he presented to the local hospital, a stool specimen was collected and the organisms seen in the figure were observed on an ova and parasite exam. Which of the following hosts is the most common reservoir for this parasite?

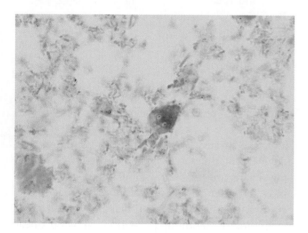

A. Beaver
B. Dog
C. Rabbit
D. Snake
E. Trout

14. Approximately 4 h after eating a meal in a neighborhood restaurant, three members of a family develop a sudden onset of nausea, vomiting, and severe abdominal cramps. Nobody is febrile, and only one family member has diarrhea. Within 24 h, the symptoms have resolved with no subsequent recurrences. Which organism is most likely responsible for this outbreak?
A. *Bacillus cereus*
B. *Campylobacter jejuni*

C. *Norovirus*
D. *Rotavirus*
E. *Shigella sonnei*

15. A 52-year-old man develops peritonitis after rupture of his appendix. After surgery for repair of the rupture, the man is treated with clindamycin and ceftazidime. Approximately 5 days later, the patient develops profuse diarrhea, abdominal cramps, and a fever of 38.5 °C. During an additional 5 days, the diarrhea worsens, with gross blood present in the stools and white plaques observed over the colonic mucosa (see figure). Which organism is most likely responsible for this patient's symptoms?

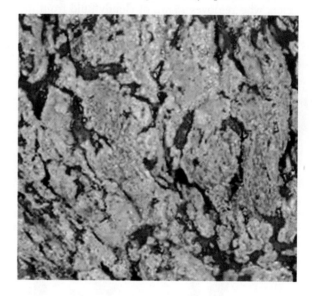

A. *Bacillus cereus*
B. *Clostridioides difficile*
C. *Escherichia coli* O157
D. *Shigella sonnei*
E. *Staphylococcus aureus*

16. A 59-year-old woman presented to the emergency department with a 3-day history of eye swelling, a frontal headache, and low-grade fevers. The woman was slowly responsive to questions on physical examination. Laboratory tests showed the patient had an elevated white blood cell count with a predominance of neutrophils and a blood glucose level of 475 mg/dL. A computed

tomography scan of the sinuses showed opacities in the ethmoid sinuses. A specimen from a sinus aspirate was collected for bacterial and fungal stains and cultures. A fungus was observed in the silver-stained material (see figure), and the mold grew in culture after 1 day. Which one of the following organisms is most likely responsible for this woman's infection?

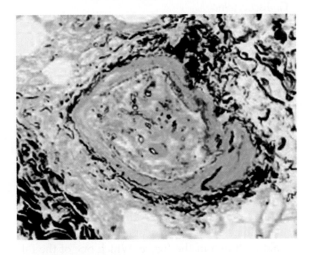

A. *Aspergillus*
B. *Bipolaris*
C. *Curvularia*
D. *Histoplasma*
E. *Rhizopus*

17. After 2 days of increasing pain during urination, a 20-year-old woman college student goes to the student health center. Upon examination, she complains of left flank tenderness and low-grade fevers. Her urine is cloudy and shows microscopic evidence of erythrocytes, pyuria, and abundant gram-positive bacteria. Her relevant past medical history is significant for no previous urinary tract infections, and she admits to being sexually active. Which organism is most likely responsible for this woman's infection?

A. *Candida albicans*
B. *Enterococcus faecalis*
C. *Neisseria gonorrhoeae*
D. *Staphylococcus aureus*
E. *Staphylococcus saprophyticus*

18. Approximately 4 weeks after a bone marrow transplant, a 42-year-old man returns to his physician with complaints of fevers and a productive sputum. The symptoms have developed during the preceding 5 days. A chest X-ray is obtained, and a cavitary lesion is observed in the upper right lobe. While the patient is in the radiology department, he has a seizure. A computed tomography scan of his head shows a mass in the right parietal area of the brain. Cultures of the sputum collected at admission and of the brain and lung tissues are performed, and after 4 days, growth of weakly staining, filamentous gram-positive rods is observed. This same organism was observed in the direct Gram stain of the tissues (see figure). The organisms also stained weakly with the acid-fast stain. Which pathogen is most likely responsible for this man's condition?

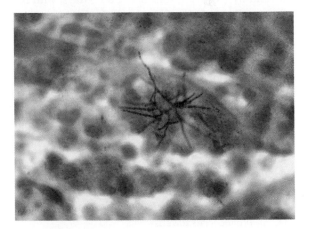

A. *Actinomyces israelii*
B. *Aspergillus fumigatus*
C. *Mycobacterium tuberculosis*
D. *Nocardia abscessus*
E. *Rhodococcus equi*

19. A 26-year-old woman living in Boston received a blood transfusion during the first trimester of her pregnancy. She had no significant travel history during her pregnancy. At birth, her infant was small and appeared to have a disproportionately small head (microcephaly). Within 2 days, the infant developed jaundice, hepatosplenomegaly, and

a petechial rash. Urine samples were found to contain cells with "owl's eye" inclusion bodies. An X-ray of the infant's head at 1 week of age showed intracranial calcifications. The infant became increasing lethargic and experienced respiratory distress progressing to seizures. The infant eventually died. Which of the following is most likely responsible for this infection?

A. *Cytomegalovirus*
B. Herpes simplex virus
C. *Rubella* virus
D. *Toxoplasma gondii*
E. Zika virus

20. An 8-year-old boy fell while playing and abraded the skin over his thigh and hip. The injury did not appear serious, and no effort was made to clean the wound or apply topical antibiotic creams. The wound over the hip worsened after 3 days, with inflammation and a small amount of purulence. That evening, the child developed a high-grade fever (40°C), headache, and a diffuse rash. By the time the child arrived at the hospital, he was hypotensive, complained of severe myalgias, and had diarrhea. After 1 more day, his skin desquamated (including over the palms and soles), and he developed renal and hepatic abnormalities. Which of the following organisms is most likely responsible for this boy's infection?

A. *Bacillus cereus*
B. *Bacteroides fragilis*
C. *Clostridium perfringens*
D. *Staphylococcus aureus*
E. *Streptococcus anginosus*

21. A 34-year-old man told his wife that for the last 3 days he had been feeling progressively worse. His illness began with a headache, mild fever, and sweats. Over time, the symptoms became more prominent, and his wife took him to the physician. The physician noted that the man had a temperature of 39°C, blood pressure of 137/85 mmHg, heart rate of 82 bpm, and respiratory rate of 25/min. This patient was previously in good health and returned from a trip to Mexico 3 weeks prior to this visit. While in Mexico, the man ate only in high-quality restaurants, although he did consume unpasteurized goat cheese. The physician ordered blood cultures for his patient, and 3 days later, the cultures were positive with very small gram-negative coccobacilli. Which one of the following organisms is most likely responsible for this patient's infection?

A. *Acinetobacter*
B. *Brucella*
C. *Escherichia*
D. *Francisella*
E. *Haemophilus*

22. A 45-year-old woman presented to her physician because she had several sores on her arm that had developed during the previous 2 weeks. The physician noted that the sores were ulcerative nodular lesions that followed the lymphatic system up her arm. Her axillary nodes were also enlarged. A specimen was aspirated from one of the lesions and a few oval, fusiform yeast cells were observed in culture. A slow-growing white mold grew in the fungal cultures of the lesions and the colonies gradually turned black. The microscopic morphology of the mold is shown in the figure. Which one of the following organisms is responsible for this woman's infection?

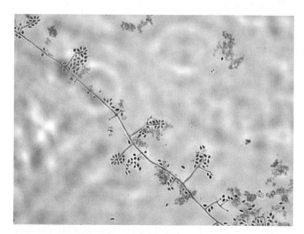

A. *Blastomyces dermatitidis*
B. *Candida albicans*
C. *Cryptococcus neoformans*
D. *Sporothrix schenckii*
E. *Trichophyton rubrum*

23. A 64-year-old man underwent intraabdominal surgery for colonic cancer. Five days after the surgery, the patient developed peritonitis for which he was treated with ceftazidime, gentamicin, and metronidazole. Although he initially responded to this therapeutic regimen, on the third night of treatment, he developed spiking fevers and abdominal tenderness. He was taken to surgery that night and 50 cc of purulent material was drained from his abdominal cavity. The material was submitted for Gram stain and culture, and blood was collected for culture. The organisms observed in the figure were grown from the aerobic and anaerobic blood cultures as well as from the purulent material. The most likely organism responsible for this infection is:

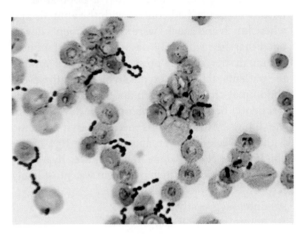

A. *Candida albicans*
B. *Enterococcus faecalis*
C. *Peptostreptococcus anaerobius*
D. *Staphylococcus aureus*
E. *Streptococcus pneumoniae*

24. A 19-year-old homosexual man was admitted for evaluation of a 2-week history of a nonproductive cough, fever, and shortness of breath. A chest radiograph was performed and demonstrated bilateral pulmonary infiltrates with both interstitial and alveolar markings. The man was HIV-positive and had a CD4$^+$ count that was less than 200 cells/mm^3. A bronchial alveolar lavage and biopsy were performed. Organisms measuring 4–5 µm were observed in the Gomori methenamine silver-stained section of the biopsy (see figure). Which organism is responsible for this man's infection?

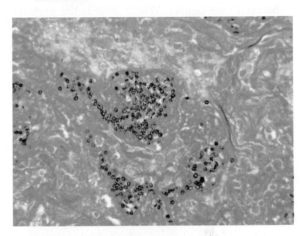

A. *Aspergillus fumigatus*
B. *Candida albicans*
C. *Cryptococcus neoformans*
D. *Histoplasma capsulatum*
E. *Pneumocystis jiroveci*

25. Approximately 36 h after a neighborhood picnic 14 people developed diarrhea, with the majority complaining of abdominal cramps. Most had low-grade temperatures and 8–10 bowel movements a day. Bloody stools affected two people. Although symptoms resolved for most of these people within 1 week, two children and one adult had to be hospitalized. One additional adult developed joint pains in the hands, ankles, and knees that persisted for 1 week. Which one of the following organisms is the most likely cause of these infections?

A. *Bacillus cereus*
B. *Campylobacter jejuni*
C. Norovirus
D. *Salmonella* enteritidis
E. *Staphylococcus aureus*

26. Three days after a 23-year-old man returned from a camping trip in Mexico, he presented to the emergency department suffering from abdominal pain,

nausea, fever, and bloody diarrhea. Stool specimens were collected and submitted to the laboratory for bacterial cultures and parasite examination. The bacterial cultures were negative but a parasite was observed (see figure). Which host is the primary reservoir for this parasite?

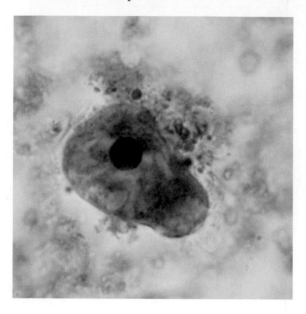

A. Cockroach
B. Dog
C. Fly
D. Human
E. Mosquito

27. A 74-year-old man was admitted to the hospital because of a 3-day history of high fever, myalgia, and chills accompanied by back pain and elimination of dark urine during the previous 12 h. His temperature was 38.5 °C, blood pressure was 120/70 mmHg, and respiratory rate was 30/min. Laboratory results included hemoglobin 131 g/L, hematocrit 0.41, serum urea 71 mg/dL, total bilirubin 4.1 mg/dL, lactic dehydrogenase 1250 U/L, and potassium 6.5 mEq/L. A urinalysis showed the presence of blood but less than five white blood cells per high-power field were seen. Within 6 h of admission into the hospital, the patient suffered a cardiac arrest and expired. Postmortem exam-

ination of tissues revealed microabscesses in the liver and gallbladder. Premortem blood cultures were positive within 6 hours of incubation for a gas-producing organism and cultures of the autopsy tissues grew the same organism. Which of the following organisms is most likely responsible for this patient's overwhelming infection?
A. *Bacteroides fragilis*
B. *Clostridium perfringens*
C. *Escherichia coli*
D. *Pseudomonas aeruginosa*
E. *Staphylococcus aureus*

28. In September 2000, an outbreak of *Escherichia coli* gastroenteritis occurred in Pennsylvania. Most of the infected patients had visited a popular dairy farm, where they had contact with the animals and where lunch and snacks were served. Patients developed diarrhea within 10 days of visiting the farm. Although the clinical presentation varied among the patients, the illness typically began with severe abdominal cramps and nonbloody diarrhea. Stools frequently became grossly bloody on day 2 or 3 of the illness. Most patients became asymptomatic within 1 week; however, approximately 10% of the children developed acute renal failure, hypertension, and seizures. Which organism was most likely responsible for these infections?
A. Enteroaggregative *E. coli*
B. Enteroinvasive *E. coli*
C. Enteropathogenic *E. coli*
D. Enterotoxigenic *E. coli*
E. Shiga toxin-producing *E. coli*

29. After returning from a trip to Arizona, a 30-year-old man experienced a respiratory illness with symptoms including a cough and fever. Approximately 1 week later, he developed red, tender nodules on his shin. His physician collected sputum specimens for stains and cultures. After 3 days of incubation at room temperature, the fungal culture grew a white filamentous mold. The microscopic morphology of the mold is shown in the figure. Which of the following is most likely responsible for this infection?

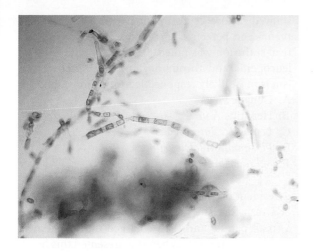

A. *Aspergillus fumigatus*
B. *Blastomyces dermatitidis*
C. *Coccidioides immitis*
D. *Histoplasma capsulatum*
E. *Sporothrix schenckii*

30. A 5-year-old boy complained to his mother that his throat hurt when he swallowed his food. The mother noted that the boy's throat was red and a whitish exudate had formed over his tonsils. The next day, a diffuse red rash developed on his chest. The mother took the boy to his pediatrician at which time the rash had spread over his neck, face, and limbs. The rash was most intense at folds of the skin. Which organism is most likely responsible for this infection?
A. *Bordetella pertussis*
B. Measles virus
C. Rubella virus
D. *Staphylococcus aureus*
E. *Streptococcus pyogenes*

31. A 23-year-old Peace Corps worker living in Africa for the previous year developed symptoms of nausea, vomiting, and diarrhea while visiting family in New York. Stool specimens were collected for bacterial culture and ova and parasite examination. The bacterial cultures were negative but the ova and parasite examination was positive for the organism shown in the figure. What is the most likely source of this woman's infection?

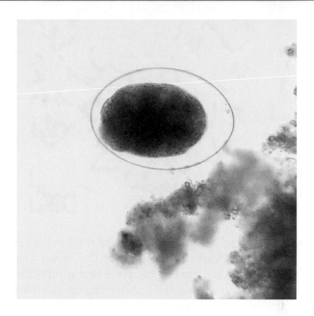

A. Consumption of uncooked pork
B. Consumption of contaminated raw vegetables
C. Direct skin penetration by infectious larvae
D. Oral exposure to the feces of an infected dog
E. Oral exposure to the feces of an infected human

32. A 42-year-old carpenter suffers a penetrating eye injury when a wooden splinter is deflected into his eye. Within 12 h of the injury, the eye is inflamed and painful. By the time the man goes to the emergency department, he has completely lost his vision in the eye. Drainage from the eye is collected on a swab and submitted for Gram stain and culture. Abundant gram-positive rods are observed on Gram stain (see figure) and within 12 h of incubation, large b-hemolytic colonies are detected on the aerobic blood agar plates. Which organism is most likely responsible for this infection?
A. *Bacillus cereus*
B. *Bacteroides fragilis*
C. *Clostridium perfringens*
D. *Corynebacterium jeikeium*
E. *Nocardia farcinica*

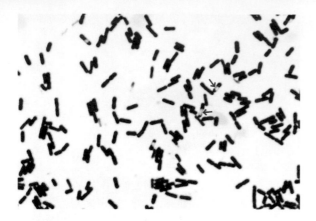

33. A 24-year-old man living in Kenya went to his local physician with the complaint that a swelling in his groin enlarged to the point that it ruptured and drained cloudy fluid. After taking a careful history, the physician discovered that the sexually active man had initially developed a small painless blister that ulcerated and then rapidly healed. Approximately 1 week later, the lymph nodes that drained the area had become enlarged. The area surrounding these swollen nodes became enlarged and tender. It was these lymph nodes that ruptured and drained purulent material. The patient felt feverish and had a headache and muscle aches. The physician made the diagnosis based on the clinical presentation and culture of the purulent material. Which organism was most likely responsible for this man's infection?
   A. *Chlamydia trachomatis*
   B. Herpes simplex virus
   C. *Klebsiella granulomatis*
   D. *Neisseria gonorrhoeae*
   E. *Treponema pallidum*

34. A 32-year-old woman presented to her family physician with a 5-day history of fevers, headaches, retro-orbital pain, myalgias, and a rash. The symptoms began 3 days after she returned from a 1-month trip to Thailand. The rash developed initially on her face and then spread over her trunk and extremities. Before her travels, she received all the appropriate vaccinations and maintained malaria prophylaxis during her trip. Physical examination showed diffuse erythroderma with blanching erythema and petechial formation. Bilateral conjunctival suffusion was noted. Laboratory tests revealed leucopenia and thrombocytopenia. Which organism is most likely responsible for this infection?
   A. Dengue virus
   B. Hepatitis A virus
   C. *Leptospira interrogans*
   D. *Plasmodium falciparum*
   E. *Salmonella typhi*

35. A resident of Wisconsin saw her physician because of a rash that she noticed on her arm. It began as a small papule and then enlarged during the next 10 days (see figure). When she presented this lesion to her physician, the involved area was 30 cm in diameter, with a flat red border and an area of central clearing. She also had a headache, low-grade fever, and myalgias. Her activities during the weeks before the rash and symptoms developed included hunting with her dog, gardening, and swimming in a local lake. Which organism is most likely responsible for this infection?

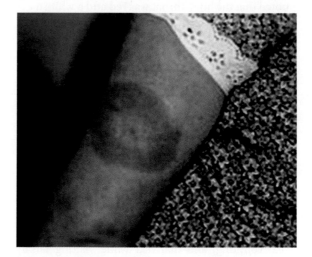

   A. *Borrelia burgdorferi*
   B. Brown recluse spider bite
   C. *Malassezia furfur*
   D. *Sporothrix schenckii*
   E. *Trichophyton rubrum*

36. A 43-year-old sexually active, HIV-positive woman living in St. Petersburg, Russia went to her physician with a 4-day history of low-grade fevers, fatigue, and a painful sore throat. A gray-colored membrane was observed over both tonsils and extended over the uvula and soft palate. Adenopathy and cervical swelling were also present. When the physician attempted to remove the membrane for culture, he noticed that the underlying mucosa was edematous and bleeding. Which organism is most likely responsible for this infection?
   A. *Bordetella pertussis*
   B. *Candida albicans*
   C. *Corynebacterium diphtheriae*
   D. *Neisseria gonorrhoeae*
   E. *Streptococcus pyogenes*

37. A 56-year-old businessman returned from China after a 1-year stay. On his return, he developed diarrhea and abdominal pain in the right upper quadrant. Examination in the hospital revealed a palpable liver and laboratory tests documented an elevation in liver enzymes. When questioned about his diet, he stated that he enjoyed eating many of the local delicacies, including raw fish and uncooked watercress. Parasite eggs were observed in the patient's stool (see figure). Which organism is most likely responsible for this patient's illness?

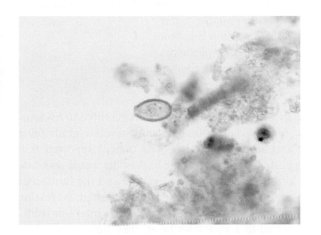

   A. *Ancylostoma duodenale*
   B. *Fasciola hepatica*

   C. *Clonorchis sinensis* (also known as *Opisthorchis sinensis*)
   D. *Paragonimus westermani*
   E. *Schistosoma mansoni*

38. A 36-year-old woman with a history of rheumatic heart disease underwent dental extractions for severely decayed teeth. Prophylactic antibiotics were not administered because of a remote history of penicillin allergy. Approximately 6 weeks after the procedure, the woman developed fevers, chills, and night sweats. After 2 weeks of these symptoms, the patient saw her physician, who noted that she had experienced a 5-kg weight loss since her last visit. Which of the following organisms is most likely responsible for this patient's infection?
   A. *Candida albicans*
   B. *Staphylococcus aureus*
   C. *Staphylococcus epidermidis*
   D. *Streptococcus mutans*
   E. *Streptococcus pneumoniae*

39. An 18-year-old male college student presented to the student health center with a sore throat, swollen cervical lymph nodes, fever, malaise, and hepatosplenomegaly. Which of the following agents is most likely responsible for this infection?
   A. Adenovirus
   B. Coxsackievirus
   C. Epstein-Barr virus
   D. Human metapneumovirus
   E. *Streptococcus pyogenes*

40. Approximately 4 h after eating a breakfast of scrambled eggs, ham, custard-filled Danish roll, and orange juice, a husband and wife developed nausea and started vomiting. They rapidly developed severe abdominal pain and diarrhea. The couple went to the local hospital and were found to be dehydrated, but had no evidence of fever, rash, or other signs. Which antibiotic should be used to treat these patients?
   A. Amoxicillin
   B. Ciprofloxacin
   C. Oxacillin
   D. Vancomycin
   E. No antibiotic

41. Approximately 2 weeks after birth, an infant developed watery discharge from both eyes. During the next few days, this discharge became purulent and the conjunctiva became erythematous (see figure). The mother returned to the hospital with the infant, and the pediatrician ordered culture and Gram stain of the discharge. No organisms were observed on Gram stain, and the culture on blood agar and chocolate agar was negative. Which of the following drugs should be used to treat this infection?

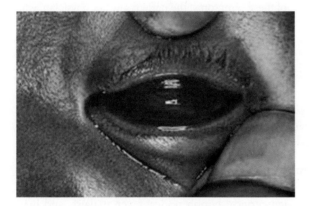

   A. Acyclovir
   B. Erythromycin
   C. Imipenem
   D. Penicillin
   E. Tetracycline

42. Approximately 3 days after attending a wedding reception in St. Louis, Missouri, 32 guests became ill with symptoms that included diarrhea, anorexia, abdominal cramping, and a low-grade fever. Cultures for bacterial and viral pathogens were negative, but coccoid forms 8–10 μm in diameter were observed when the stool specimens were stained with an acid-fast stain. Which organism is most likely responsible for these infections?
   A. *Candida*
   B. *Cryptosporidium*
   C. *Cyclospora*
   D. *Cystoisospora*
   E. *Microsporidia*

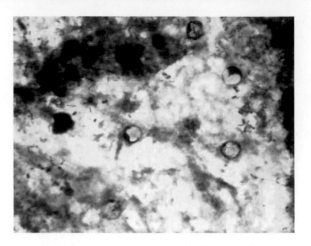

43. In late 2001 and early 2002, four infants residing in Staten Island, New York became ill with the same bacterial pathogen. The infants were between the ages of 3 weeks and 18 weeks. All had been in good health following uneventful pregnancies. Two infants were breast-fed, and two were formula-fed. Upon presentation to the hospital, all infants were irritable, lethargic, and constipated. Two infants had sluggishly reactive pupils, and two were described as having loss of facial expression. Three of the infants required mechanical ventilation. Specimens of blood, stool, urine, and cerebrospinal fluid were collected for microbiological testing. Which organism was most likely responsible for these infections?
   A. *Campylobacter jejuni*
   B. *Clostridium botulinum*
   C. Herpes simplex virus
   D. Lymphocytic choriomeningitis virus
   E. *Salmonella choleraesuis*

44. In August, a 26-year-old man presented to his family physician with complaints of a low-grade fever and severe headaches. The patient reported that blisters developed at the back of his throat and base of his tongue 1 week previously and the headaches began shortly after the blisters appeared, increasing in severity over the last 5 days. The man was transferred to a local hospital where a lumbar puncture was performed. The cell counts and chemistry for the cerebrospinal fluid were: 177 cells with 81%

lymphocytes, a normal glucose (54 mg/dL) and elevated protein (60 mg/dL). No organisms were observed on Gram stain and bacterial and fungal cultures were negative. After 2 weeks, the patient's headaches gradually decreased in frequency and intensity. The most likely cause of this patient's symptoms is which of the following organisms?

A. Coxsackievirus A
B. *Cryptococcus neoformans*
C. Herpes simplex virus
D. *Naegleria fowleri*
E. *Streptococcus pneumoniae*

45. During a military conflict in Somalia, soldiers developed a febrile illness characterized by the abrupt onset of fever with rigors, severe headache, myalgias, arthralgias, lethargy, photophobia, and coughing. A petechial rash developed 4 days into the illness and then faded 1 to 2 days later when the symptoms waned. Splenomegaly and hepatomegaly were also present. After 10 days, the symptoms recurred. The tentative diagnosis for these soldiers was relapsing fever, which was confirmed by serology. Which vector is most likely responsible for transmission of this disease?

A. Flea
B. Hard tick
C. Louse
D. Mite
E. Mosquito

46. Three patients presented to an inner city hospital with infections subsequently demonstrated to be caused by the same organism. The first patient, a 23-year-old female prostitute, presented with a temperature of 38.5 °C, hypotension, icterus, pulmonary rales, and muscle tenderness. The second patient, a 38-year-old man, had a temperature of 38.5 °C, icterus, mild upper quadrant tenderness, and muscle tenderness. The third patient, a 28-year-old man, had flulike symptoms, a low-grade fever, and muscle tenderness. The first and third patients had cut their feet on glass in a city alley, whereas the second patient cut his hand on glass in an alley. The patients had not been in contact with each other, and no one

had a significant travel history. Two of the patients developed acute renal failure in the second week of hospitalization; one patient developed meningitis. A fourth patient was subsequently reported to the public health department with a similar illness. One common feature for all four patients was a history of swimming in a city reservoir 7–10 days before their illness developed. Which organism is most likely responsible for these illnesses?

A. Hepatitis A virus
B. *Leptospira interrogans*
C. *Mycobacterium marinum*
D. *Naegleria fowleri*
E. *Vibrio vulnificus*

47. A 22-year-old man presents to the emergency department with complaints of eye pain and blurred vision during the preceding day. He did not remember an eye injury but had been wearing contact lenses for an extended period when the eye pain started. The patient also admitted to cleaning his contact lenses with tap water. Examination of the eye revealed ulceration of the cornea. Bacterial cultures of the eye were negative; however, Giemsa stains of the eye scrapings revealed an organism (see figure). Which of the following organisms is most likely responsible for this infection?

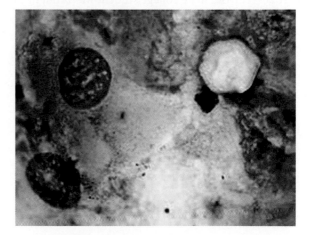

A. Acanthamoeba
B. Dientamoeba

C. Entamoeba
D. Isospora
E. Microsporidia

48. A 60-year-old woman living in Connecticut presented to her physician with a 5-day history of high fevers (up to 40 °C), headaches, myalgias, and malaise. She remembered that 12 days before the start of her illness she removed two engorged ticks from her legs. Leukopenia and thrombocytopenia were documented at the time she was admitted into the hospital. During the course of her illness, no evidence of a rash developed. The fever, however, was persistent despite intravenous treatment with ceftazidime and vancomycin, and she became increasingly confused and somnolent. Bacterial cultures of blood, cerebrospinal fluid, and stool were negative. Giemsa stains of her peripheral blood demonstrated intracellular organisms in the granulocytic cells. Which organism is most likely responsible for this infection?
    A. *Anaplasma phagocytophilum*
    B. *Babesia microti*
    C. *Coxiella burnetii*
    D. *Plasmodium vivax*
    E. *Rickettsia rickettsii*

49. A 20-year-old male college student was brought to the student health center by his girlfriend. Upon physical examination, the patient was found to be obtunded, with a temperature of 39 °C, blood pressure 104/52 mmHg, and heart rate of 148 bpm. He had a stiff neck and generalized petechial rash with two areas of purpura. Cerebrospinal fluid was collected. The opening pressure was 180 mm H_2O, white blood cells 4300/mm^3 with 91% neutrophils, glucose 10 mg/dL, and protein 755 mg/dL. A Gram stain and culture of the cerebrospinal fluid was performed with both tests positive for the organism seen in the figure. Which organism is most likely responsible for this patient's infection?
    A. *Cryptococcus neoformans*
    B. *Haemophilus influenzae*
    C. *Listeria monocytogenes*
    D. *Neisseria meningitidis*
    E. *Streptococcus pneumoniae*

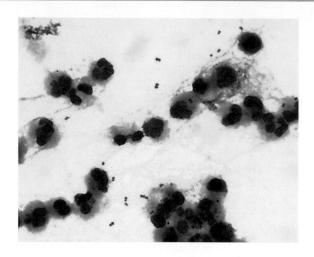

50. A 61-year-old man presents to his physician with diarrhea, abdominal pain, and a nonproductive cough. The diagnosis of multiple myeloma was made 2 years prior to this episode, and 1 month before his current illness began, he underwent a bone marrow transplant. Induced sputum and blood are collected for bacterial culture and stool specimens are collected for bacterial culture and ova and parasite examination. The sputum and stool cultures are negative but the blood culture is positive for *Escherichia coli*. The ova and parasite examination is also positive for an organism (see figure). Which parasite is most likely responsible for this patient's illness?

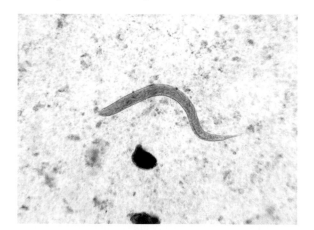

    A. Ancylostoma
    B. Ascaris
    C. Necator
    D. Strongyloides
    E. Trichinella

ANSWERS

1. **Correct answer: B. Hepatitis A vaccine.**
   The patient had serologic and clinical evidence of an acute hepatitis A virus infection. This virus is spread person-to-person by fecal contamination. Although immune serum has been used historically to control spread of infections, hepatitis A vaccine is now preferred.

2. **Correct answer: D. Tularemia.**
   Francisella tularensis (the etiologic agent of tularemia) is highly infectious, capable of penetrating unbroken skin. This is a significant health hazard for both physicians and laboratory personnel. *Histoplasma* and *Coccidioides* are significant risks for laboratory personnel when the mold form of these fungi grow in the laboratory; however, the yeast form of *Histoplasma* and the spherule form of *Coccidioides,* that are present in the patient's clinical specimens, are not infectious. The diagnosis of *Borrelia burgdorferi* infections is primarily by serology, and *Entamoeba histolytica* in stool specimens is not considered a health risk if the specimens are appropriately handled.

3. **Correct answer: B. *Candida parapsilosis*.**
   Each of the fungi listed in this question exist as yeasts in the patient; however, only *C. parapsilosis* can grow in blood cultures in 2 days. This yeast is also associated with hyperalimentation, so isolation in this immunocompromised patient is not unusual. *Malassezia furfur* is also associated with

hyperalimentation but it would not be isolated in traditional blood cultures because it requires lipids for growth. *Cryptococcus neoformans* is recovered in blood cultures but it typically requires 3–5 days before growth is detected. Both *Blastomyces dermatitidis* and *Histoplasma capsulatum* can grow in blood cultures but must be incubated for 2 weeks or longer.

4. **Correct answer: E. *Nocardia farcinica*.**
   Only *Nocardia* and *Mycobacterium* will stain with the modified acid-fast stain. *Nocardia* characteristically forms long, branching, partially staining acid-fast rods. Mycobacteria are typically shorter with minimal branching and stain uniformly. *Actinomyces* can resemble *Nocardia* with long, branching rods but these organisms do not stain acid-fast.

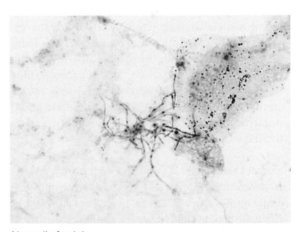

Nocardia farcinica.

5. **Correct answer: D. Herpes simplex virus.**
   The lesions are characteristic of herpes gladiatorum and oral herpes, diseases caused by herpes simplex virus. The disease is spread when one person's vesicular lesion (usually orofacial) comes into contact with another person's skin. Similar lesions are not produced by the other viruses listed in this question.

6. **Correct answer: B. *Legionella* pneumophila.**
   L. pneumophila does not stain well with the Gram stain so microscopy is typically negative. Traditional media also does not support the growth of *Legionella* so cultures are also negative.

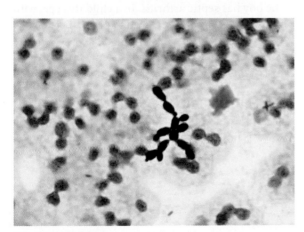

Candida parapsilosis.

Specialized media supplemented with cysteine and iron is required. *Klebsiella* will be observed on the Gram stain and grows readily on conventional bacterial media. *Mycobacterium* will stain with the acid-fast stain. *Histoplasma* would not be observed in the Gram stain or acid-fast stain, but will grow in fungal cultures. Influenza virus infections are typically not observed during the warm months of the year.

7. Correct answer: E. *Pasteurella*.
   Pasteurella multocida is commonly associated with animal bite wounds, particularly cat bites. Cats can inflict a deep puncture wound that is difficult to clean adequately. *Capnocytophaga* are also associated with animal bites but these are long, thin, gram-negative bacilli. *Fusobacterium* is also long and thin but is a strict anaerobe. *Eikenella* resembles *Pasteurella* but is associated with human bite wounds and not animal bites. *Escherichia* is not associated with bite wounds. With the exception of *Escherichia*, the other bacteria listed in this question reside in the mouths of humans (*Capnocytophaga*, *Eikenella*, and *Fusobacterium*) or animals (*Pasteurella*) and are commonly associated with bite wounds. Although these are gram-negative bacteria, many of the infections can be treated with penicillin.

8. Correct answer: A. *Blastomyces dermatitidis*.
   B. dermatitidis appears as yeast in tissue and generally grows after 2 weeks in culture as a mold. *Histoplasma capsulatum* has a similar growth pattern although the yeast cells are typically much smaller than *Blastomyces*. Additionally, blastomycosis is characterized by the predilection to disseminate, producing characteristic skin lesions. Infection with *Sporothrix schenckii* is also characterized by the development of skin lesions but these are primary infections associated with the introduction of the fungus directly through skin penetration. *Candida albicans* can cause skin lesions but it would grow more rapidly in culture. *Mycobacterium marinum* characteristically causes skin lesions but these are also associated with direct penetration of the skin; also, the acid-fast stain would be positive for *M. marinum* infections.

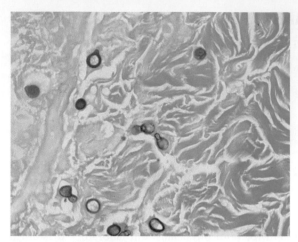

Blastomyces dermatitidis.

9. Correct answer: B. *Listeria monocytogenes*.
   Although *L. monocytogenes* is most likely the bacterium that caused the meningitis, all five of the listed bacteria can cause meningitis. *Escherichia coli* and group B *Streptococcus* (*Streptococcus agalactiae*) are primarily restricted to babies less than 1 month of age; however, *E. coli* is a gram-negative rod and *S. agalactiae* is a gram-positive coccus. The other three bacteria can cause meningitis in all age groups although *Neisseria meningitidis* is most common in young adults, while *Listeria* and *Streptococcus pneumoniae* are primarily observed in the young and the very old. Only *Listeria* is a small gram-positive rod and the organism grows slowly both in the patient and in culture.

10. Correct answer: D. *Staphylococcus aureus*.
    The boy has septic arthritis. In a child this age, with no evidence of an open wound from the fall, the most common cause of septic arthritis is *S. aureus*. The Gram stain results are consistent with this diagnosis. *Staphylococcus epidermidis* resides on the skin surface and has a similar Gram stain appearance but is not associated with septic arthritis. The other organisms listed are also not associated with septic arthritis unless there is an open traumatic wound.

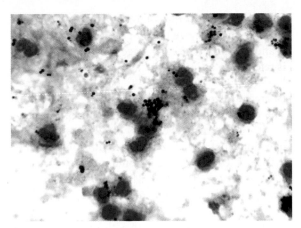

Staphylococcus aureus.

11. Correct answer: E. Candidiasis.

The organisms observed in the microscopic examination are yeast cells, so a *Candida* infection is the most likely diagnosis. *Neisseria gonorrhoeae* would appear as gram-negative diplococci. *Chlamydia trachomatis* are intracellular bacteria and would appear as iodine-staining inclusions in the infected cell. *Trichomonas vaginalis* is a flagellated parasite. Bacterial vaginosis represents an alteration of the vaginal microbiome, with a shift from a predominance of gram-positive rods (i.e., lactobacilli) to a mixture of anaerobic species.

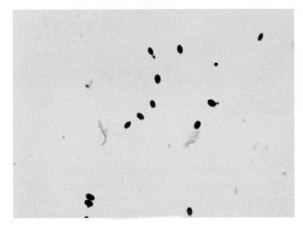

Candidiasis.

12. Correct answer: D. *Streptococcus pneumoniae*.

Patients that are asplenic are at increased risk of developing overwhelming infections with encapsulated organisms. The spleen is responsible for producing opsonizing antibodies, required for the removal of encapsulated organisms such as *S. pneumoniae*,

Haemophilus influenzae, and *Neisseria meningitidis*. In the absence of a functional spleen, infection with these organisms can reach a magnitude that allows the organisms to be observed directly in blood specimens. The vast majority of these infections are caused by *S. pneumoniae*. Observation of gram-positive cocci in pairs in the blood confirms the diagnosis.

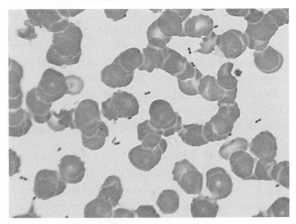

Streptococcus pneumoniae.

13. Correct answer: A. Beaver.

The organism in the figure is *Giardia lamblia*. *Giardia* has a worldwide distribution, with streams and lakes contaminated in mountainous areas. The sylvan distribution is maintained in reservoir animals such as beavers and muskrats. In this setting, giardiasis is acquired through the consumption of inadequately treated contaminated water. The other animals listed in the answers to this question (dog, rabbit, snake, and trout) have not been implicated in disease caused by this parasite.

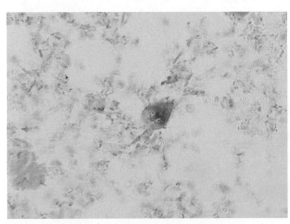

Giardia lamblia.

14. Correct answer: A. *Bacillus cereus.*

The clinical presentation of this disease is consistent with food poisoning caused by *B. cereus.* Disease is mediated by a heat-stable enterotoxin. *B. cereus* can grow in contaminated foods, releasing the enterotoxin. Subsequent reheating of the food does not inactivate the enterotoxin. Because the enterotoxin is present in the food, the incubation period between ingestion and disease and the duration of symptoms is short. Each of the other organisms listed produces gastroenteritis 1 to 3 days after ingestion of the contaminated foods. The delay occurs because the organisms must grow in the intestines before they invade the intestinal mucosa or produce enteric toxins. Diseases caused by these other bacteria and viruses are self-limiting, but symptoms may persist for up to 1 week after onset.

15. Correct answer: B. *Clostridioides difficile.*

All five organisms in the answers to this question can cause gastrointestinal disease; however, the important clue is that the symptoms developed after the patient started antibiotics. β-lactam antibiotics and clindamycin are most commonly associated with disease caused by *C. difficile.* The antibiotics suppress the bacteria normally present in the gastrointestinal tract and allow proliferation of *C. difficile,* which may have been present in the intestine or acquired during hospitalization. The presence of white plaques over the colonic mucosa is consistent with the more severe form of disease, pseudomembranous colitis. The early stage of *C. difficile* disease is referred to as "antibiotic-associated diarrhea."

16. Correct answer: E. *Rhizopus.*

The organism in the figure is a nonseptate mold (a zygomycetes). The only mold listed in this question that is nonseptate is *Rhizopus.* Other zygomycetes that cause human disease include *Absidia, Cunninghamella, Mucor, Rhizomucor,* and *Saksenaea.* These molds are ubiquitous, and exposure for most people is inconsequential. Some individuals, such as patients with uncontrolled diabetes mellitus, are at increased risk for infections. Rhinocerebral mucormycosis (invasion of a zygomycetes into the sinuses and then to the orbit or brain) is a particular concern in diabetic patients in acidosis. This disease is fatal unless promptly treated.

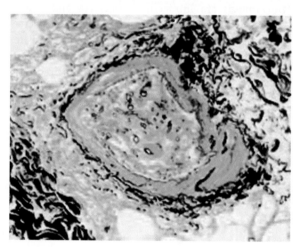

Rhizopus.

17. Correct answer: E. *Staphylococcus saprophyticus.*

This patient's clinical illness is consistent with a urinary tract infection (UTI). It could be restricted to the bladder (cystitis) or more likely involve the kidneys (acute pyelonephritis). The latter is indicated by the flank pain (over the kidney) and fever. *S. saprophyticus* causes UTIs primarily in young, sexually active women. This organism can also produce upper tract infection with urinary tract stone formation due to production of urease by the

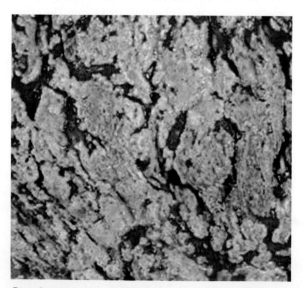

Pseudomembranous colitis caused by *Clostridioides difficile.*

bacteria, leading to alkalization of the urine and mineral precipitation. The Gram stain is consistent with a *Staphylococcus* infection. This would also be consistent with *Staphylococcus aureus* but UTIs with this organism are less common unless the patient is also bacteremic with *S. aureus*. *Enterococcus faecalis* is also a gram-positive coccus that can cause UTIs but this typically is in patients who have been treated with broad-spectrum antibiotics and are either catheterized or have a history of urinary tract manipulations. *Candida albicans* will stain gram-positive but is much larger than bacteria and would not be mistaken for bacteria. *Neisseria gonorrhoeae* is a gram-negative diplococci.

18. Correct answer: D. *Nocardia abscessus*.
An infection with *N. abscessus* typically presents as a bronchopulmonary infection, with dissemination to the central nervous system or subcutaneous tissues as a common complication. These bacteria are gram-positive but characteristically stain poorly. *Nocardia* have mycolic acids in their cell wall and are weakly acid-fast. *Actinomyces israelii* can resemble *Nocardia* but does not stain with the acid-fast stain. *Mycobacterium tuberculosis* is strongly acid-fast but does not form long filaments. *Rhodococcus equi* is partially acid-fast and does cause cavitary pulmonary disease, but does not typically disseminate to the brain and the morphology resembles cocci (as implied by the name) or short rods. *Aspergillus fumigatus* is a mold that produces cavitary pulmonary disease.

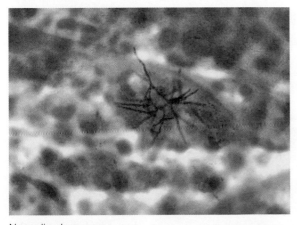

Nocardia *abscessus*.

19. Correct answer: A. Cytomegalovirus.
The most frequent causes of congenital infection are the so-called TORCH agents (*Toxoplasma*, rubella virus, cytomegalovirus, and herpes simplex virus). Cytomegalovirus, the only agent associated with owl's eye inclusion bodies, is the most common viral cause of congenital malformation. The mother likely suffered a primary asymptomatic cytomegalovirus infection as a result of her blood transfusion and transmitted the virus to her baby. Infants infected with herpes simplex virus may have vesicular lesions but would not have calcifications. Infants infected with rubella virus usually suffer from cataracts and deafness. Congenital infections with Zika virus are well-documented but this woman did not live in an area where viral transmission through an infected mosquito has been documented.

20. Correct answer: D. *Staphylococcus aureus*.
This boy had toxic shock syndrome produced by *S. aureus*. Toxic shock syndrome is characterized by multiorgan dysfunction, skin desquamation, and shock. *Bacteroides fragilis* and *Clostridium perfringens* can produce overwhelming disease (myonecrosis) that can be rapidly fatal but would not present with a rash or desquamation. *Bacillus cereus* is associated with diarrheal disease and eye infections following trauma. *Streptococcus anginosus* is associated with focal abscess formation.

21. Correct answer: B. *Brucella*.
This man had an infection with *Brucella*, most likely with *Brucella melitensis*, which is associated with contaminated dairy products. This is a slow-growing, gram-negative coccobacillus. *Francisella* and *Haemophilus* can also resemble this organism on Gram stain, although neither is associated with goat cheese. *Francisella* infections most commonly follow exposure to infected ticks or rabbits, and *Haemophilus* infections are typically in the very young or elderly. *Acinetobacter* and *Escherichia* would not be confused for *Brucella* on Gram stain.

22. Correct answer: D. *Sporothrix schenckii*.
This woman has an infection with the dimorphic fungus *S. schenckii*. The mold lives in soil rich in organic material. Most infections are acquired when the fungus is introduced into the cutaneous tissues

by mild trauma, usually associated with gardening. At body temperature, the fungus replicates as a yeast and has been referred to as "cigar-shaped." Typically, relatively few yeast cells are observed in the clinical specimens. At 25 °C to 30 °C the fungus grows as a dematiaceous or pigmented mold. The delicate "rosette" arrangement of the conidia (round, fruiting structures on the thin hyphae) is characteristic of *Sporothrix* (suggesting the dangers of rose gardening). *Candida* and *Cryptococcus* exist only in the yeast form and *Trichophyton* only as a mold. *Blastomyces* is a dimorphic fungus but the yeast and mold forms do not resemble *Sporothrix*.

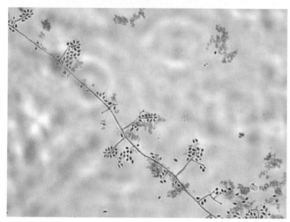

Sporothrix schenckii.

23. Correct answer: B. *Enterococcus faecalis.*
    Organisms responsible for peritonitis have demonstrated an ability to produce disease in the intestinal tract (i.e., they have specific, relevant virulence factors). Even though many different species of bacteria are present in the intestines, relatively few produce peritonitis. *Enterococcus* organisms, both *E. faecalis* and *Enterococcus faecium*, can cause peritonitis. The Gram stain result for the patient is consistent with this organism. Two additional organisms that commonly cause peritonitis are *Escherichia coli* (which is treated effectively with ceftazidime) and *Bacteroides fragilis* (which is treated with metronidazole). Yeasts such as *Candida albicans* could also be responsible for infection in this setting; however, the organism would not grow anaerobically. *Peptostreptococcus anaerobius* is associated with polymicrobic abdominal infections, but this organism would not grow aerobically. Streptococci and staphylococci are uncommon

causes of peritonitis in this setting. As can be seen in the figure, the Gram stain of *Enterococcus* can be confused with *Streptococcus pneumoniae*.

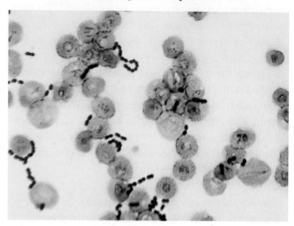

Enterococcus faecalis.

24. Correct answer: E. *Pneumocystis jiroveci.*
    This patient had *Pneumocystis* pneumonia, a common infection in HIV-AIDS patients. *P. jiroveci*, like all yeasts, will stain with silver stains. This fungus must be distinguished from *Candida albicans* and the yeast forms of other fungi. *C. albicans* rarely causes pulmonary infections, so this organism is less likely than *P. jiroveci* to be responsible for the patient's infection. *Aspergillus fumigatus* does not form yeast-like cells. *Cryptococcus neoformans* causes pulmonary infections, particularly in immunocompromised patients; however, the cells are slightly larger and are typically surrounded by a capsule. The yeast form of *Histoplasma* is smaller and typically intracellular.

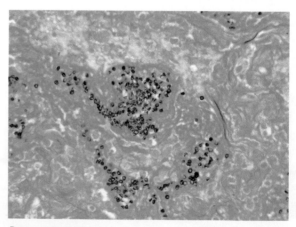

Pneumocystis jiroveci.

25. Correct answer: B. *Campylobacter jejuni.*
All of the organisms listed in this question can cause diarrheal disease. *Bacillus cereus* and *Staphylococcus aureus* are intoxications, with their toxins ingested with previously contaminated foods. The most common presentation for disease caused by these two organisms is a rapid onset of symptoms (typically 4h), acute diarrhea and abdominal cramps, and resolution within 24h. Norovirus is the most common virus associated with diarrheal disease, and *Campylobacter* and *Salmonella* are the most common bacteria. Although each can produce similar symptoms, the reactive arthritis observed in one patient is primarily a complication of *Campylobacter* infections.

26. Correct answer: D. Human.
The parasite observed in the figure is the trophozoite form of *Entamoeba histolytica*, the etiologic agent of amebiasis. Patients infected with *E. histolytica* pass noninfectious trophozoites and infectious cysts in their stools. The trophozoites cannot survive in the external environment or when transported through the stomach. Therefore, the main source of water and food contamination is the asymptomatic carrier who passes cysts. Cockroaches and flies can serve as vectors of this parasite by transferring the cysts from human feces to food or water. Dogs do not serve as reservoirs, and mosquitoes have not been implicated as vectors.

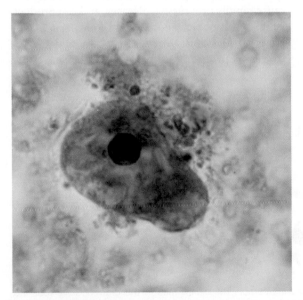

Entamoeba histolytica.

27. Correct answer: B. *Clostridium perfringens.*
Massive hemolysis is a rare but well-recognized complication of a *C. perfringens* infection, which this patient had. It is surprising that this complication is not seen more commonly, in light of the variety of hemolytic toxins produced by this organism. The most important is alpha toxin, a lecithinase that lyses erythrocytes, platelets, leukocytes, and endothelial cells. This toxin can produce enhanced vascular permeability and results in massive hemolysis and bleeding. Although the other organisms listed in this question produce hemolytic toxins, none have been associated with the massive hemolysis that was seen in this patient.

28. Correct answer: E. Shiga toxin–producing *Escherichia coli.*
All five groups of *E. coli* in the answer to this question have been implicated as causes of gastroenteritis. Infections with enterotoxigenic *E. coli*, enteropathogenic *E. coli*, and enteroaggregative *E. coli* are generally restricted to the small intestine, whereas infections with Shiga toxin-producing *E. coli* and enteroinvasive *E. coli* primarily involve the colon. The patients in this report had colitis, with or without blood. Ten percent of the patients (children) developed hemolytic uremic syndrome, which is characterized by acute renal failure, microangiopathic hemolytic anemia, thrombocytopenia, hypertension, and central nervous system manifestations. Shiga toxin-producing *E. coli* (formerly called enterohemorrhagic *E. coli*), but not enteroinvasive *E. coli*, is frequently associated with hemolytic uremic syndrome in children.

29. Correct answer: C. *Coccidioides immitis.*
This man had coccidioidomycosis. This fungus is endemic in the southwestern states of the United States, with infections common in Arizona. Most exposures result in an asymptomatic infection; however, progressive pulmonary disease and meningitis can occur. The mold form of this dimorphic fungus grows in nature and is highly contagious. The arthroconidia (barrel-shaped spores seen in the figure) can be readily dispersed in winds and drift for hundreds of miles. Inhalation of these spores can initiate infection. The form of the fungus seen in patients is that of a thick-walled spherule filled with

endospores. None of the other fungi listed in the answers to this question can produce arthroconidia.

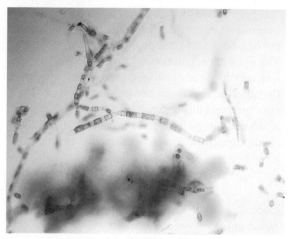

Coccidioides immitis.

30. Correct answer: E. *Streptococcus pyogenes.*

This is a classic presentation of scarlet fever caused by *S. pyogenes* (group A *Streptococcus*). Infection initially develops as pharyngitis, although a wound infection may occur. The distribution of the rash and the more intense inflammation along the skin folds (Pastia sign) is characteristic of the scarlatiniform rash. *Bordetella pertussis* produces a primary infection of the throat and emits a toxin that mediates the systemic signs of disease (pertussis or whooping cough); however, the clinical presentation of the rash is not consistent with *B. pertussis.* Measles and rubella viruses can initiate infection as an upper respiratory tract infection that disseminates as characterized by a rash, but the rash is a maculopapular rash and does not resemble scarlet fever. *Staphylococcus aureus* can also present as a rash in toxic shock syndrome but it is typically followed by desquamation, and the clinical illness is much more severe with multiorgan failure.

31. Correct answer: C. Direct skin penetration by infectious larvae.

This woman was infected with a hookworm, either *Ancylostoma duodenale* or *Necator americanus.* The eggs of these two parasites are indistinguishable. Eggs are shed in the feces of an infected patient. If the eggs are deposited on shady, well-drained soil, they can hatch and mature into infectious larvae.

The larvae then penetrate unbroken skin (usually bare feet), migrate to the lungs, and find their way to the small intestine. *Strongyloides* is the other important nematode that initiates infections in humans by penetrating the skin.

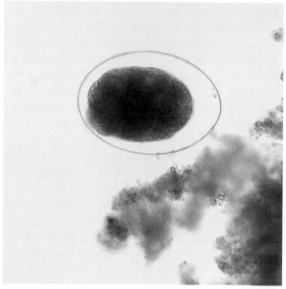

Hookworm.

32. Correct answer: A. *Bacillus cereus.*

Both *B. cereus* and *Clostridium perfringens* are spore-forming organisms found in nature, can cause rapidly progressive diseases, and can produce large, β-hemolytic colonies on blood agar plates. However, *B. cereus* grows aerobically and *C. perfringens* is an anaerobic organism. *Corynebacterium*

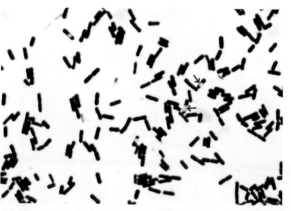

Bacillus cereus. The clear areas in the gram-positive rods are unstained spores (arrows).

jeikeium colonizes the skin surfaces and, although it could be isolated in an eye specimen, it would not be associated with this type of infection. *Nocardia farcinica* is also found in nature and is gram-positive but is not associated with rapidly progressive eye infections. *Bacteroides fragilis* is an anaerobic gram-negative rod.

33. Correct answer: A. *Chlamydia trachomatis*.
The patient had lymphogranuloma venereum caused by *C. trachomatis*. The infection is endemic in Africa, Asia, and South America and is sporadically reported in North America, Australia, and Europe. The disease is caused by four specific serotypes of *C. trachomatis*: serotypes L1, L2, L2a, and L3. Adenopathy ("bubo") with ulcer formation is characteristic of the disease. Herpes simplex virus produces a painful ulcer at the site of initial infection. The swollen, ulcerating lymph nodes seen in lymphogranuloma venereum are not characteristic of herpes infections. *Klebsiella granulomatis* is not culturable. *Neisseria gonorrhoeae* can be cultured on chocolate agar and specialized media (e.g., Thayer-Martin) but does not present as described in this patient. *Treponema pallidum* (the etiologic agent of syphilis) produces a painless ulcer, is not characterized by ulcerating lymph nodes, and does not grow in culture. *C. trachomatis* can be cultured in tissue culture cells (an intracellular pathogen); however, the most common test is nucleic acid amplification.

34. Correct answer: A. Dengue virus.
Infections with dengue virus can range from asymptomatic to a life-threatening hemorrhagic fever. Most infections are characterized by a 4- to 7-day incubation period followed by an acute onset of fever, headache, retro-orbital pain, myalgias, and rash. Disease is typically self-limiting after a 6- or 7-day course, although progression to dengue hemorrhagic fever and shock syndrome can occur. Infection with hepatitis A virus, *Leptospira interrogans*, *Plasmodium falciparum*, and *Salmonella* Typhi can all produce febrile illnesses in travelers to developing countries. Hepatitis A can initially present as a mild flu-like illness with fever, headache, myalgias, and malaise. Symptoms will progress to development of dark urine followed by pale stools and yellow discoloration of the skin and mucous membranes. Development of a rash is not characteristic. Symptomatic *L. interrogans* infections are typically characterized by high fevers, myalgias, and headaches. Conjunctival suffusion may be present. A rash is not commonly seen. *P. falciparum* would present as a febrile illness with nausea, vomiting, and diarrhea. This disease is unlikely with the history of compliant malaria prophylaxis. *S. typhi* infections are characterized by fever, headache, myalgias, and malaise. Although a rash may develop, it is not a prominent feature of the infection.

35. Correct answer: A. *Borrelia burgdorferi*.
This woman's symptoms are a classic description of erythema migrans, a rash that develops in the primary stage of Lyme disease. The rash initially develops at the site of the tick bite. The rash will disappear after a few weeks, and other transient lesions may subsequently appear. It is common to have no history of a tick bite at the time of presentation because infection most commonly develops following exposure to the nymph stage of the hard. The hard tick in this stage is the size of a poppy seed and likely would not be noticed. A spider bite would have a more aggressive stage of development with localized necrosis. *Malassezia furfur* and *Trichophyton rubrum* produce localized skin manifestations but not the systemic symptoms observed in this woman. *Sporothrix* produces ulcerative, nodular lesions along the lymphatics (not like this woman's presentation) and systemic symptoms.

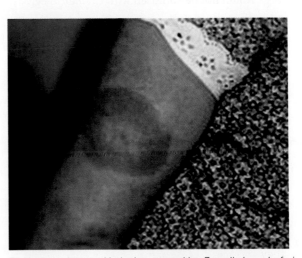

Erythema migrans skin lesion caused by *Borrelia burgdorferi*.

36. Correct answer: C. *Corynebacterium diphtheriae*.
This patient's disease is respiratory diphtheria, which is characterized by an abrupt onset of malaise, a sore throat, exudative pharyngitis, and a low-grade fever. A firm, adherent pseudomembrane consisting of bacteria, lymphocytes, plasma cells, and fibrin will develop over the tonsils and adjacent structure. *Bordetella pertussis*, *Neisseria gonorrhoeae*, and *Streptococcus pyogenes* can produce pharyngitis, but none of these organisms are associated with pseudomembrane formation. *Candida albicans* produces oral thrush, most commonly observed in immunocompromised patients such as HIV-AIDS patients. Again, a pseudomembrane would not be observed with *Candida* infections. Diphtheria has been eliminated in many countries with childhood vaccination but is still seen in some countries such as Russia where vaccination is not widespread.

37. Correct answer: C. *Clonorchis sinensis* (also known as *Opisthorchis sinensis*).
C. sinensis is the Chinese liver fluke. This patient's travel history and diet indicate that he could have been infected with this organism or *Fasciola hepatica*, the sheep liver fluke. *C. sinensis* is associated with consumption of infected raw fish and *F. hepatica* with uncooked watercress. The diagnosis is made by examination of the stool for characteristic eggs. The eggs of *C. sinensis* are much smaller than the *F. hepatica* eggs. The other parasites listed in the question are not associated with hepatitis, and their eggs would not be confused with *C. sinensis* eggs.

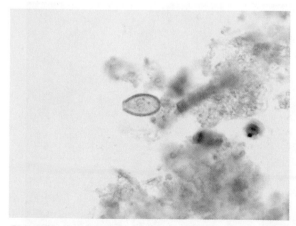

Clonorchis sinensis.

38. Correct answer: D. *Streptococcus mutans*.
This patient had subacute bacterial endocarditis, which is characterized by an indolent onset and vague symptoms of poor health developing over weeks to months. *S. mutans* is a member of the viridans group of streptococci and is a normal resident of the upper respiratory tract. It has the ability to adhere to the surface of teeth as well as damaged heart valves. It is recognized that patients with preexisting damaged heart valves (e.g., rheumatic heart disease) are at significant risk for developing valvular infections unless prophylactic antibiotics are administered before dental procedures. The other organisms listed in the answers to this question are members of the upper respiratory tract and could theoretically be responsible for endocarditis. However, *Candida albicans* is an uncommon cause of endocarditis; *Staphylococcus aureus* is more commonly associated with a rapidly developing course of disease (i.e., acute endocarditis); *Staphylococcus epidermidis* is associated with subacute diseases but those typically involving a surgical cardiac procedure such as placement of an artificial heart valve; and *Streptococcus pneumoniae* is an uncommon cause of endocarditis and almost always presents in an acute form.

39. Correct answer: C. Epstein-Barr virus.
The patient's clinical history is consistent with Epstein-Barr virus infection or infectious mononucleosis. Adenovirus is a common cause of pharyngitis, with or without conjunctivitis, but would not be associated with hepatosplenomegaly. Coxsackievirus and human metapneumovirus are common causes of upper respiratory tract infections ("common colds"), and *Streptococcus pyogenes* is the most common cause of bacterial pharyngitis, but none of these organisms would produce hepatosplenomegaly.

40. Correct answer: E. No antibiotic.
The most likely cause of this food poisoning is *Staphylococcus aureus*. Staphylococcal food poisoning is produced by preformed toxins present in food. Viable bacteria may not be in the food at the time it is consumed because reheating the food

after preparation can kill the staphylococci without affecting the heat-stable toxin or its activity. For this reason, antibiotic therapy would not alter the clinical course of this condition and is not recommended.

41. Correct answer: B. Erythromycin.
This child had inclusion conjunctivitis caused by *Chlamydia trachomatis*. The infection is acquired at birth during passage through an infected birth canal. After a 2- to 3-week incubation period, the infant develops symptoms as described in this case. Pneumonitis may also develop. *C. trachomatis* lacks a peptidoglycan layer in the cell wall, so β-lactams antibiotics (e.g., penicillin, imipenem) are ineffective in treating infections caused by this organism. Erythromycin and newer macrolide antibiotics (e.g., azithromycin) are the drugs of choice for treating this infection. Tetracyclines are not recommended for infants, and resistance has been found against this antibiotic. Acyclovir is an antiviral drug used to treat herpes virus infections which is not what this infant had.

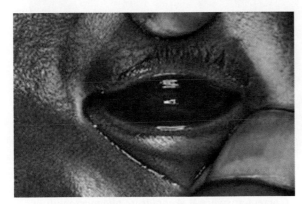

Inclusion conjunctivitis caused by *Chlamydia trachomatis*.

42. Correct answer: C. *Cyclospora*.
Of the organisms listed in the answers to this question, all are acid-fast except *Candida*. The easiest way to differentiate the acid-fast parasites is by their size: microsporidia are 1–2 μm in diameter; *Cryptosporidium* is 4–6 μm; *Cyclospora* is 8–10 μm; and *Cystoisospora* is 10–19 μm wide and 20–30 μm long.

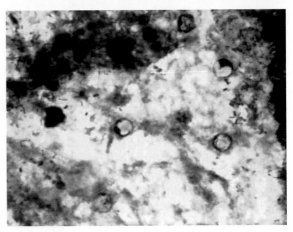

Cyclospora.

43. Correct answer: B. *Clostridium botulinum*.
This case describes a somewhat unusual outbreak of infant botulism because none of the children had a history of ingestion of honey or other contaminated food products. Consumption of honey is not recommended for infants less than 12 months of age because it can be contaminated with spores from *C. botulinum*. The infants lived in an area where construction was underway, and they were exposed to dust contaminated with *C. botulinum* spores. *C. botulinum* is commonly isolated from soil samples. Although the epidemiology of this outbreak is unusual, the clinical presentation is common and should have alerted the medical staff. Botulism should be suspected in infants less than 1 year of age who are constipated and have weakness in sucking, swallowing, or crying. Progressive muscle weakness and respiratory failure are symptoms of advanced disease. All of these infants' symptoms were effects of the botulinum toxin that blocks neurotransmission at peripheral cholinergic synapses by preventing release of the neurotransmitter acetylcholine. Although each of the other pathogens listed in this question can cause disease in neonates, none would produce this clinical picture.

44. Correct answer: A. Coxsackievirus A.
This patient had aseptic meningitis. Enteroviruses including the coxsackieviruses are the most common cause of viral meningitis during the summer months. The blisters in the patient's throat and

mouth are consistent with a preceding coxsackievirus A infection. Specific diagnosis of coxsackievirus A infection is most commonly made by molecular methods such as polymerase chain reaction amplification of viral nucleic acids. If bacteria such as *Streptococcus pneumoniae* were responsible for this patient's infection, the progression of disease would have been more rapid and the cerebrospinal fluid profile would have been different (i.e., predominance of polymorphonuclear leukocytes, low glucose, and elevated protein). *Cryptococcus neoformans* can cause a similar clinical picture; however, without treatment the yeast would have been seen on Gram stain and would have grown on both the bacterial and fungal media. Herpes simplex virus can produce vesicular lesions and aseptic meningitis as seen in this patient; however, this diagnosis is less likely because the patient would have been much sicker. *Naegleria fowleri* can cause a primary meningoencephalitis; however, the disease is rapidly fatal and the amoeba would be observed in the cerebrospinal fluid upon careful examination.

45. Correct answer: C. Louse.
These soldiers had louse-borne epidemic relapsing fever caused by *Borrelia recurrentis*. This disease is spread person-to-person by infected lice, with humans the only reservoirs. Lice ingest the *B. recurrentis* during a blood meal, and the bacteria multiply in the hemolymph of the parasite. Infection is transmitted when the louse is crushed on the skin surface (bacteria are not present in the saliva or feces of the lice). Fleas, mites, and mosquitoes are not infected with *B. recurrentis*. Soft ticks are the vectors of endemic relapsing fever, and hard ticks are the vectors of Lyme disease.

46. Correct answer: B. *Leptospira interrogans*.
Leptospirosis is typically an asymptomatic infection. For patients who develop clinically apparent disease, the onset of symptoms generally develops 1–2 weeks after exposure to the bacteria. The initial presentation is a flu-like illness with fever and myalgias. These may remit after 1 week or progress to a more advanced disease, such as meningitis or a generalized illness with headache, rash, vascular collapse, thrombocytopenia, hemorrhage, and hepatic and renal dysfunction. The reservoirs for

Leptospira infections are rodents, particularly rats, as well as dogs and farm animals. The bacteria can colonize the renal tubules of infected animals and be shed in urine. Human infections are most commonly acquired by contact with contaminated water (e.g., standing water, lakes).

47. Correct answer: A. *Acanthamoeba*.
Acanthamoeba species can produce a devastating keratitis that is difficult to treat and frequently leads to enucleation of the eye. The keratitis is usually associated with eye trauma that occurred before contact with contaminated soil, dust, or water. In this patient's situation, the eye trauma is likely related to contact lens use that can abrade the surface of the cornea. The use of contaminated water to clean the contact lenses can introduce the amoeba onto them. The other parasites listed in the answers to this question are not associated with eye infections.

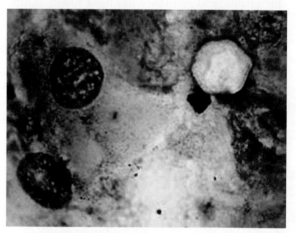

Acanthamoeba.

48. Correct answer: A. *Anaplasma phagocytophilum*.
A. phagocytophilum (formerly *Ehrlichia phagocytophila*) is the etiologic agent of human anaplasmosis (previously called human granulocytic ehrlichiosis). Clinically, it is difficult to differentiate *A. phagocytophilum* infections from *Rickettsia rickettsii* infections, although a rash is less commonly seen in *A. phagocytophilum* infections. In addition, ticks are the vectors for *A. phagocytophilum* and *R. rickettsii*, the etiologic agent of Rocky Mountain spotted fever. The observation of intracellular bacteria (i.e., morula) in peripheral blood granulocytes is useful

for distinguishing between these two organisms. Infected blood cells are observed more frequently with human anaplasmosis than with monocytic ehrlichiosis. Despite this positive result, the diagnostic tests of choice for anaplasmosis are nucleic acid amplification and serology. *Coxiella burnetii* is a related intracellular organism that causes infections most commonly by the airborne route (although ticks can be responsible for some infections). *Babesia microti* and *Plasmodium vivax* cause blood infections but infect erythrocytes and not granulocytes.

49. Correct answer: D. Neisseria *meningitidis.*
All of the organisms listed in the answers to this question can cause meningitis. The clinical picture is consistent with bacterial meningitis, so it is unlikely that *Cryptococcus neoformans* would cause meningitis in a previously healthy person. Furthermore, the Gram stain is inconsistent with *Cryptococcus* (a fungus). The most common causes of meningitis in college students are *N. meningitidis* and *Streptococcus pneumoniae. N. meningitidis* is a gram-negative diplococci with sides flattened against each cocci, and *S. pneumoniae* is a gram-positive diplococci with the cells arranged end-to-end. The Gram stain and clinical presentation for this patient is consistent with *N. meningitidis. Haemophilus influenzae* is a gram-negative rod that causes meningitis in unvaccinated children ages 3 months to 5 years. *Listeria monocytogenes* is a gram-positive rod that causes meningitis in the very young and the elderly.

50. Correct answer: D. Strongyloides.
This patient has an infection with *Strongyloides stercoralis.* The larvae of the parasite are able to penetrate skin, enter the circulatory system, and pass through the lungs. The worms are coughed up, swallowed, and then develop into adults in the small intestine. Eggs are deposited in the intestinal mucosa, where they hatch, releasing the larvae. Larvae and not eggs are detected in the stool specimens. Autoinfections can occur in immunocompromised patients. In this situation, the larvae in the stool develop into the infectious filariform larvae and repenetrate the intestines, initiating their migratory path from the circulatory system to the lungs, and then to the small intestine. Autoinfections are characterized by perforation of the intestines when the larvae penetrate the intestinal wall to the circulatory system and pneumonitis when the worms migrate through the lungs. Passage through the intestinal wall is the likely reason for bacteremia with *Escherichia.* Hookworms have the same developmental cycle, but eggs and not larvae are found in the stool specimens. Larvae for *Ascaris* or *Trichinella* would not be observed in clinical specimens.

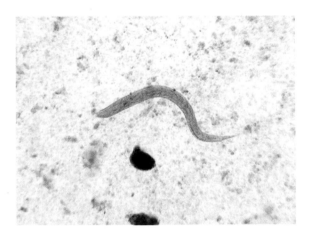

Strongyloides stercoralis.

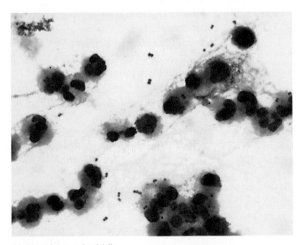

Neisseria meningitidis.

INDEX

Note: Page numbers followed by *f* indicate figures, *t* indicate tables, and *b* indicate boxes.

A

A-B exotoxin, *Corynebacterium diphtheriae* and, 28
Abscess(es)
  brain. (*see* Brain abscess)
  Nocardia species and, subcutaneous, 34*b*
  renal, pathogens of, 6–8*t*
Acanthamoeba duodenale, 267*f*
Acanthamoeba spp., 148*t*, 153*b*, 267, 267*f*, 280
Acid-fast bacteria, 30–36, 30*b*
  Mycobacterium avium complex, 34, 34*b*
  Mycobacterium leprae, 33–34, 33*b*
  Mycobacterium tuberculosis, 32–33, 32*b*
  Nocardia species, 34–36, 34*b*
Acid-fast organisms, 30–32, 31*t*
Acid-fast stain, 2
Acinetobacter baumannii, 38–39*t*, 44–45, 44*b*, 44*f*
  pneumonia, 188*b*
Acquired immune deficiency syndrome (AIDS), in Los Angeles, first report of, 93*b*
Actinomyces, 64
Actinomycosis, 64
  pelvic, 69*b*
Acute cerebellar ataxia, 96*b*
Acute hepatitis, hepatitis E virus and, 111
Acute HSV-2 proctitis, 215*b*
Acute meningitis, 213
Acute rheumatic fever, *Streptococcus pyogenes*, 238*b*
Acute rotavirus infection, 200*b*
Acyclovir, 90*t*
Adefovir, 89*t*
Adenoviridae, 85–86*t*
Adenovirus, 107, 116, 116*b*
Adenovirus gastroenteritis in immunocompromised child, 202*b*

Adenovirus 14
  pathogenic, 107*b*
  pneumonia, 193*b*
Adult inclusion conjunctivitis, 82*b*
Aerobic bacteria, 5
Aerobic fermentative Gram-negative rods, 49–58, 49*b*
  Escherichia coli, 51–52, 51*b*, 51*f*
  Klebsiella pneumoniae, 50–51*t*, 52–53, 53*b*, 53*f*
  Proteus mirabilis, 50–51*t*, 53–54, 53*b*
  Salmonella species, 54–55, 54*b*, 54*f*
  Shigella species, 55–56, 55*b*
  Vibrio cholerae, 57–58, 57*b*
  Yersinia pestis, 50–51*t*, 56–57, 56*b*
Aerobic Gram-negative cocci and coccobacilli, 37–48, 37*b*, 38–39*t*
  Acinetobacter baumannii, 44–45, 44*b*, 44*f*
  Bordetella pertussis, 45–46, 45*b*
  Brucella species, 47–48, 47*b*
  Eikenella corrodens, 40–41, 41*b*
  Francisella tularensis, 46–47, 46*b*
  Haemophilus influenzae, 42–43, 42*b*, 42*f*
  Kingella kingae, 41, 41*b*
  Moraxella catarrhalis, 41–42, 41*f*, 42*b*
  Neisseria gonorrhoeae, 38–39, 38*b*, 38*f*
Aerobic Gram-positive cocci, 12–23, 12*b*
  Enterococcus, 15, 15*t*, 22–23, 22*b*
  β-hemolytic streptococci, 14, 14*t*, 17–20
  Staphylococcus, 12, 12*t*
  Streptococcus, 12, 12*t*, 14
  viridans streptococci, 14, 14*t*, 21–22, 21*b*
Aerobic Gram-positive rods, 24–29, 24*b*
  Bacillus anthracis, 25–27, 25*b*
  Bacillus cereus, 24*t*, 25–27, 26*b*, 27*f*
  clinically important species of, 24*t*
  Corynebacterium diphtheriae, 28–29, 28*b*
  Listeria monocytogenes, 27–28, 27*b*, 28*f*

Aerobic nonfermentative Gram-negative rods, 59–62, 59*b*
  Burkholderia cepacia, 59*t*, 61, 61*b*
  Pseudomonas aeruginosa, 59*t*, 60–61, 60*b*, 60*f*
  Stenotrophomonas maltophilia, 61–62, 62*b*, 62*f*
African sleeping sickness, 157, 157*b*
Agranulocytosis, EBV infectious mononucleosis associated with, 99*b*
AIDS in Los Angeles, first report of, 192*b*
Allergic aspergillosis, 138*b*
Alternaria, 138*t*, 139*f*
Amantadine rimantadine, 90*t*
Aminoquinoline analogs, 145*t*
Amoeba, 142*t*
  free-living, 153–154
Anaerobic bacteria, 5, 63–70, 63*b*, 63–64*t*
  Bacteroides fragilis, 68–70, 69*b*
  Clostridioides difficile, 67–68, 67*b*
  Clostridium botulinum, 65–66, 65*b*
  Clostridium perfringens, 66–67, 66*b*, 68*f*
  Clostridium tetani, 64–65, 64*b*
Anal caner, 117
Anal carcinoma, 118*b*
Anamorph, 119
Anaplasma phagocytophilum, 79*t*, 268, 280–281
Anaplasmosis, human, clinical case of, 83*b*
Ancylostoma duodenale, 161*t*, 163*b*
Angioinvasion, 138*b*
Anthrax, 25
Anthrax-like pulmonary disease, *Bacillus cereus* and, 26*b*
Antibacterial agents, 8, 8–11*t*
Antibiotic-associated diarrhea, 63–64, 67*b*. See also *Clostridioides difficile*
  pathogens of, 6–8*t*

Antifungal agents, 121, 122t
Antihelminth agents, 145t
Antimetabolite, 8–11t
Antiprotozoal agents, 145t
Antiviral agents, 89
  for hepatitis virus infections, 89t
  for herpesvirus infections, 90t
  for HIV infections, 89t
  for respiratory infections, 90t
Arenaviridae, 85–86t
Arthritis
  Haemophilus influenzae and, 42b
  Neisseria gonorrhoeae, 250b
  pathogens of, 6–8t
  reactive, 72b
  septic, *Kingella kingae* and, 41b
Arthroconidia, 130
Arthropods, 142t, 180, 180t
Ascariasis, 163b
  hepatic, 167b
Ascaris lumbricoides, 161t, 163b
Aseptic meningitis complicating acute
      HSV-2 proctitis, 215b
Aspergillosis
  allergic, 138b
  invasive, 139b
Aspergillus fumigatus, 137–138, 137f,
    138b, 273
Astrovirus, 115–116, 115b
Asymptomatic carriage
  Cryptosporidium spp., 150b
  Cyclospora cayetanensis, 150b
  Cystoisospora belli, 151b
  Entamoeba histolytica, 149b
Asymptomatic infections, 118b
Avermectines, 145t

B

Babesia microti, 148t, 155b, 281
Babesiosis, 155b
Bacillary angiomatosis, pathogens of,
    6–8t
Bacillus, 24
Bacillus anthracis, 24t, 25–27, 25b
  disease with epsis, 241b
Bacillus cereus, 24t, 25–27, 26b, 27f, 198,
    258, 263, 272, 276–277
  food poisoning, 199b
  traumatic endophthalmitis, 29b, 248b
Bacteremia
  blood transfusion-related, 56
  Escherichia coli, 242b

Bacteremia *(Continued)*
  Listeria, 29b
  Mycobacterium catheter associated,
    245b
  Tsukamurella, 244b
Bacteria, 1–2t, 2, 5–8, 198, 235. *specific*
    bacteria
  acid-fast, 30–36, 30b
  aerobic, 5
  anaerobic, 5, 63–70, 63b, 63–64t
  antibacterial agents, 8, 8–11t
  classifications of, 5–6, 6t
  Gram-negative, 2, 6t
  Gram-positive, 2, 5t
  intracellular, 78–83, 78b
  role in disease, 6–8, 6–8t
  spiral-shaped, 71–77, 71b, 71t
Bacteroides fragilis, 63–64t, 68–70, 69b,
    198, 273
  necrotizing fasciitis, 224b
Beaver, 258, 258f, 271
Benzimidazoles, 145t
Bile salts, resistance to, 50
Bipolaris, 138t
Bite wounds, pathogens of, 6–8t
Black piedra, 123t
Blastomyces dermatitidis, 128t, 129–130,
    129b, 129f, 256, 256f, 270
Blastomycosis, 128t, 129
  central nervous system, 133b
  South American, 129
Blindness, from *Chlamydia trachomatis*,
    82b
Blood disease, due to parasites,
    143–144t
Blood nematodes, 165–167, 165t
  antiparasitic agents for, 145–147t
Blood protozoa, 148t
  antiparasitic agents for, 145–147t
Blood transfusion-related bacteremia,
    56
Blood trematodes, 168–169t, 172–174
  antiparasitic agents for, 145–147t
Boceprevir, 89t
Bone marrow disease, due to parasites,
    143–144t
Bone marrow transplant, CMV
    pneumonia after, 99b
Bordetella pertussis, 38–39t, 45–46, 45b
  outbreak in healthcare workers,
    184b
  whooping cough, 184b

Borrelia burgdorferi, 71t, 75–76, 75b,
    75f, 264, 264f, 277
Botulism, 65b
Brain abscess
  Nocardia species and, 34b
  pathogens of, 6–8t
Bronchial infections, 187
Bronchiolitis, respiratory syncytial virus
    and, 105
Bronchitis
  Moraxella catarrhalis and, 42b
  pathogens of, 6–8t
Bronchopneumonia, *Moraxella*
    catarrhalis and, 42b
Bronchopulmonary disease, *Nocardia*
    species and, 34b
Brucella sp., 47–48, 47b, 260, 273
Brucella melitensis, 38–39t, 47f
  sepsis, 242b
Brucellosis, 47b
  Brucella species and, 47b
Brugia malayi, 165t
Bubonic plague, 56b
Bunyaviridae, 85–86t
Burkholderia cepacia, 59t, 61, 61b
Burkholderia cepacia complex, 61
Burkholderia cepacia pulmonary
    infection, 190b
Burkholderia pseudomallei, 60
Burkitt lymphoma, Epstein-Barr virus
    and, 98b
Burns, infections of, pathogens of, 6–8t

C

Calabar swellings, *Loa loa* and, 166b
Caliciviridae, 85–86t
Campylobacter fetus, septicemia, 240b
Campylobacter jejuni, 71t, 72–73, 72b,
    72f, 261, 275
  enteritis and Guillain-Barré
    syndrome, 77b, 203b
Candida albicans, 134–136, 134t, 135b,
    135f, 208, 273
  keratitis following cataract surgery,
    249b
Candida glabrata, 134t
Candida krusei, 134t
Candida parapsilosis, 134t, 255, 255f,
    269
Candida tropicalis, 134t
Candidemia, 139b
  in immunocompetent woman, 243b

Candidiasis, 257, 257*f*, 271
Capnocytophaga, 270
Capsid, 85
Carbuncles, 221*t*
  pathogens of, 6–8*t*
Cardiovascular infections, 235
Cat-associated tularemia, 48*b*
Catheter-related *Candida auris* sepsis, 245*b*
CD4 T cells, HIV virus and, 92
Cellulitis, 17*b*, 66*b*, 221*t*
  Haemophilus influenzae and, 42*b*
  Nocardia species and, 34*b*
  pathogens of, 6–8*t*
Cell wall, disruption of, antibiotics for, 8–11*t*
Central nervous system
  blastomycosis, 133*b*, 217*b*
  disease of, due to parasites, 143–144*t*
  infections, 213–220
  lymphoma, Epstein-Barr virus and, 98*b*
Cervical adenitis, *Mycobacterium avium* complex and, 34*b*
Cervical cancer, 118*b*
Cervicitis, pathogens of, 6–8*t*
Cestodes, 142*t*, 175–179, 175*b*
  intestinal, 176–178, 176*t*
  tissue, 176*t*, 178–179
Chickenpox, 96, 96*b*
Chitin, 119
Chlamydia trachomatis, 78*b*, 78*t*, 82–83, 82*b*, 264, 271, 277
  pelvic inflammatory disease and Reiter syndrome, 211*b*
  pneumonia in newborn infants, 83*b*, 197*b*
  trachoma, 249*b*
Chlamydophila pneumoniae, 79*t*
Chlamydophila psittaci, 79*t*
Cholangitis, caused by *Clonorchis sinensis*, 174*b*, 254*b*
Chromoblastomycosis, 127*t*
Chronic granulomatous disease (CGD), 61
Chronic obstructive pulmonary disease (COPD), 187
Chronic Q fever, 81*b*
Cidofovir, 90*t*
*Clonorchis sinensis*1, 2, 3. *See Opisthorchis sinensis*
  cholangitis caused by, 174*b*
  egg of, 169*f*

Clostridioides difficile, 63–64*t*, 67–68, 67*b*, 198, 258, 258*f*, 272
  colitis, 69*b*, 206*b*
Clostridium, 63–64
Clostridium botulinum, 63–64*t*, 65–66, 65*b*, 266, 279
  infection, 219*b*
Clostridium perfringens, 63–64*t*, 66–67, 66*b*, 68*f*, 198, 262, 275
  food poisoning, 199*b*
  gastroenteritis, 69*b*, 200*b*
  sepsis, 239*b*
Clostridium septicum, sepsis with occult malignancy, 247*b*
Clostridium tetani, 63–64*t*, 64–65, 64*b*
  infection, 219*b*
CMV pneumonia post-bone marrow transplant, 190*b*
Coagulase-negative staphylococci, 13
Cocci
  aerobic Gram-negative, 37–48, 37*b*, 38–39*t*
  aerobic Gram-positive, 12–23, 12*b*
  Gram-positive, 64
Coccidia, 149–151
Coccidioides immitis, 128*t*, 130–131, 130*f*, 131*b*, 263, 263*f*, 275–276
Coccidioides posadasii, 128*t*, 130–131, 131*b*
Coccidioidomycosis, 128*t*, 130, 133*b*, 195*b*
Coccobacilli, aerobic Gram-negative, 37–48, 37*b*, 38–39*t*
Colitis
  Clostridioides difficile, 69*b*, 206*b*
  pseudomembranous, 67*b*
Common colds, 182, 182*t*
Congenital cytomegalovirus (CMV), 217*b*
Congenital syphilis, 74*b*, 226*b*
Conidia, 3
Conjunctivitis
  adult inclusion, 82*b*
  neonatal, 82*b*
  pathogens of, 6–8*t*
Corneal blindness, herpes simplex virus and, 95*b*
Coronaviridae, 85–86*t*
Coronaviruses, 102–103, 103*b*, 187
Corynebacterium, 24
  contaminated blood cultures with, 246*b*

Corynebacterium diphtheriae, 24*t*, 28–29, 28*b*, 265, 278
COVID-19 pandemic, 225*b*, 233*b*
Coxiella burnetii, 78*t*, 81–82, 82*b*, 281
  endocarditis, 237*b*
  clinical case, 83*b*
Coxsackievirus A, 267, 279–280
Croup, parainfluenza viruses and, 104
Cryptococcal brain abscess, in HIV patient, 216*b*
Cryptococcosis, 139*b*, 232*b*
Cryptococcus neoformans, 136–137, 136*b*, 136*f*, 269
Cryptosporidiosis, 159*b*, 203*b*
Cryptosporidium spp., 149, 150*f*, 151*b*
Curvularia, 138*t*
Cutaneous anthrax, *Bacillus anthracis* and, 25*b*
Cutaneous blastomycosis, 231*b*
Cutaneous diphtheria, *Corynebacterium diphtheriae* and, 28*b*
Cutaneous fungi, 123–127, 123*b*
  dermatophytosis, 123–125, 127*b*
  fungal keratitis, 125–126
  lymphocutaneous sporotrichosis, 123, 126–127, 126*b*
Cutaneous leishmaniasis, 157*b*
Cutaneous manifestations, viruses responsible for, 87*t*
Cyclospora, 266, 266*f*, 279
Cyclospora cayetanensis, 148*t*, 150*b*, 150*f*
Cyclospora infection, in immunocompetent traveller, 204*b*
Cysticercosis, 176*t*
Cystitis, 208
  pathogens of, 6–8*t*
Cystoisospora belli, 148*t*, 151*b*
Cytokines, in HIV, 92
Cytomegalovirus (CMV), 94–95*t*, 97–98, 97*t*, 260, 273
  congenital, 97*b*
  pneumonia, 97*b*
    post-bone marrow transplant, 99*b*
  retinitis, 97*b*
Cytotoxin, 67

D

Delta retroviruses, 91*t*, 92
Dematiaceous mold, 119
Dengue virus, 264, 277
Dermatophytosis, 123–125, 229*b*
  in immunocompromised host, 127*b*

Dialysis-associated peritonitis, pathogens of, 6–8t
Diamidines, 145t
Diarrhea
 antibiotic-associated, 63–64, 67b
  pathogens of, 6–8t
 rotavirus and, 113
Dimorphic fungi, 3, 119
 systemic, 128–133, 128b, 128t
  Blastomyces dermatitidis, 129–130, 129b, 129f
  Coccidioides immitis, 130–131, 130f, 131b
  Coccidioides posadasii, 130–131, 131b
  Histoplasma capsulatum, 131–133, 132b, 132f
Diphtheria, 28
 cutaneous, *Corynebacterium diphtheriae* and, 28b
 respiratory, *Corynebacterium diphtheriae* and, 28b
Diphyllobothriasis, 179b, 207b
Diphyllobothrium latum, 175b, 176t
 egg of, 175f
Dipylidium caninum, 175, 176t, 178b
Disseminated disease
 herpes simplex virus and, 95b
 Mycobacterium avium complex and, 34b
Disseminated histoplasmosis, 133b, 233b
Disseminated leishmaniasis, 157b
Disseminated nocardiosis, 35b, 215b
DNA viruses, 85, 85–86t
Drug-resistant giardiasis, 159b
Drug-resistant giardiasis infection, in AIDS patient, 204b
Drug-resistant *Mycobacterium tuberculosis*, 35b, 191b

E

Early-onset neonatal disease, *Listeria monocytogenes* and, 27b
Echinococcosis, 179b
 in pregnant woman, 196b
Echinococcus granulosus, 176t, 178, 179b
Echinococcus multilocularis, 176t
Ehrlichia chaffeensis, 78t, 80–81, 80b
Ehrlichia phagocytophila. See Anaplasma phagocytophilum
Ehrlichiosis, human monocytic, 80b

Eikenella corrodens, 37–38t, 40–41, 41b
 bite wound infections, 234b
Elephantiasis, 165t
Empyema, pathogens of, 6–8t
Encephalitis, 96b, 213
 granulomatous amebic, 153b
 herpes simplex virus and, 95b
 pathogens of, 6–8t
 viruses responsible for, 88t
Endocarditis
 Coxiella burnetii, 237b
  clinical case, 83b
 Enterococcus faecalis, 236b
 Kingella kingae, 237b
 Lactobacillus, 64, 69b, 237b
 pathogens of, 6–8t
 Staphylococcus aureus and, 23b, 236b
 Staphylococcus epidermidis, 236b
 Staphylococcus lugdunensis, 236b
 Streptococcus mutans and, 23b
 subacute, *Kingella kingae* and, 41b
Endogenous infection(s), 3, 134
Endophthalmitis, 248b
 pathogens of, 6–8t
 traumatic, *Bacillus cereus*, 29b
Entamoeba histolytica, 148t, 149b, 149f, 198, 269
Entecavir, 89t
Enteric hepatitis viruses, 108
Enteritis
 Campylobacter jejuni, 77b
 necrotizing, 66b
Enterobacteriaceae, 49, 50–51t
 Escherichia coli, 51–52, 51b, 51f
 Klebsiella pneumoniae, 50–51t, 52–53, 53b, 53f
 Proteus mirabilis, 50–51t, 53–54, 53b
 Salmonella species, 54–55, 54b, 54f
 Shigella species, 55–56, 55b
 Vibrio cholerae, 57–58, 57b
 Yersinia pestis, 50–51t, 56–57, 56b
Enterobiasis, 161b
Enterobius vermicularis, 161b, 161t
Enterococcus, 12, 12t
 important, 15, 15t, 22–23, 22b
Enterococcus faecalis, 15t, 261, 261f, 273
 endocarditis, 236b
Enterococcus faecium, 15t, 22f
Enterocolitis, 151b
Enterohemorrhagic *Escherichia coli* (EHEC), 205b

Enterotoxigenic *Escherichia coli* gastroenteritis, 203b
Enterotoxin, 67
Epidermophyton floccosum, 124f
Epidural abscess, 213
Epiglottitis, 182, 182t
 Haemophilus influenzae and, 42b
Epstein-Barr virus (EBV), 94–95t, 98–99, 98b, 117, 117t, 265, 278
 infectious mononucleosis associated with agranulocytosis, 99b, 251b
 lymphoma IN HIV patient, 217b
Ergosterol, 119
Erysipelas, 17b
 pathogens of, 6–8t
Erythromycin, 266, 266f, 279
Escherichia coli, 50–51t, 51–52, 51b, 51f, 208
 bacteremia, 242b
 meningitis in neonate, 214b
 urinary tract infections, 209b
Eukaryotic organisms, 3
Eumycotic mycetoma, 127t
Exanthema subitum, 99
Exogenous infection(s), 3, 134
External otitis, 182
Extraintestinal amebiasis, 149b
Extrapulmonary tuberculosis, *Mycobacterium tuberculosis* and, 32b
Eye disease, due to parasites, 143–144t
Eye infections
 herpes simplex virus and, 95b
 Pseudomonas aeruginosa, 248b
 traumatic, *Bacillus cereus* and, 26b
Eye worm, 166b

F

Facultative anaerobes, 2, 5
Famciclovir, 90t
Fasciola hepatica, 168–169t, 170
Fascioliasis, 174b, 254b
Fasciolopsis buski, 168–169t, 169
 egg of, 169f
Fatal *Corynebacterium diphtheriae* infection, 184b
Febrile seizures, 99
Filariasis, 165t
Filoviridae, 85–86t
Flaccid paralysis, 65
Flagellate, 142t, 151–153
Flatworms. *See* Trematodes

Flaviviridae, 85–86*t*, 110
Flea, 180*t*
Flukes. *See* Trematodes
Fly, 180*t*
Folic acid antagonists, 145*t*
Folliculitis, 221*t*
    pathogens of, 6–8*t*
    Pseudomonas, 62*b*
Food-borne botulism, 65*b*
Food intoxication, pathogens of, 6–8*t*
Food poisoning, 66*b*
    staphylococcal, 23*b*, 278–279
Foscarnet, 90*t*
Francisella tularensis, 38–39*t*, 46–47,
        46*b*, 269
    pneumonia, 195*b*
    ulceroglandular tularemia, 230*b*
        cat-associated, 230*b*
Fulminant sepsis, 20*b*
Fulminant septicemia, *Streptococcus
        pneumoniae* and, 239*b*
Fungal keratitis, 123
Fungi, 1–2*t*, 3, 119–121
    antifungal agents, 121, 122*t*
    classification of, 119–120, 120*t*
    cutaneous and subcutaneous,
        123–127, 123*b*
    opportunistic. (*see* Opportunistic
        fungi)
    role in disease, 120–121, 120–121*t*
    systemic dimorphic, 128–133, 128*b*,
        128*t*
    yeast-like, 137
Furuncles, 221*t*
    pathogens of, 6–8*t*
Fusariosis, 139*b*, 245*b*
Fusarium, 138*t*, 139*f*
Fusobacterium, 270

G

Ganciclovir, 90*t*
Gastric adenocarcinoma, 73*b*
Gastritis, 73*b*, 198
    pathogens of, 6–8*t*
Gastroenteritis, 69*b*
    Bacillus cereus and, 26*b*
    bacterial, 72, 72*b*
    Clostridium perfringens, 69*b*
    Listeria, 29*b*
    pathogens of, 6–8*t*
Gastrointestinal anthrax, *Bacillus
        anthracis* and, 25*b*

Gastrointestinal symptoms, viral
        infections, 88
Gastrointestinal tract infections,
        198–207
Gastrointestinal viruses, 113–116, 113*b*
    adenovirus, 116, 116*b*
    astrovirus, 115–116, 115*b*
    norovirus, 114–115, 114*b*, 116*b*
    rotavirus, 113–114, 114*b*, 116*b*
    sapovirus, 114–115, 114*b*
Genital caner, 117
Genital herpes infection, in patient with
        diabetes mellitus, 210*b*
Genital infections, 208
    herpes simplex virus and, 95*b*
Genital ulcers, 208
    pathogens of, 6–8*t*
Genitourinary tract disease, due to
        parasites, 143–144*t*
Genitourinary tract infections, 118*b*,
        208–212
Germs, 3
Giardia duodenalis, 148*t*, 152*b*, 152*f*
Giardiasis, 152*b*
    drug-resistant, 159*b*
Glomerulonephritis, acute, 17*b*
Glucan, 119
Gonococcal arthritis, 250*b*
Gonorrhea, *Neisseria gonorrhoeae* and,
        38*b*
Gram-negative bacteria, 2, 6*t*
Gram-negative rods
    aerobic fermentative, 49–58, 49*b*
        Escherichia coli, 50–51*t*, 51–52,
            51*b*, 51*f*
        Klebsiella pneumoniae, 50–51*t*,
            52–53, 53*b*, 53*f*
        Proteus mirabilis, 50–51*t*, 53–54,
            53*b*
        Salmonella species, 54–55, 54*b*,
            54*f*
        Shigella species, 55–56, 55*b*
        Vibrio cholerae, 57–58, 57*b*
        Yersinia pestis, 50–51*t*, 56–57, 56*b*
    aerobic nonfermentative, 59–62, 59*b*
        Burkholderia cepacia, 59*t*, 61, 61*b*
        Pseudomonas aeruginosa, 59*t*,
            60–61, 60*b*, 60*f*
        Stenotrophomonas maltophilia,
            61–62, 62*b*, 62*f*
Gram-positive bacteria, 2
Gram-positive cocci, 64

Gram-positive rods, aerobic, 24–29, 24*b*
    Bacillus anthracis, 25–27, 25*b*
    Bacillus cereus, 24*t*, 25–27, 26*b*, 27*f*
    clinically important species of, 24*t*
    Corynebacterium diphtheriae, 28–29,
        28*b*
    Listeria monocytogenes, 27–28, 27*b*,
        28*f*
Gram stain, 5
Granuloma, 31
Granulomatous amebic encephalitis,
        153*b*
Granulomatous infections, pathogens
        of, 6–8*t*
Group A *Streptococcus*, 182
Guillain-Barré syndrome, 72*b*, 77*b*, 97*b*

H

Haemophilus influenzae, 38–39*t*, 42–43,
        42*b*, 42*f*, 281
    meningitis caused by, 214*b*
    pneumonia caused by, 48*b*, 187*b*
    type B epiglottitis, 185*b*
Health care workers, pertussis outbreak
        in, 48*b*
Heart disease, due to parasites, 143–144*t*
Helicobacter pylori, 71*t*, 73–74, 73*b*, 198
    peptic ulcers, 200*b*
β-Hemolytic streptococci, 14, 14*t*, 17–20
Hemolytic uremic syndrome, 55*b*, 205*b*
Hepadnaviridae, 85–86*t*
Hepatic ascariasis, 253*b*
Hepatic cells, hepatitis B virus and, 109
Hepatitis A infections, 252*b*
Hepatitis A vaccine, 255, 269
Hepatitis A virus, 108*t*, 109, 109*b*
Hepatitis B infections, 252*b*
Hepatitis B virus, 108*t*, 109–110, 109*b*,
        117*t*
Hepatitis C infections, 253*b*
Hepatitis C virus, 108*t*, 110–111, 110*t*,
        111*b*, 117*t*
Hepatitis D virus, 108*t*, 109–110, 109*b*
Hepatitis E virus, 108*t*, 111–112, 111*b*
Hepatitis viruses, 108–112, 108*b*
    hepatitis A virus, 108*t*, 109, 109*b*
    hepatitis B virus, 108*t*, 109–110, 109*b*
    hepatitis C virus, 108*t*, 110–111, 110*t*,
        111*b*
    hepatitis D virus, 108*t*, 109–110, 109*b*
    hepatitis E virus, 108*t*, 111–112, 111*b*
    infections of, antiviral agents for, 89*t*

Herpes labialis, herpes simplex virus and, 95*b*
Herpes simplex virus, 256, 269
　neonatal, 99*b*
　type 1 (HSV-1), 94–95*t*, 95–96
　type 2 (HSV-2), 94–95*t*, 95–96
Herpesviridae, 85–86*t*
Herpesvirus infections, antiviral agents for, 90*t*
Herpes zoster ophthalmicus, 96*b*
Heterophile antibodies, 98*b*
Histoplasma capsulatum, 128*t*, 131–133, 132*b*, 132*f*, 269
Histoplasmosis, 128*t*, 131, 189*b*
　disseminated, 133*b*
H5N1 avian influenza, 107*b*, 193*b*
Hodgkin disease, 216*b*
Hookworm
　infections, 163*b*
　infectious larvae of, direct skin penetration by, 263, 276
Hortaea werneckii, 123*t*
Host, of trematodes
　intermediate, 168
　primary, 168
H proteins, 50
HPV-associated nasopharyngeal carcinoma, 118*b*
HPV-associated oropharyngeal carcinomas, 185*b*
HPV type 16 penile cancer, 212*b*
HSV-1 gingivostomatitis, 185*b*
Human
　as *Entamoeba histolytica* host, 262, 262*f*, 275
　as nematode host, 160
Human adult T-cell leukemia virus type 1 (HTLV-1), 117*t*
Human granulocytic anaplasmosis, 228*b*
Human herpesviruses, 94–100, 94*b*
　alpha herpesviruses, 95
　beta herpesviruses, 95
　gamma herpesviruses, 95
　human herpesvirus 6 (HHV-6), 94–95*t*, 99–100
　　exanthem subitum, 226*b*
　human herpesvirus 7 (HHV-7), 94–95*t*, 99–100
　human herpesvirus 8 (HHV-8), 94–95*t*, 99–100, 117*t*
　human pathogens of, 94–95*t*

Human immunodeficiency virus (HIV), 88, 91–93, 91*b*, 93*b*
　and amebic liver abscess, 207*b*
　HIV-1, 92–93
　　group M, 92
　　transmission of, 92
　HIV-2, 92
　　laboratory diagnosis of, 92
　incidence of, 91
　infections of, antiviral agents for, 89*t*
Human metapneumovirus, 106–107, 106*b*
Human monocytic ehrlichiosis, 80*b*, 243*b*
Human papillomavirus (HPV), 117–118, 117–118*b*, 117*t*
Hyaline mold, 119
Hymenolepis diminuta, 176*t*, 177
　egg of, 177*f*
Hymenolepis nana, 175, 176*t*, 177, 178*b*
　egg of, 177*f*
　infection in pregnant woman, 207*b*
Hyperinfection, *Strongyloides*, 167*b*
Hyphae, 3, 119

I

Idoxuridine, 90*t*
Immunoassays, for HIV diagnosis
　laboratory-based, 92
　rapid point-of-care, 92
Impetigo, 221*t*
　pathogens of, 6–8*t*
Inclusion conjunctivitis, adult, 82*b*
India ink, 136*b*
Infant botulism, 65*b*, 69*b*, 219*b*
Infant pneumonia, 82*b*
Infections
　disseminated, *Neisseria gonorrhoeae* and, 38*b*
　due to *Bacteroides fragilis*, 69*b*
　eye. (*see* Eye infections)
　opportunistic. (*see* Opportunistic infections)
　orofacial, herpes simplex virus and, 95*b*
　prosthetic-associated, pathogens of, 6–8*t*
　respiratory. (*see* Respiratory infections)
　urogenital, from *Chlamydia trachomatis*, 82*b*

Infectious mononucleosis, 97*b*
　Epstein-Barr virus and, 98*b*
　associated with agranulocytosis, 99*b*
Influenza A, 103–104
Influenza B, 103–104
Influenza C, 103–104
Influenza viruses, 103–104, 104*b*, 107*b*
Inhalation anthrax (bioterrorism), 29*b*, 241*b*
　Bacillus anthracis and, 25*b*
Inhalation botulism, 65*b*
Insect vector, blood nematodes, 165
Integrase strand inhibitors, 89*t*
Intestinal amebiasis, 149*b*
Intestinal *Bacillus anthracis* disease, with sepsis, 29*b*
Intestinal cestodes, 176–178, 176*t*
　antiparasitic agents for, 145–147*t*
Intestinal nematodes, 160–165, 160*t*
　antiparasitic agents for, 145–147*t*
Intestinal protozoa, 148*t*
　antiparasitic agents for, 145–147*t*
Intestinal tract disease, due to parasites, 143–144*t*
Intestinal trematodes, 168–169*t*, 169–170
　antiparasitic agents for, 145–147*t*
Intracellular bacteria, 78–83, 78*b*
　bacteria related to, 79*t*
　　Chlamydia trachomatis, 78*b*, 78*t*, 82–83, 82*b*
　　Coxiella burnetii, 78*t*, 81–82, 82*b*
　　Ehrlichia chaffeensis, 78*t*, 80–81, 80*b*
　　Rickettsia rickettsii, 78–79*b*, 78*t*, 79–80
Invasive aspergillosis, in renal transplant patient, 190*b*
Invasive cervical carcinoma, 212*b*

K

K antigens, 50
Kaposi sarcoma, 99
　in HIV patients, 232*b*
Keratitis, 153*b*
　fungal, 123
　pathogens of, 6–8*t*
Kingella kingae, 38–39*t*, 41, 41*b*
　endocarditis, 237*b*
Klebsiella pneumoniae, 50–51*t*, 52–53, 53*b*, 53*f*

Klebsiella pneumoniae pneumonia, 188*b*
Klebsiella pneumoniae-producing
    carbapenemases (KPC), 52

L

Lactobacillus, 208
    bacteremia, 240*b*
    endocarditis, 64, 69*b*, 237*b*
Lactose, fermentation of, 50
Lamivudine, 89*t*
Laryngeal carcinoma, 118*b*
Laryngitis, 182, 182*t*
Late-onset neonatal disease, *Listeria*
    monocytogenes and, 27*b*
Legionella pneumophila, 256, 269–270
Leishmaniasis
    cutaneous, 157*b*
    disseminated, 157*b*
    mucocutaneous, 157*b*
    visceral, 157*b*
Leishmania spp., 148*t*, 156, 157*b*
Lentivirus, 91*t*
Lepromatous leprosy, 31
    Mycobacterium leprae and, 33*b*
Leprosy
    lepromatous, 31*t*, 33*b*
        Mycobacterium leprae and, 33*b*
    tuberculoid, 31
Leptospira interrogans, 267, 280
Leptospira species, 71*t*, 76–77, 76*b*
Leptospirosis, 76, 76*b*, 250*b*, 280
    in triathlon participants, 77*b*
Lethal toxins, 66, 66*b*
Lice, 180*t*
Lipid A, 50
Lipopolysaccharide (LPS), 50
Listeria, 24
    gastroenteritis and bacteremia, 29*b*,
        204*b*
Listeria meningitis, in
        immunocompromised man, 29*b*,
        215*b*
Listeria monocytogenes, 24*t*, 27–28, 27*b*,
        28*f*, 257, 270, 281
Liver cirrhosis, 254*b*
Liver disease, due to parasites, 143–144*t*
Loa loa, 166*b*
Loa loa infection, 249*b*
Loiasis, 166*b*
Louse, 267, 280
Lower respiratory tract infections, 187
    case studies, 187–197*b*

Lung disease, due to parasites, 143–144*t*
Lyme disease, 75, 75*b*, 224*b*
Lymphatics, due to parasites, 143–144*t*
Lymphocutaneous disease, *Nocardia*
        species and, 34*b*
Lymphocutaneous sporotrichosis, 123,
        126–127, 126*b*
Lymphogranuloma venereum, 82*b*, 211*b*
Lymphoproliferative disease, Epstein-
        Barr virus and, 98*b*

M

Malaria, 154*b*, 159*b*, 243*b*
Malassezia, 137*t*
Malassezia furfur, 123*t*, 124*f*, 269
    infections, 227*b*
Medical microbiology
    microbial classification, 1–2*t*
    overview of, 2–3
Melioidosis, 60
Meningitis, 20*b*, 136, 213
    aseptic, complicating acute HSV-2
        proctitis, 99*b*
    Haemophilus influenzae and, 42*b*,
        214*b*
    Listeria, in immunocompromised
        man, 29*b*
    Neisseria meningitidis, 40*b*
    pathogens of, 6–8*t*
    Streptococcus pneumoniae, 214*b*
    viruses responsible for, 88*t*
Meningococcal disease, 40*b*
Meningococcemia, *Neisseria*
        meningitidis, 40*b*
Merkel cell polyomavirus, 117*t*
MERS-CoV, 102–103
    infection, 194*b*
Microbes
    classification of, 1–2*t*
    good *versus* bad, 3
Microbiome, 3
Microsporidia, 137*t*
Microsporum canis, 124*f*
Miscellaneous infections, 248–254
Mite, 180*t*
Molds, 3, 119
Moraxella catarrhalis, 38–39*t*, 41–42,
        41*f*, 42*b*
Moraxella catarrhalis
        bronchopneumonia, 188*b*
Morulae, 80
Mosquito, 180*t*

Mucocutaneous leishmaniasis, 157*b*
Mucorales, 138*t*
Mucormycosis
    in COVID-19 patient, 233*b*
    subcutaneous, 127*t*
Muscle disease, due to parasites,
        143–144*t*
Mycetoma, *Nocardia* species and, 34*b*
Mycobacteria
    "rapid-growing," 30
    slow-growing, 30
Mycobacterial infections associated with
        nail salons, 222*b*
Mycobacterium and *pneumocystis*
        lymphadenitis, 232*b*
Mycobacterium avium, 34, 34*b*
Mycobacterium avium complex, 31*t*, 32*f*,
        34, 34*b*
Mycobacterium avium infection, in
        AIDS patient, 191*b*
Mycobacterium avium-intracellular
        (MAI) infection, in HIV patient,
        251*b*
Mycobacterium catheter associated
        bacteremia, 245*b*
Mycobacterium leprae, 31*t*, 33–34, 33*b*
Mycobacterium leprae infection, 228*b*
Mycobacterium tuberculosis, 31*f*, 31*t*,
        32–33, 32*b*
    drug-resistant, 35*b*
Mycolic acids, 30
Myocarditis, 235
    pathogens of, 6–8*t*
    viruses responsible for, 88*t*
Myonecrosis, 66*b*

N

Naegleria fowleri, 280
Naegleria spp., 148*t*, 153*b*
Nail salons, mycobacterial infections
        associated w, 35*b*
Nasopharyngeal carcinoma, Epstein-
        Barr virus and, 98*b*
Necator americanus, 161*t*, 163*b*
Necrotizing cellulitis, pathogens of, 6–8*t*
Necrotizing enteritis, 66*b*
Necrotizing fasciitis, 221*t*, 223*b*
    Bacteroides fragilis, 224*b*
    Pasteurella multocida, 223*b*
    pathogens of, 6–8*t*
    streptococcal, 17*b*
    Streptococcus pyogenes, 223*b*

Neisseria gonorrhoeae, 37–38*t*, 38–39, 38*b*, 38*f*, 271
  arthritis, 250*b*
  urethritis, 210*b*
Neisseria meningitidis, 37–38*t*, 39–40, 39*f*, 40*b*, 268, 268*f*, 281
  pneumonia, 194*b*
  sepsis, 241*b*
Nematodes, 142*t*, 160–167, 160*b*, 160*t*
  in blood, 165–167, 165*t*
  intestinal, 160–165, 160*t*
  tissue, 167
Neonatal conjunctivitis, 82*b*
Neonatal HSV infection, 228*b*
Neurocysticercosis, 179*b*, 218*b*
Neurosyphilis, 74*b*
Nitrofurans, 145*t*
Nitromidazoles, 145*t*
Nocardia abscessus, 259, 259*f*, 273
Nocardia farcinica, 255*f*, 256, 269
Nocardia species, 31*t*
  acid-fast stain of, 35*f*
  Gram stain of, 35*f*
Noninflammatory intestinal infections, 198
Non-nucleoside reverse transcriptase inhibitors, 89*t*
Nonsuppurative diseases, 17
Normal flora, 3
Norovirus, 114–115, 114*b*, 201*b*
  outbreak, 116*b*
  transmission on cruise ship, 201*b*
Novel viruses, 103–104
Nucleic acid amplification tests
  for *Chlamydia trachomatis*, 82*b*
  for HIV diagnosis, 92
Nucleic acid synthesis, inhibition of, 8–11*t*
Nucleoside and nucleotide reverse transcriptase inhibitors, 89*t*

O

Oculoglandular tularemia, *Francisella tularensis* and, 46*b*
Onchocerca volvulus, 166*b*
  in onchocerciasis, 165*t*
Onchocerciasis, 166*b*, 227*b*
Onychomycosis, 123
Opisthorchis sinensis, 265, 265*f*, 278
O polysaccharide, 50
Opportunistic fungi, 134–139, 134*b*
  Aspergillus fumigatus as, 137–138, 137*f*, 138*b*

Opportunistic fungi *(Continued)*
  Candida albicans and related species as, 134–136, 134*t*, 135*b*, 135*f*
  Cryptococcus neoformans as, 136–137, 136*b*, 136*f*
Opportunistic infections
  Bacillus cereus, 26*b*
  HIV virus, 92
Opportunistic molds, 138
Orientia scrub typhus, 225*b*
Orientia tsutsugamushi, 79*t*
Orofacial infections, herpes simplex virus and, 95*b*
Oropharyngeal caner, 117
Orthomyxoviridae, 85–86*t*
Oseltamivir, 90*t*
Osteomyelitis, pathogens of, 6–8*t*
Otitis externa, pathogens of, 6–8*t*
Otitis media, 20*b*, 182, 182*t*
  pathogens of, 6–8*t*
  respiratory syncytial virus and, 105
Outer membrane, 5

P

Paecilomyces, 138*t*
Painless ulcer, 82*b*
Papillomaviridae, 85–86*t*
Paracoccidioides brasiliensis, 129
  infection, 231*b*
Paracoccidioidomycosis, 129
Paragonimiasis, 174*b*, 196*b*
Paragonimus westermani, 168–169*t*, 170, 171*b*
Parainfluenza viruses (PIV), 104–105, 105*b*
  in neonatal intensive care unit, 197*b*
Paralysis
  flaccid, 65
  spastic, 64
Paramyxoviridae, 85–86*t*, 104
Parasites, 1–2*t*, 3, 141–145
  antiparasitic agents for, 144–145, 145–147*t*
  classification of, 141–143, 142*t*
  role in disease, 143–144, 143–144*t*
Paronychia, pathogens of, 6–8*t*
Parvoviridae, 85–86*t*
Pasteurella, 256, 270
Pasteurella multocida, necrotizing fasciitis, 223*b*
Pathogens, opportunistic, 59*t*
Pelvic actinomycosis, 69*b*, 211*b*
  Chlamydia trachomatis, 211*b*

Pelvic inflammatory disease, 83*b*, 211*b*
Penciclovir, 90*t*
Penicilliosis, 129
Penile carcinoma, 118*b*
Peptic ulcers, 73*b*
Peptostreptococcus anaerobius, 274
Pericarditis, 235
  pathogens of, 6–8*t*
  viruses responsible for, 88*t*
Peritonitis, pathogens of, 6–8*t*
Pertussis, *Bordetella pertussis* and, 45*b*
Pertussis toxin, 45*b*
Phaeohyphomycosis, subcutaneous, 127*t*
Pharyngitis, 17*b*, 182, 182*t*
  pathogens of, 6–8*t*
Phase I variants, of *Coxiella burnetii*, 81
Phase II variants, of *Coxiella burnetii*, 81
Phosphocholine analog, 145*t*
Picornaviridae, 85–86*t*
Picornavirus family, 109
Piedraia hortae, 123*t*
Piperazine, 145*t*
Plague, 56
Plasmodium spp., 148*t*, 154, 154*b*, 154*f*
Plasmodium vivax, 281
Pneumocystis, 137*t*
Pneumocystis jiroveci, 137*f*, 261, 261*f*, 274
Pneumocystis pneumonia, in newly diagnosed HIV/AIDS patient, 192*b*
Pneumonia, 96*b*
  Chlamydia trachomatis, in newborn infants, 83*b*
  CMV, post-bone marrow transplant, 99*b*
  infant, 82*b*
  Neisseria meningitidis and, 40*b*
  pathogens of, 6–8*t*
  Streptococcus pneumoniae and, 20*b*, 23*b*
Pneumonic plague, 56*b*
Pneumonic tularemia, *Francisella tularensis* and, 46*b*
Polyomaviridae, 85–86*t*
Polysaccharide capsule, 136
Poxviridae, 85–86*t*
Primary amebic meningoencephalitis, *Naegleria* spp. in, 153*b*
Primary fungal infection, 221*t*

Proctitis
  HSV-2, aseptic meningitis
    complicating, 99*b*
  pathogens of, 6–8*t*
Proglottids, 175
Prokaryotic organisms, 2
Propionibacterium, shunt infected with, 69*b*
Prostatitis, 208
  pathogens of, 6–8*t*
Prosthetic-associated infection,
    pathogens of, 6–8*t*
Protease inhibitors, for HIV infections, 90*t*
Proteus mirabilis, 50–51*t*, 53–54, 53*b*
  urinary tract infection, 209*b*
Protozoa, 3, 141, 142*t*, 148–159, 148*t*, 149*b*
"Pseudoappendicitis,", 56
Pseudomembranous colitis, 67*b*
Pseudomonas, 60
Pseudomonas aeruginosa, 59*t*, 60–61, 60*b*, 60*f*, 182, 223*b*
  ear infection, 186*b*
  eye infection, 248*b*
  pneumonia, 189*b*
Pseudomonas folliculitis, 62*b*, 223*b*
Psittacosis, 195*b*
  in previously healthy man, 83*b*
Pulmonary disease, *Mycobacterium avium* complex and, 34*b*
Pyelonephritis, 208
  pathogens of, 6–8*t*
Pyoderma, 17*b*

Q

Q (query) fever, 81, 81*b*

R

Reactive arthritis, 72*b*
Reinfection, in patient with SARS-COV-2, 194*b*
Reiter syndrome, 83*b*, 211*b*
Renal abscess, pathogens of, 6–8*t*
Renal calculi, pathogens of, 6–8*t*
Reoviridae, 85–86*t*
Respiratory diphtheria, 183*b*
  Corynebacterium diphtheriae and, 28*b*
Respiratory infections
  antiviral agents for, 90*t*
  viruses responsible for, 87–88*t*

Respiratory syncytial virus (RSV), 105–106, 105*b*
  infection, 197*b*
Respiratory viruses, 101–107, 101*b*
  adenovirus, 107
  coronaviruses, 102–103, 103*b*
  human metapneumovirus, 106–107, 106*b*
  influenza viruses, 103–104, 104*b*, 107*b*
  parainfluenza viruses, 104–105, 105*b*
  respiratory syncytial virus, 105–106, 105*b*
  rhinoviruses, 101–102, 102*b*
Retinitis, CMV, 97*b*
Retroviridae, 85–86*t*, 91, 91*t*
Rhabdoviridae, 85–86*t*
Rheumatic fever, acute, *Streptococcus pyogenes* associated with, 17*b*, 23*b*
Rhinoviruses, 101–102, 102*b*
Rhizopus, 139*f*, 259, 259*f*, 272
Rhodococcus equi, 273
  pulmonary infection, 191*b*
Rhodotorula, 137*t*
Ribavirin, 90*t*
Rickettsia akari, 79*t*
Rickettsialpox, 224*b*
  in New York City, clinical case of, 83*b*
Rickettsia prowazekii, 79*t*
  epidemic typhus, 225*b*
Rickettsia rickettsii, 78–79*b*, 78*t*, 79–80
Rickettsia typhi, 79, 79*t*
  murine typhus, 225*b*
River blindness, 166*b*
RNA viruses, 85, 85–86*t*
Rocky Mountain spotted fever, 78*b*, 80*b*, 224*b*
Rods
  Gram-negative. (*see* Gram-negative rods)
  Gram-positive. (*see* Gram-positive rods)
Rotavirus, 113–114, 114*b*, 116*b*
  severe infection in infant, 116*b*

S

Salmonella gastroenteritis, 206*b*
Salmonella species, 54–55, 54*b*, 54*f*, 275
Salmonella typhi infection, 242*b*
  clinical case in, 54*f*, 58*b*
Sandfly, 157*b*

Sapovirus, 114–115, 114*b*
SARS-CoV, 102–103
SARS-CoV-2, 194*b*, 225*b*, 233*b*
SARS infection, 107*b*, 193*b*
Scarlet fever, 17*b*
Scedosporium, 138*t*
Schistosoma haematobium, 168–169*t*, 172*f*, 173*b*
  infection in Italian family, 212*b*
Schistosoma japonica, 168–169*t*, 173*b*
Schistosoma mansoni, 168–169*t*, 172*b*
Schistosomiasis, 174*b*, 218*b*
Scolex, 175
Seizures, febrile, 99
Sepsis, 235
  Bacillus anthracis disease with, 241*b*
  Brucella melitensis, 242*b*
  catheter-related *Candida auris*, 245*b*
  Clostridium perfringens, 239*b*
  Clostridium septicum, with occult malignancy, 247*b*
  intestinal *Bacillus anthracis* disease with, 29*b*
  Neisseria meningitidis, 241*b*
  pathogens of, 6–8*t*
  Streptococcus gallolyticus, 246*b*
  Vibrio vulnificus, 239*b*
  Yersinia pestis, 242*b*
Septic arthritis, *Kingella kingae* and, 41*b*
Septic shock
  staphylococcal, 23*b*
  staphylococcal furuncle, 222*b*
  Streptococcus pyogenes, 223*b*
Septic thrombophlebitis, pathogens of, 6–8*t*
Septum, 119
Serology
  for *Ehrlichia chaffeensis*, 80*b*
  for Q (query) fever, 81*b*
  for *Rickettsia rickettsii*, 80*b*
Severe rotavirus infection, in infant, 200*b*
Severe sepsis, 235
Shiga toxin *Escherichia coli* (STEC), 205*b*
Shiga toxin-producing *Escherichia coli* (STEC) infections, 262, 275
Shigella gastroenteritis, in gay males, 205*b*
Shigella infections, in day-care centers, 205*b*

Shigella species, 55–56, 55*b*
Shigellosis, 55*b*
Shingles, 96
Shunt
  infected with *Cutibacterium*
      (*Propionibacterium*) acnes,
      216*b*
  infected with *Propionibacterium*, 69*b*
Simeprevir, 90*t*
Sinusitis, 20*b*, 182, 182*t*
  Moraxella catarrhalis and, 42*b*
  pathogens of, 6–8*t*
Skin and soft tissue infections, 221–234
Skin disease, due to parasites, 143–144*t*
Skin lesions, 221
Sofosbuvir, 90*t*
Somatic O polysaccharides, 50
South American blastomycosis, 129
Spastic paralysis, 64
Spiral-shaped bacteria, 71–77, 71*b*, 71*t*
  bacteria related to, 71*t*
  Borrelia burgdorferi, 75–76, 75*b*, 75*f*
  Campylobacter jejuni, 71*t*, 72–73,
      72*b*, 72*f*
  Helicobacter pylori, 73–74, 73*b*
  Leptospira species, 76–77, 76*b*
  Treponema pallidum, 74–75, 74*b*, 74*f*
Spleen disease, due to parasites,
    143–144*t*
Splenomegaly, 254*b*
Spores, 119
Sporothrix schenckii, 126, 126*f*, 260,
    260*f*, 273–274
Sporotrichosis, 230*b*
  lymphocutaneous, 123, 126–127,
      126*b*
Sporozoan, 142*t*
Spotted fever group, 79
Staphylococcal food poisoning,
    199*b*
Staphylococcal furuncle and septic
    shock, 222*b*
Staphylococcal scalded skin syndrome
    (SSSS), 222*b*
Staphylococcal toxic shock syndrome,
    238*b*
Staphylococcus, 12, 12*t*
  food poisoning by, 23*b*
  group B disease in neonate, 19*b*
  important, 13
  septic shock, 23*b*
  toxic shock syndrome, 23*b*

Staphylococcus aureus, 13, 13*f*, 13*t*,
    15–17, 15*b*, 182, 198, 235, 257,
    257*f*, 260, 270, 273
  endocarditis, 23*b*, 236*b*
  pneumonia, 192*b*
  scalded skin syndrome, 222*b*
Staphylococcus epidermidis, 13*t*, 270
  endocarditis, 236*b*
Staphylococcus lugdunensis, 13*t*
  endocarditis, 236*b*
Staphylococcus saprophyticus, 13*t*, 208,
    259, 272–273
  urinary tract infection, 209*b*
Stenotrophomonas infection, 240*b*
Stenotrophomonas maltophilia, 61–62,
    62*b*, 62*f*
Streptococcus, 12, 12*t*
  β-hemolytic, 14, 14*t*, 17–20
  important, 14
  toxic shock syndrome, 17*b*, 23*b*
  viridans, 14, 14*t*, 21–22, 21*b*
Streptococcus agalactiae, 14*t*, 19, 19*b*
Streptococcus agalactiae disease, in
    neonate, 214*b*
Streptococcus anginosus, 14*t*
  abscesses, 233*b*
Streptococcus dysgalactiae, 14*t*
Streptococcus dysgalactiae pharyngitis,
    183*b*
Streptococcus gallolyticus, 14–15*t*
  sepsis, 246*b*
Streptococcus mitis, 14*f*, 14–15*t*
Streptococcus mutans, 14–15*t*, 265, 278
  endocarditis caused by, 23*b*
  subacute endocarditis, 246*b*
Streptococcus pneumoniae, 14–15*t*,
    20–21, 20*b*, 20*f*, 257, 257*f*, 271
  fulminant septicemia, 239*b*
  meningitis, 214*b*
  pneumonia, 23*b*, 189*b*
Streptococcus pyogenes, 14*t*, 17, 17*b*, 263,
    276
  acute rheumatic fever associated with,
      23*b*, 238*b*
  necrotizing fasciitis and septic shock,
      223*b*
  pharyngitis and scarlet fever, 183*b*
Streptococcus salivarius, 14–15*t*
Strongyloides hyperinfection, 167*b*, 251*b*
Strongyloides stercoralis, 161*t*, 164*b*,
    164*f*, 268, 268*f*, 281
  in *Strongyloides* hyperinfection, 167*b*

Strongyloidiasis, 164*b*
Subacute endocarditis, 235
  Streptococcus mutans, 246*b*
Subacute endocarditis, *Kingella kingae*
    and, 41*b*
Subcutaneous abscesses, *Nocardia*
    species and, 34*b*
Subcutaneous fungi, 123–127, 123*b*
  dermatophytosis, 123–125, 127*b*
  fungal keratitis, 123
  sporotrichosis, lymphocutaneous,
      123, 126–127, 126*b*
Subcutaneous infections, other, 127
Subcutaneous mucormycosis, 127*t*
Subcutaneous phaeohyphomycosis, 127*t*
Subcutaneous tissue disease, due to
    parasites, 143–144*t*
Subdural empyema, pathogens of, 6–8*t*
Sulfated naphthylamine, 145*t*
Superantigens, 12
Suppurative diseases, 17
Suppurative myositis, 66*b*
Surgical wounds, pathogens of, 6–8*t*
Swine flu, 103–104
Sylvatic plague, 56*b*
Syphilis, 74, 74*b*
Systemic disease, due to parasites,
    143–144*t*

T

Taenia, egg of, 175*f*
Taenia saginata, 175, 176*t*
Taenia solium, 176*t*
Talaromyces (*Penicillium*) *marneffei*, 129
Talaromyces marneffei infection, in
    HIV/AIDS patient, 229*b*
Tapeworms. *See* Cestodes
Telaprevir, 90*t*
Teleomorph, 119
Tenofovir, 90*t*
Tetanospasmin, 64
Tetanus, 63–64, 64*b*
Tetrahydropyrimidine, 145*t*
Thiazolides, 145*t*
Tick, 180*t*
Tick-borne borrelia relapsing fever, 226*b*
Tick-borne relapsing fever, outbreak
    of, 77*b*
Tinea barbae, 125*t*
Tinea capitis, 125*t*
  in adult woman, 127*b*, 229*b*
Tinea corporis, 125*t*

Tinea cruris, 125*t*

Tinea nigra, 123*t*

Tinea pedis, 125*t*

Tinea unguium, 125*t*

Tinea versicolor, 123*t*, 127*b*

  in immunocompetent woman, 227*b*

Tissue cestodes, 176*t*, 178–179

  antiparasitic agents for, 145–147*t*

Tissue nematodes, 167

  antiparasitic agents for, 145–147*t*

Tissue protozoa, 148*t*

  antiparasitic agents for, 145–147*t*

Tissue trematodes, 168–169*t*, 170–172

  antiparasitic agents for, 145–147*t*

Togaviridae, 85–86*t*

TORCH agents, 273

Toxic shock syndrome, 273

  staphylococcal, 17*b*, 23*b*

  streptococcal, 23*b*

Toxins, lethal, 66, 66*b*

Toxoplasma gondii, 148*t*, 156*b*

Toxoplasmosis, 156*b*

  in woman with Hodgkin disease, 216*b*

Trachoma, 82*b*

Trachomatous trichiasis (TT), 249*b*

Traumatic endophthalmitis, *Bacillus cereus*, 29*b*

Traumatic wounds, pathogens of, 6–8*t*

Trematodes, 142*t*, 168–174, 168*b*, 168–169*t*

  blood, 168–169*t*, 172–174

  intestinal, 168–169*t*, 169–170

  tissue, 168–169*t*, 170–172

Treponema pallidum, 71*t*, 74–75, 74*b*, 74*f*, 277

  neurosyphilis, 220*b*

  syphilis, 210*b*

Trichinella spiralis, 167*b*

Trichinosis, 167*b*

Trichomonas vaginalis, 148*t*, 153*b*, 271

Trichophyton rubrum, 124*f*, 277

Trichosporon spp., 123*t*, 137*t*

Trichuriasis, 162*b*

Trichuris trichiura, 161*t*, 162*b*

Trifluridine, 90*t*

Trimethoprim-sulfamethoxazole (TMPSMX), 61

Trypanosoma brucei, 148*t*, 157, 157*b*

Trypanosoma cruzi, 148*t*, 157*b*

Trypanosomiasis, 159*b*, 244*b*

Tsetse flies, 157*b*

Tsukamurella, bacteremia, 244*b*

Tuberculoid leprosy, 31

  Mycobacterium leprae and, 33*b*

Tuberculosis, *Mycobacterium tuberculosis* and, 32*b*

Tularemia, 255, 269

  cat-associated, 48*b*

  oculoglandular, *Francisella tularensis* and, 46*b*

  pneumonic, *Francisella tularensis* and, 46*b*

  ulceroglandular, *Francisella tularensis* and, 46*b*

U

Ulceroglandular tularemia, *Francisella tularensis* and, 46*b*

Ulcer, painless, 82*b*

Upper respiratory tract infections, 118*b*, 182–186

  case reports, 183–186*b*

Urban plague, 56*b*

Urethritis, 153*b*, 208

  pathogens of, 6–8*t*

Urinary tract infections (UTIs), 208, 209*b*

  Escherichia coli, 209*b*

  Proteus mirabilis, 209*b*

  Staphylococcus saprophyticus, 209*b*

Urogenital infections, from *Chlamydia trachomatis*, 82*b*

Urogenital protozoa, 148*t*

  antiparasitic agents for, 145–147*t*

  Trichomonas vaginalis in, 153*b*

V

Vaccine, hepatitis A, 255, 269

Vaginitis, 153*b*

  pathogens of, 6–8*t*

Valacyclovir, 90*t*

Valganciclovir, 90*t*

Varicella, 96, 229*b*

Varicella-zoster virus (VZV), 94–95*t*, 96–97, 96*b*

Veillonella, 64

Vibrio cholerae, 57–58, 57*b*

Vibrio cholerae gastroenteritis, 202*b*

Vibrionaceae, 49–50, 50–51*t*

  Vibrio cholerae, 57–58, 57*b*

Vibrio parahaemolyticus, gastroenteritis, 202*b*

Vibrio vulnificus sepsis, 239*b*

Viral diarrhea, rotavirus and, 113

Viral entry inhibitors, 89*t*

Viridans streptococci, 14, 14*t*, 21–22, 21*b*

Virus(es), 1–2*t*, 2, 85, 87–89, 198

  classification of, 85

  DNA, 85, 85–86*t*

  respiratory, 101–107, 101*b*

  responsible for cutaneous manifestations, 87*t*

  responsible for meningitis and encephalitis, 88*t*

  responsible for pericarditis and myocarditis, 88*t*

  responsible for respiratory infections, 87–88*t*

  RNA, 85, 85–86*t*

  role in disease, 87–89

Visceral leishmaniasis, 157*b*

Vulvovaginitis, 208

W

Warts, 117, 118*b*

Weil disease, 76*b*

White piedra, 123*t*

Wound botulism, 65*b*

Wuchereria bancrofti, 165*t*

Y

Yeast-like fungi, 137

Yeasts, 3, 119

Yersinia pestis, 50–51*t*, 56–57, 56*b*

  sepsis, 242*b*

Z

Zanamivir, 90*t*

Zoonotic disease, 25

Zoster, 96, 96*b*, 229*b*